POPULAR CULTURE IN COUNSELING, PSYCHOTHERAPY, AND PLAY-BASED INTERVENTIONS

Lawrence C. Rubin, PhD, LMHC, RPT-S, is a Professor of Counselor Education at St. Thomas University in Miami, Florida, where he teaches a variety of counseling courses and directs the Mental Health Counseling program. A licensed psychologist and mental health counselor, as well as a registered play therapist supervisor in private practice, Dr. Rubin specializes in clinical supervision and play therapy as well as the assessment and treatment of children, teens, and families. His research interests lie at the intersection of psychology and popular culture, and as such, he has published a previous volume with Springer entitled *Using Superheroes in Counseling and Play Therapy*. Dr. Rubin is also the editor of *Food for Thought: Essays on Eating and Culture*, and *Psychotropic Drugs and Popular Culture: Essays on Medicine, Mental Health and the Media*, the latter of which won the 2006 Ray and Pat Browne Award for best edited volume from the Popular Culture Association. He is an unabashed pop-culture junkie.

Popular Culture in Counseling, Psychotherapy, and Play-Based Interventions

Lawrence C. Rubin, PhD, LMHC, RPT-S
Editor

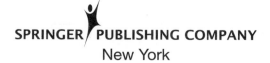

SPRINGER PUBLISHING COMPANY
New York

Springer Publishing Company, LLC
11 West 42nd Street
New York, NY 10036
www.springerpub.com

Acquisitions Editor: Sheri W. Sussman
Production Editor: Julia Rosen
Cover design: Mimi Flow
Composition: Apex Publishing, LLC

08   09   10/   5   4   3   2   1

Library of Congress Cataloging-in-Publication Data

Popular culture in counseling, psychotherapy, and play-based interventions / [edited by] Lawrence C. Rubin.
   p. ; cm.
Includes bibliographical references and index.
ISBN 978-0-8261-0118-1 (alk. paper)
   1. Child psychotherapy.   2. Adolescent psychotherapy.   3. Popular culture—Therapeutic use.   I. Rubin, Lawrence C., 1955–
[DNLM: 1. Psychotherapy—methods.   2. Adolescent.   3. Child.
4. Counseling—methods.   5. Mass Media.   6. Play Therapy—methods.
WS 350.2 P831 2008]

RJ504.P65   2008
616.89'1653—dc22   2008000725

Printed in the United States of America by Bang Printing.

For Randi, Zachary and Rebecca

Contents

PART IV: Video and Board Games

PART V: Television

PART VI: Sports

Contributors

Gregory B. Barker, PhD, received his doctorate in School/Clinical Child Psychology from the University of Virginia in 1981. For over 25 years he has specialized in working with children and adolescents in residential, hospital, college counseling, and school settings. For 17 years Dr. Barker consulted to the Bard College Counseling Center and is currently a school psychologist in the Rondout Valley public schools. He also has a private practice in Rhinebeck, New York, where he specializes in working with families and children.

Leya Barrett, MSW, LCSW, is the Family Therapist on Program I, "The Field of Dreams," at Onarga Academy, where she specializes in the treatment of adolescents with sexual behavior problems. As a licensed clinical social worker, she is always increasing her experience with expressive arts activities and finding new ways to bring treatment alive for her clients. She has presented at national conferences for professionals who treat children with sexual behavior problems and at international play therapy conferences. In addition, she has coauthored (along with three of her Onarga Academy colleagues) a chapter in *Using Superheroes in Counseling and Play Therapy,* edited by Lawrence Rubin. The use of pop culture in counseling and play therapy is a natural fit for Barrett, who has a special place in her heart for 1980s pop culture.

Jan M. Burte, PhD, MSCP, is a Licensed Psychologist who has taught and lectured nationally and internationally on hypnosis for the past 20 years. He is a past director of the Milton H. Erickson Institute of Long Island, past president of the New York Society of Clinical Hypnosis, and a Certified and Approved Consultant in Clinical Hypnosis (ASCH). Dr. Burte has been published in numerous journals and books, and has appeared on radio and television discussing the applicability of hypnosis for a wide range of patients and conditions. In addition, Dr. Burte is a Certified Sex Therapist (AASECT), a Diplomate in Pain Management (AAPM), and holds a postdoctoral master's degree in Clinical Psychopharmacology. He is an adjunct professor at Nova Southeastern University and is in private practice in Boca Raton, Florida.

David A. Crenshaw, PhD, ABPP, RPT-S, is a Board Certified Clinical Psychologist by the American Board of Professional Psychology and a Registered Play Therapist Supervisor by the Association for Play Therapy. He is founder and director of the Rhinebeck Child and Family Center in Rhinebeck, New York. He is a cofounder and currently the president of the New York Association for Play Therapy. He is the author of several books on child and adolescent psychotherapy, including *Evocative Strategies in Child and Adolescent Psychotherapy* (2007) and *Therapeutic Engagement of Children and Adolescents: Play, Symbol, Drawing and Storytelling Strategies* (2008).

Nancy Davis, LCSW, RPT-S, is a Licensed Clinical Social Worker and a Registered Play Therapist Supervisor. She is a therapist in private practice at Child and Family Counseling, LLC, in Crawfordsville, Indiana. She has over 20 years of clinical experience working with children, teenagers, and adults. She served on the board of directors for the Indiana Association for Play Therapy from 1995 to 2000 and the National Association for Play Therapy, 2001–2007. She was president of the Association for Play Therapy in 2003–2004. Nancy grew up in a very musical family. Her mother, Beth Pickard, with whom she cowrote the chapter, was an elementary and a college music teacher and instilled in her a love of music. She has three children, each of whom is involved in music. The beat goes on!

Pamela Dickinson, MA, earned her master's degree in Counselor Education from the Department of Educational Leadership and Counseling at Old Dominion University, Norfolk, Virginia. Her work using characters such as Basil Henderson, who are drawn from fiction and other popular culture sources, to illustrate diagnosis skills, approaches to case conceptualization, and methods of treatment planning, emerged from her own study and practice of diagnostic, conceptualization, and treatment planning skills while pursuing her graduate education.

Thelma Duffey, PhD, is professor of counseling and is also counseling program director at the University of Texas at San Antonio. Dr. Duffey spearheaded efforts to establish the Association for Creativity in Counseling, the newest division within the American Counseling Association, and has served as founding president for the association. She is also editor for the *Journal of Creativity in Mental Health.* Dr. Duffey has received awards for teaching and service and more recently received two international awards during the 2006 American Counseling Association convention in Montreal: the Professional Development Award by the American

Counseling Association and the Counseling Vision and Innovation Award by the Association for Counselor Education and Supervision. Her book, *Creative Interventions in Grief and Loss Therapy: When the Music Stops, a Dream Dies* was published in 2007.

George Enfield, MHR, Med, PCC, is an independently Licensed Counselor in the state of Ohio, where he currently works with preadolescent boys and infants and toddlers. He has been working with children since 1993 and has a broad range of experiences in individual and family counseling, in both inpatient and outpatient group settings. This broad spectrum of experience has taught him that clients provide both the language and desire to work on their own issues and it is our job as clinicians to hear them and adapt what we know about counseling to them so that they are able to make the most of the treatment.

Dora Finamore, EdD, is a professor at Northcentral University and has worked as a psychotherapist for the past 25 years. She is a Registered Play Therapist and founding editor of the Florida Play Therapy Association Newsletter. Dr. Finamore has served on the task force for ethics and policy for the Association for Play Therapy. She is a teacher of play therapy, child psychology, positive psychology, cognitive psychology, and peace and social justice studies. She has been published numerous times and has worked extensively with clients and professionals on parenting, grief, and trauma. Her research interests are learned helplessness, positive psychology, resilience, and personality. Her most recent publication is on resilience.

Danny Fingeroth was the longtime Group Editor of Marvel Comics' *Spider-Man* line, was consultant on early versions of what was to become the 2002 *Spider-Man* movie, and has written many comic books for Marvel and other companies. He is the author of *Superman On the Couch: What Superheroes Really Tell Us About Ourselves and Our Society* (2004) and of *Disguised as Clark Kent: Jews, Comics and the Creation of the Superhero* (2007). Fingeroth has spoken about comics and popular culture at venues including The Smithsonian Institution and Comic-Con International, San Diego, as well as on National Public Radio's *All Things Considered* and NBC's *Today Show,* and has written about them for publications including *The Los Angeles Times* and *The Baltimore Sun.* He teaches comics and graphic novel writing and appreciation at New York University and The New School. His *Rough Guide to Graphic Novels* will be published in 2008.

Loretta Gallo-Lopez, MA, LMHC, RPT-S, is a Licensed Mental Health Counselor and Certified Supervisor, a Registered Play Therapist and Supervisor, and a Registered Drama Therapist and Board Certified

Trainer in private practice in Tampa, Florida. Her practice is focused on providing effective, creative treatment interventions for children, adolescents, and families. She specializes in helping individuals, families, and groups with issues related to mood, anxiety, and behavioral disorders, trauma and loss, and developmental disabilities. Her work has been published in major play therapy and creative arts therapy texts and she is coeditor of the book *Play Therapy with Adolescents* (2005).

Melonie Grosser, PCCs, Professional Clinical Counselor Supervisor, works as both an agency clinician and play therapist in private practice. She is an adjunct instructor at Raymond Walters College and an assistant professor at Embry Riddle Aeronautical University. She is the mother of two grown daughters, Alisha and Lauren, and the grandmother of Lilly. After over 20 years as a former military spouse, she calls Cincinnati, Ohio, her home. She is currently the president of the Ohio Play Therapy Association and is a registered play therapist supervisor.

Linda B. Hunter, PhD, the clinical director for the all-volunteer Association for Community Counseling, has been working professionally with children and families since 1983. Dr. Hunter is a Psychologist (licensed in Hawaii), Marriage and Family Therapist (licensed in California), a Social Sorker (licensed in Florida), a Play Therapist-Supervisor (RPT-S), and a clinical member of the International Society for Sandplay Therapists (ISST). She is the author of *Images of Resiliency: Troubled Children Create Healing Stories in the Language of Sandplay* (1998) and articles about the use of play and sandplay therapy with culturally diverse populations published in *Child Welfare, The Journal of Sandplay Therapy,* and books on play therapy. She has used play and sand tray therapy with a wide range of clients of varying cultures and nationalities, both here and abroad.

Harry Livesay, LCSW, a Licensed Clinical Social Worker and Professional of the Healing Arts (LPHA) for the Mental Health and Mental Retardation Authority of Harris County, Texas, received his master's degree from the University of Houston Graduate School of Social Work. His interest in the therapeutic benefits of board games was a result of his clinical work for a school-based health center in the Houston Area, providing counseling and therapeutic play activities for students between the ages of 5 and 18, and their families. He has been an avid comic book and toy collector for the past 40 years and has written on the use of superheroes in counseling with children and adolescents, in the *International Journal of Play Therapy,* and in the recent Springer volume, *Using Superheroes in Counseling and Play Therapy.*

Kelly E. MacDonald, LPC, spent 10 years working in advertising and public relations, where primarily she marketed public health campaigns and other human service programs, before earning a master's degree in Counseling from the Department of Educational Leadership and Counseling, Old Dominion University, in Norfolk, VA. She is a Licensed Professional Counselor and a National Certified Counselor. Her counseling caseload has included children, adolescents, young adults, and families. She has practiced in residential settings, academic environments, and outpatient settings.

William McNulty, LCSW-C, RPT-S, is a Licensed Clinical Social Worker and Registered Play Therapist-Supervisor. He works in Rockville, Maryland, at the Reginald S. Lourie Center for Infants and Young Children as a therapist in the outpatient clinic and the Therapeutic Nursery Program. He has also been a board member of the Maryland/District of Columbia Play Therapy Association since 2003. He received his master's degree in Psychology from Salisbury State University and his master's in Social Work from the University of Maryland, Baltimore. He wishes to thank his wife for her interest, support, and guidance in writing his chapter.

Beth Pickard, BS, earned her Bachelor of Science Degree in Education and Master of Arts in Education from Ball State University. She has taught general music in the Anderson Community Schools for 28½ years, retiring in 2000. Earning a master of science in Music Technology in 1998 from Indiana University, she taught various music classes in the IU School of Music and the IU School of Education at IUPUI 1997–2007. She directed the Young Scholars Program for the IU School of Education at IUPUI from 2001 to 2007 and served as the Music Technology Chair for the Indiana Music Educators from 1997 to 2007. Music has always been a very important part of her life and she plays the piano, the guitar, the cello, the mountain dulcimer, and various other folk instruments.

Robert Poole, BS, is the unit coordinator of Program 1, "Field of Dreams," at the Onarga Academy. He holds a bachelor's degree in Psychology from Eureka College, alma mater of President Ronald Reagan. In 2007, Robert coauthored "A Super Milieu: Using Superheroes in the Residential Treatment of Adolescents With Sexual Behavior Problems," a chapter in the volume *Using Superheroes in Counseling and Play Therapy* (edited by Lawrence C. Rubin). Little did he know that the weekly trips to the movies during his high school years would cultivate the opportunity to use movies and pop culture to assist clients in his future career. Now as he watches movies, his mind continually finds messages and themes that can assist in client treatment.

Scott Riviere, MS, LPC, RPT-S, is a Licensed Professional Counselor who has worked exclusively with children, adolescents, and their families since 1990. He founded Louisiana's first Play Therapy Institute called K.I.D.Z., Inc., and also founded Healing Kidz, a nonprofit organization committed to the healthy development of children. He is a registered play therapist-supervisor and is also approved to supervise interns seeking to obtain their state counseling license. He has developed a variety of therapeutic products and is a published author in the books *Adolescent Play Therapy,* and *Short Term Play Therapy with Children* (2nd edition). He has been recognized as an international speaker and is a sought-out presenter at national and state conferences. He is available to do training and supervision nationwide and can be reached at Callkidz@aol.com.

Karen Robertie, MS, LCPC, is the Clinical Supervisor of Program 1, "The Field of Dreams," at the Onarga Academy, a residential facility for adolescents with sexual behavior problems. A licensed clinical therapist of over 20 years, she continually strives to integrate the expressive arts into her clinical work with trauma victims. She has presented trainings on using play therapy with children with sexual behavior problems at local, regional, national, and international conferences for play therapists, and those who specialize in treating children with sexual behavior problems. In addition, she has coauthored (along with three of her Onarga Academy colleagues) a chapter in *Using Superheroes in Counseling and Play Therapy,* edited by Lawrence Rubin. A child of the TV generation, she is a fount of pop culture information.

Lisa Saldaña, LMHC, RPT-S, is a Licensed Mental Health Counselor and Registered Play Therapist-Supervisor in Miami, Florida; director of training at The Institute for Child & Family Health, Inc.; and a practitioner in a private practice where she works with children, adolescents, and adults. She is a past president of both the national Association for Play Therapy and its Florida branch. Her first credit card purchase in 1979 was an enormous Betamax VCR and a small color television. *The Wizard of Oz* was on television, and she was determined to have her own copy to watch as often as she wished. Saldaña and her husband, Neal, have a daughter, Toni, who inherited her love of reading and is currently a Peace Corps volunteer in Benin. Their son, Geoff, inherited her love of animation, fantasy, and graphic novels.

Alan M. "Woody" Schwitzer, PhD, is a Licensed Clinical Psychologist, and associate professor of Educational Leadership and Counseling at Old Dominion University in Norfolk, Virginia. He is editor of the *Journal of College Counseling* and recipient of the American College Counseling Association's Outstanding Contributions to Professional Knowledge Award.

Recent books include *Skills and Tools for Today's Counselors and Psychotherapists: From Natural Helping to Professional Counseling* and *Promoting Student Learning and Student Development at a Distance: Student Affairs Concepts and Practices for Televised Instruction and Other Forms of Distance Education.* He also is an independent practitioner and consultant. He lives near the Lafayette River with his wife, dog, and john-boat.

Deidre Skigen, LMHC, is a Licensed Mental Health Counselor who maintains a private practice in Miami, Florida, providing individual, family, and group psychotherapy, workshops, and seminars. She has also worked in the Dade County Public School System with severely emotionally disturbed children and their families, was one of the founding group facilitators for the Children's Bereavement Center, assisting children and their families through the grieving process, and has also served as an adjunct professor of psychology.

Laura Sullivan, MS, is a Licensed Marital and Family Therapist currently in a private practice of 12 years in Mooresville, Indiana. With two children of her own and over 20 years of experience in social services assisting individuals and families in distress, she recognizes the value of playfulness in work and life. As a faculty member, she incorporates play into her facilitation of adult education in psychology, sociology, and critical thinking at the University of Phoenix in Indianapolis. She enjoys writing stories for kids and inventing games as creative expression in her work.

Heather Trepal, PhD, LPC, is an assistant professor in the Department of Counseling and Educational Psychology at the University of Texas at San Antonio. She received her doctorate in counseling and human development from Kent State University. Her research focuses on self-injurious behaviors, at-risk youth, women's issues, gender issues in counseling, and the use of technology in counselor education and supervision. She currently serves as a trustee on the executive board for the Association of Creativity in Counseling (ACC).

Ryan Weidenbenner, MS, the Senior Sexuality Therapist working with children with sexual behavior problems at the Onarga Academy, holds two master's degrees from Illinois State University, one in Psychology and one in Counseling, as well as a liberal arts degree from Wabash College. These creative influences are readily apparent in his therapeutic work with the Onarga clients, and his lifelong appreciation of comic books, role-playing games, and movies has been instrumental in developing creative therapeutic interventions at Onarga. In 2007, he coauthored "A Super Milieu: Using Superheroes in the Residential Treatment of Adolescents with Sexual Behavior Problems," a chapter in Lawrence Rubin's 2006 publication, *Using Superheroes in Counseling and Play Therapy.*

Foreword

I'M A STRANGER HERE, MYSELF

What do I do? I'm a key figure in an ongoing government charade. An annoyance to my superiors. A joke among my peers. "Spooky," they call me. Spooky Mulder. Whose sister was abducted by aliens when he was a kid. Who now chases little green men with a badge and a gun, shouting to the heavens and anyone who'll listen that the fix is in. That our government's hip to the truth and a part of the conspiracy. That the sky is falling and when it hits it's gonna be the shitstorm of all time.

—Fox Mulder,
The X-Files: Fight the Future, 1998

The title of this foreword was the working title for many of director Nicholas Ray's films. (His other favorite was *The Gun Under My Pillow.*) These movies would later see release as *Rebel Without a Cause, They Live By Night, Bigger Than Life,* and many others. It wasn't until the making of a 1975 documentary about Ray that the title *I'm a Stranger Here, Myself* was actually used. The sense of alienation both working titles convey is a common one in popular culture.

The *X-Files* movie quote, another declaration of alienation, is possibly the most succinct summation of a complex character's raison d'être ever used in a movie. We learn everything about Mulder here—his history, his tragedies, his personality. A pity that most people don't speak in such concentrated bites.

All this is by way of saying that who we are or aren't—alienated or not—is, for many of us, largely defined by our relationship to popular culture.

It's not exactly a secret that pop culture is a veritable force of nature that fuels multibillion dollar businesses—not to mention our very

---

Foreword to *Popular Culture in Counseling, Psychotherapy, and Play-Based Interventions,* copyright © 2008 Danny Fingeroth.

imaginations. For some, pop culture is the only culture they know, for others, an occasional guilty pleasure. Still, even the most sophisticated of us can probably recite the lyrics to the theme songs of at least a few TV shows and can't help but be diverted by the sight of a movie star walking down the street.

But, as the frantic caricature on *The Simpsons* is fond of saying, "What about the children?" In other more serious words, and more to the point of this book, *Popular Culture in Counseling, Psychotherapy, and Play-Based Interventions,* what is the effect of this pop culture saturation on kids and teenagers? And how can the power of pop culture be "harnessed for good," as scientists in B-movies are fond of saying?

After all, it can't be denied, even by this lifelong entertainment professional, that, unmediated by a reasonably healthy environment, a pure diet of popular culture can leave kids with some weird ideas about life that may eventually require professional intervention.

That's where Lawrence Rubin and his collaborators on this book can provide some important insights about using popular culture to treat kids, teens, and adults, whatever the source of their problems. After all, with so many people, layman and professional, willing to blame popular culture for the ills of our society, it's only fitting that same pop culture be used to tackle some of those same problems. That is the admirable, albeit highly challenging, task that Rubin and colleagues have taken on here, as in *Using Superheroes in Counseling and Play Therapy* (Springer Publishing Company, 2007).

Of course, by daring to access the pop culture arena in order to treat children and adolescents, you risk becoming therapeutic trespassers in a world that these kids have carefully arranged for you to not be welcomed in. Much of pop culture, especially for young people, has to do with the creation of identity, of assuming and discarding selves as if they were articles of clothing, and often enacting the fantasies involved with that development outside of the view or control of parental figures—including therapists. The heroes of pop culture therefore become role models, coming up with solutions to the challenges of life that may seem too much for kids, their parents, and their "official" teachers in school.

For instance, *24*'s Jack Bauer is ruthless, even to the point of using torture to get information from adversaries—and yet we have the impression that he's really some kind of peaceful idealist, forced by circumstance to do what he does, his motivation ultimately being love—of country, of family, and especially of justice. Like the classic superheroes, who are in essence vigilantes, we want to feel that, through Jack (no one thinks of him as anything but his first name) we will be able to know how and when to use power wisely—which also assumes the important-to-kids idea that we actually have the ability to accrue some power, to achieve some control over our lives.

So pop culture is a dual (at least) edged sword. Abused, it can enable us to flee down rabbit holes of fantasy. Used correctly—whatever that means to you—it can inspire us, help us through tough times, teach us about ourselves, and help us move to the next level of development.

As a kid, I had a certain understanding of Kurt Vonnegut's concept—articulated in *Slaughterhouse Five*—of simultaneously living in various eras—"Billy Pilgrim has become unstuck in time"—as a convenient method to allow the story Vonnegut was telling to jump back and forth in time. Today, as a middle-aged adult, I experience this phenomenon on a daily basis, as no doubt the middle-aged Vonnegut was doing when he wrote the book. Oftentimes, all the periods of my life seem as if they're occurring simultaneously in the present: the "me" of my childhood, the "me" in high school, the "me" that dated my college girlfriend, who later became my ex-wife, the "me" that's remarried and raising young children now, and who is watching as they become inundated in the seas of popular culture, especially on television, and registering how that makes me feel and behave.

Every time I see an ad extolling the pleasures of a home theater system, I roll my eyes. The last thing I or my family (or anyone else) needs is a more pleasurable TV viewing experience. It would be as if I were a heroin addict being offered a purer form of the drug, or a painless needle. Sure, it'd be more convenient—but it would also be a quicker route to self-destruction. For many, TV is an addictive drug, comforting, educational, but, like alcohol or food, one that needs to be doled out wisely. The same can be said for many of the pop culture delivery systems of our age.

With my own children, twin 5-year-old boys, one of whom is on the autism spectrum, I see how popular culture can be used and also abused. With each kid, it has different benefits and pitfalls.

My "spectrum son," while improving weekly in his dealings with other humans, often identifies more intimately with the television screen than he does with many people. While some of us may joke about how the TV was an extra family member when we were growing up, for my son, it truly is. For most people, TV is like coffee—if you go off it for a day or two, your equilibrium will restore itself. For a child on the autism spectrum such as mine, who echoes and repeats things he's heard on TV—some with understanding, some without—the relationship to TV is more complex. What makes it especially complex is the good it can do. For example, the kid makes incredible clay sculptures based on imagery he sees on TV.

My other, "typically" developing son certainly loves TV too much, if not too wisely, much as his parents do. But he is capable of playing without it, alone or with other kids, in a highly imaginative, creative way. Of course, many of the elements of his imagination are branded, licensed characters.

Kids are the proverbial empty vessels, filled with the culture around them—filtered through their own personalities. So, for instance, as

Spider-Man learned the hard way that, "with great power, there must also come—great responsibility," kids and teens also learn some version of this lesson. While few people ever get great power in political or cultural terms, we all acquire or become prey to power on lesser levels that may have the effect of great power. An abusive parent, a manipulative child, a sadistic boss—all these people may not be able to order an invasion of a foreign country, but they can and do utilize power over others, with the consent, spoken or unspoken, of those over whom they wield it. So, in that sense, use of power—or its abuse—is a daily occurrence. You don't have to be bitten by an irradiated spider and face a clinically insane human octopus to know this. And popular culture is where many of us learn to deal with power relationships.

You don't need me to tell you that one of the ways that power is ideally wielded responsibly is in the therapeutic relationship. Interestingly, as that relates to popular culture, the image most people—even sophisticated people—have about therapy and therapists comes largely from pop culture. When one first makes the decision to embark on some kind of psychotherapy, one is also entering into a dialogue with the notions embedded in our heads by the popular portrayals of therapy and therapists. I have a feeling the same is true on the other side of the couch or desk. Therapists, I would imagine, must determine what being a therapist means, both to themselves as well as to their clients. Each therapist's definitions are likely informed—as much as by teachers and other therapists he or she has encountered—by Robin Williams in *Good Will Hunting,* Judd Hirsch in *Ordinary People,* or even Billy Crystal in *Analyze This*; to say nothing of Dr. Melfi and her peers (especially Peter Bogdanovich's Dr. Kupferberg and Sully Boyar's Dr. Caligari, sans cabinet) in *The Sopranos,* and a hundred other pop culture shrinks we all know and love/hate.

Teens and children are also familiar with these archetypes. The popular notion of a Viennese accented Freud-like (if not Freudian) character with a beard regularly appears in kids' entertainment, since that figure has become as ubiquitous as the snotty rich girl, the dumb jock, the weird nerd, and so on, in popular culture.

I would imagine that having to deal with these preconceptions about psychotherapists, while possibly annoying to a therapist, must also be potentially quite useful, especially in dealing with children, teens, and even adults. You can show them that, while people (such as therapists) may have some characteristics that are "typical" of one or more groups, people are also individuals, with problems that can be named and dealt with.

Because of these psychotherapist-pop-culture figures, and because our society tends to see human misbehavior as nature- and environment-based—as opposed to the work of demons—most people are open to the uses of psychology even if it "isn't for me." So even the clichéd images of therapists in pop culture can serve a purpose. The trick, it seems to me, is to convince people—kids, especially—that therapy isn't only for the really screwed up or the deranged; that most of us need, at one time or another, some guidance in our lives, guidance of a type that our friends and family can't provide because they're just too close to us, and that they also don't have the training to provide.

Most people who have jobs supervising others feel that they spend part of their time playing psychiatrist. In my case, as a supervising editor, I was constantly juggling the often wildly divergent needs of my staff, other staffers, and a crew of freelancers. Some of these people were easy to deal with, others, not so much. Some of the difficult people were ones who legitimately had needs that were at odds with those of the company or of other freelancers. But there were those who seemed to generate conflict just for the sake of generating conflict. On some level, of course, the workplace is all about people from different cultural and family backgrounds being forced to work together. That's the reason for the popularity of TV shows and movies about the workplace, such as those set in hospitals or police precincts. In effect we all have to be diplomats and therapists. And in a supervisory position, it's not merely a matter of convenience or preference to get along with others. If your team or teams don't work well together, everyone's livelihood is at stake, not to mention their mental health.

So as I was practicing amateur therapy in the workplace, I would often apply, for better or worse, what I had learned from popular culture. In retrospect, this seems to me to go back to Lawrence Rubin's idea of guided popular culture viewing/reading as important in therapeutic environments. Every work of art or popular culture has meaning, often several, and multiple messages. People can experience the same work and come away from it with opposite messages—often connected to the worldview they bring to the experience. So it would seem to me to be the extremely valuable role of the therapist to extract from the works experienced all of the possible lessons the works contain—and not turn a blind eye to the "wrong" ones' lessons, but deal with them head on—thereby giving them the tools they need to help young people develop the more positive elements of their personalities.

For example, one could watch *Star Wars,* and come away with many different lessons. One would be, of course, that might makes right, that destroying things that menace you will set you free. On the other hand, the more positive lesson of the film is that we all have within us great potential that can be realized and directed toward positive ends.

As another example, the *Godfather* movies are also powerful pop culture totems, especially relating to family relationships. On the positive side, they're brilliant family dramas, played out in operatic terms, with the mob figures so powerfully delineated that real-world mobsters started behaving like characters from the movies after having become mesmerized and immersed in the first two films.

The films' Corleone family members and their relationships are written and acted with such unerring skill that most people watching the films find themselves identifying with one or the other of the Corleone brothers, or with adopted brother Tom Hagen, or with sister Connie. Everyone has, at some time, been the wild and crazy child, the angry, resentful child, the good child with, we fear, the capacity for evil beneath the socially acceptable façade.

Interestingly, the *Godfather* films have become some of the most powerful family dramas of our age, bringing the mob families' drama to the level of Shakespeare or opera (both of which, though considered highbrow now, were, at the time of their original presentation, considered TV-like popular culture). The *Godfather* movies take the extreme highs and lows of family life and extend them to a worldview that, in the case of even the "noble" Corleones, is essentially a justification for cynical, violent, criminal activity.

Still, a fictional world that is so well known and so moving to so many must surely have a therapeutic use, even as a cautionary tale. Has there ever been so moving a father-son scene as when Marlon Brando's Don Vito Corleone warns son Michael (Al Pacino) about who he can and can't trust in upcoming intermob negotiations? Vito expresses tearful regret that his son has to engage in the ugly business of organized crime, that Michael has inherited his mantle of leadership. "I never wanted this for you, Michael. It should have been 'Senator Corleone,' 'Governor Corleone.' There just wasn't enough time." And what does Michael reply? Why, what every father would want his son to say after a confession of failure: "We'll get there, Pop." And when Michael says, "We'll get there," he doesn't just mean the Corleone family, he means, by extension, every immigrant group, and beyond that, every person who ever chased a dream. "We'll get there." And, expressed beneath that is yet another meaning, the idea that Michael's children won't have to be gangsters, that they'll "get there," to a promised land where they can be just Americans, just regular people, without the life-warping burden of the power and responsibility of running a criminal empire. Perhaps "We'll get there" can even be taken to refer to arriving at a state of psychological health, where one's inner and outer life can finally be in some kind of balance.

Of course, without proper guidance—internal or external—the message of *The Godfather*, like the message of *Star Wars*, could be interpreted by a child or adolescent as: "Nobody messes with the toughest, most ruthless kid on the block. So if you're not going to be that kid, you're screwed." These aren't just issues for kids in therapy, but for our society as a whole. How and when is it okay to kick ass? How and when is it okay to turn the other cheek? How can we feel good about ourselves no matter which of those two we have done, and how can we really mean it—not just rationalize either excess aggression or excess passivity?

Ultimately, therapists using popular culture in treatment will face the same dilemma that creators of these works find themselves up against. Can popular culture, something that can be, and often is, used to appeal to the worst in human nature—the easiest solutions to complex problems, the not-too-subtle imprecations to buy stuff, the codification of ethnic and gender stereotypes—possibly be interpreted and enhanced to be a stealth launching system for positive values—to even inoculate patients and therapists alike against the abuses inherent in the content of popular culture? The premise of this entire book is, of course, that they can. I think you'll find fascinating, as I did, how Lawrence Rubin and the other writers in this collection put that theory into practice.

Danny Fingeroth
Author of *Superman on the Couch: What Superheroes Really Tell Us About Ourselves and Our Society* (2004); past Group Editor of the *Spider-Man* books at Marvel Comics.
November, 2007

Acknowledgments

It is not uncommon for a therapist to query a client regarding the client's earliest memory, as such might provide valuable insights for self-understanding. As I organized my thoughts for this volume, I tried to recall my earliest popular culture memory. It was the song, "Itsy Bitsy Teeny Weeny Yellow Polka-Dot Bikini," by Brian Hyland, which dates to my then-burgeoning awareness of the inescapable sights, sounds, objects, and people that comprise popular culture. In retrospect, the litany of my interests, possessions, passions, and subsequent low-brow collecting obsessions reads like confessions of a baby boomer pop culture junkie, which I guess it is. To name a few: Beatles albums, Schwinn Stingray bicycles, a twice-built, 5-foot tall replica of the Saturn V rocket, baseball cards, Aurora monster models of Frankenstein, Wolfman, and Dracula, beer cans, melamine (aka Melmac) dishes, Chuck Taylor Converse Hi Top sneakers, superhero and Archie comic books, paint-by-number "artwork," Heywood-Wakefield mid-century modern furniture, and Disney movies . . . and don't forget three 1970s Volvo 1800s, aka Roger Moore's cool sports car on the 1960s television show, *The Saint*.

I've long since sold off my baseball cards; and my monster models, precious Saturn V rockets, and comic books are slowly decomposing in some faraway landfill along with the childhood memories and possessions of a legion of others. However, I still wear Cons, love superheroes, ride around the neighborhood on my Stingray, and type this work while at the desk of my retro furniture. For me, the stuff of popular culture is clearly about a romanticized tie to my past, but it still pervades every aspect of my current life in innumerable ways. It is for this reason that it made sense for me to ask: In what ways have I and the other therapists you will meet in this volume tapped into the stuff of popular culture as a resource for self-understanding, healing, and growth? I deeply thank each of them for doing so.

I wish to thank, first and foremost, my parents, Esther and Herbert, who in their innocent efforts to indulge or perhaps pacify me unknowingly contributed to my love of all things popular, beginning with Thursday night visits with Dean Martin and Sundays on the Ponderosa with Ben Cartwright and the boys. And then there is my wife Randi, always loving and supportive and ever indulgent of both my enduring and quixotic passions, and who at the time of this writing was trying to maintain her thin veil of support as I contemplated a Superman tattoo. I must acknowledge my wonderful and wonder-filled children Zachary and Rebecca, who have inherited my passion for all things popular, and who are currently building their own childhood memories, complete with Spider-Man, Barbie, Tony Hawk video games, Jessie McCartney concert stubs, and yes, even a frightening fascination with Paris and Brittney. Thanks to Sheri W. Sussman, Senior Vice President/Editorial at Springer Publishing, for once again venturing forth into new territory. And finally, I wish once again, to thank the many fine clinicians who gave of their creativity, time, and patience with my incessant editorial demands in the preparation of this book.

Introduction

Popular Culture As a Resource for Growth and Change

Lawrence C. Rubin

A depressed and disillusioned 32-year-old scours a popular song lyric Web site so that she can clearly articulate and communicate painful feelings of loss.

A 9-year-old boy who struggles to control anger dramatically describes and reenacts the most recent episode of Naruto, a Japanese anime character who has a destructive force within him.

A lonely and alienated 23-year-old college senior spends hours in the cyber World of Warcraft in attempts to connect with others and experience the power she feels denied in her day-to-day life.

—From the author's clinical casework, 2005–2007

Aside from their place as fixtures in contemporary American popular culture, what do Naruto, the World of Warcraft, the Billboard Hot 100,[1] and as we shall soon see, *The Sopranos, Harry Potter,* MySpace.com, the *Wizard of Oz,* and perennial board game favorite Candy Land have in common? An answer to this question begs an even more compelling one for clinicians: "How can such a seeming diversity rise to a level of coherence and therapeutic applicability?" In order to answer these questions, I will first identify important issues related to an understanding of popular culture, and then address its potential relevance for clinicians as a means of fostering communication with clients and as a therapeutic resource for self-expression, awareness, healing, and growth.

POPULAR CULTURE 101

> To be articulate and discriminating about ordinary affairs and information
> is the mark of an educated [person].
>
> (Marshall McLuhan)[2]

In the spirit of clinical inquiry, I would like to begin this discussion by posing a simple question. What comes to mind when you think of the concept of 'popular culture'?

Did you focus on the latest anticipated installment of the newest superhero or action hero movie in production and the inevitable avalanche of related toys, footwear, and food products? Or did you reflect on some imponderable Internet bidding frenzy over a piece of food bearing the likeness of the Virgin Mary? Perhaps you attempted to make sense of why thousands across the country sacrificed a night's sleep and a week's pay to purchase the newest techno-neato gadget. Or maybe you eagerly anticipated the morning news in order to discover whether the hot dog eating record was still intact or the paparazzi captured a super-celeb in a compromising position.

Then again, perhaps your popular culture sensibilities were loftier than these seemingly banal examples, and you reflected instead on the unique musical hybrid called Afropop, contemplated the dystopian-postapocalyptic trend in popular literature, successfully connected the dots linking modern art to medieval graffiti, or wondered whether or not McLuhan's media-driven global community would bring humanity together or push it into the abyss of a postmodern dark age.

In either case, whether your attention thrashed around in the shallows or probed the depths, you have entered the broad, rich, and multilayered realm of popular culture. In order to appreciate popular culture, one must first define culture, which for the purpose of this discussion is the global, historic, and evolving self-definition of a people, comprising accumulated knowledge, a worldview, art, and customs that are passed down from one generation to the next (Nye, 1971). In a sense, culture is an unfolding dramatic saga. Popular culture, on the other hand, is a series of seemingly disparate snapshots, taken from the everyday lives of those same people, captured at specific moments in time and at times in compromising positions. Just as physical anthropologists seek to weave together the story of a society from the objects it has left behind, those who appreciate and study popular culture work in the present attempt to unlock the attitudes, assumptions, and practices of a people through an appreciation of its icons, defined as "admired artifacts, external expressions of internal convictions; everyday things that make every day meaningful"

(Fishwick, 2002, p. 47). While icons have historically been reserved for and preserved in churches and monasteries, the objects and practices that comprise popular culture may be found on television screens, in fast food stores, and along superhighways—both real and virtual. If culture is a drama unfolding, popular culture comprises the interstices. It may even be feasible to analogize culture with the dramatic, and that which is popular with the lighthearted or humorous.

Unlike the historically broader and often unyielding nature of culture that is received as legacy, popular culture is an index of change, which according to Browne is "all those elements of life which are not narrowly intellectually or creatively elitist and which are generally, though not necessarily disseminated through the mass media . . . and consists of the spoken and printed word, sound, pictures, objects and artifacts" (Browne, 2006, p. 21). When one thinks of popular culture, words such as fads, folksy, and fleeting may come to mind, and it has even been suggested that it is as old as humanity itself, since "culture has always been popular, thriving on formula, archetypes and stereotypes . . . cyclic, repetitive and powerful" (Fishwick, 2002, p. 3). However, who is to decide what is trivial and what is important?

In this context, a perennial debate among scholars has centered on the tension between those who consider popular culture studies to be a diminutive form, a red-headed stepchild of cultural studies, and those who consider it to be a valid and legitimate field of study in its own right. Neal (1995) argues that cultural fragmentation resulting from both human and technological forces creates societal angst in which the boundaries between good and evil, chaos and order, and the sacred and profane blur. Popular, or "mass" culture as Neal calls it, which is reflected in collective memories expressed through art and music, "provides individuals with frameworks for locating their present lifestyles along a continuum somewhere between the 'best possible' and 'worst possible' of all social worlds" (p. 122). In this sense, that which is popular, or readily embraced and often made available through mass production and/or the media, is a unifying force. Its study chronicles the breaking down and building up of societies.

Others point out that the popular is "marked by hierarchies of artistic value, with European high art and the philosophical aesthetics of Western ruling classes set against the entertainment that people purchase from the commercial world" (Miller & McHoul, 1998, p. 3). In this vein, that which is considered to be culturally elite (a Mozart symphony, a Marxist treatise, or a painting by Picasso) derives its power from the spiritual and theoretical, and is to be judged from a distance. High culture in this regard can be appreciated only by those formally educated in the subtleties and nuances of beauty and perfection (Harrington & Bielby, 2001). Unlike high culture, which is inventive, creative, inspirational, deeply evocative, and attributable to a specific individual, popular or low culture is formulaic, contrived, impersonal, and commercial (Cawelti, 2001; Nye, 1971). Its products range from, among other things, branded breakfast cereals, mass-produced art, movies and movie-based giveaways, and board, video, and Internet games, to comic books as well as sports memorabilia and celebrities.

POPULAR CULTURE CAN HELP

What significance, you may wonder, does the foregoing discussion have for those outside of the field of popular culture studies? Its concepts and theories seem better suited to academic discussion than to clinical application. Beyond the clinician's passing interest in a client's clothing or food choice, the music, movies, or video games she enjoys, or sports figure he admires, is there a meaningful way to integrate popular culture into counseling and psychotherapy? The answer is yes, and it resides within a therapeutic triangle composed of the client, the therapist, and the objects, personages, and activities of everyday life, of which they are both consumers—co-consumers so to speak. Conceptualized this way, the various mediums through which popular culture flows, including movies, board games, music, literature, television, and the Internet move from the realm of commodity to that of therapeutic resource and shall be referred to as *popular culture intervention*. It is important to note that this is not a model of therapy, per se, but instead a means of broadening the clinician's already established theoretically based clinical repertoire.

According to Kidd (2007), popular culture serves a variety of functions, including defining norms for behavior, establishing social boundaries, providing a set of rituals that increase solidarity, producing innovation, and serving as an impetus of social change. In this regard, clients as consumers of popular culture may choose to align their values with those whom they encounter on a television show or movie, give voice to their thoughts and feelings as they relate to the lyrics of a song, or establish boundaries between themselves and others by identifying with the ideals and behavior of a popular sports or political figure. Even a client's clothing choice may have iconic significance, be it a T-shirt or a tattoo bearing the likeness of a favorite superhero.

Children may identify with the main character in a popular action movie, and in so doing, experiment with alternate ways of expressing themselves. Young and impressionable audiences are often directly targeted by merchandising and media advertising campaigns, and popular cartoon and real-life heroes promote values and ideologies that may either be consistent or discrepant with their own burgeoning worldviews, thus providing the opportunity to express and resolve a developmental tension. Even the rarified world of Disney contains numerous characters whose stories and adventures convey very clear messages for proper and improper ways of living.

A recent Kaiser Family Foundation survey entitled "Talking with Kids about Tough Issues" (2001) noted that children and teens are turning to sources other than their parents for information about complicated topics such as alcohol, drugs, sex, and violence. In fact, they noted that 26% of surveyed children between the ages of 8 and 11, and 37% of surveyed teens in the 12–15-year age range, turned to television and movies for information on these topics. Whatever the sociological reason, and for better or for worse, young people consume popular culture as a means to learn about life. It makes sense, therefore to use this already established link in the counseling room.

Working with urban youth, Mattingly noted that "a child's beloved [popular culture] character can offer a kind of narrative shadow, a cultural resource that children, families and healthcare professionals readily turn to in the task of creating socially shared meaning, especially the sort of meaning that has to do with trying to positively shape a child's future" (2006, p. 494). Her idea that the icons and narratives of popular culture function as a lingua franca or primary language for young people places an obligation on the clinician to learn the language.

In today's society, the Internet, cable television, and the media make it possible to instantly access the world in order to indulge in a startling barrage of images, sounds, and narratives from around the corner or across the planet. With the advent of devices such as the Blackberry, iPhone, or computer terminal at the corner library, a veritable portal to events and people lies at one's fingertips. Today's clinicians must acknowledge the instantaneity and accessibility of information, stimulation, and entertainment available and be ready to harness it therapeutically. Clinician Ron Taffel notes that in order to be prepared to work with 21st-century clients, she must "check out the TV shows most adults reflexively stay clear of . . . take in movies they would naturally avoid, and become acquainted with music they may even have moral objections to" (2005, p. 35). Taffel often invites clients to bring music and discuss their popular culture interests, including their favorite video games, books, and comics, and quotes one of his clients who argued, "If you don't know what any of this is about, it's impossible to have an intelligent conversation with us" (p. 35).

Along similar lines, albeit from outside of the clinical world, Steven Johnson, in his provocative volume *Everything Bad Is Good for You,* identifies a new generation of consumers most unique to the electronic age whom he calls "screenagers." He notes that today's 10-year-old is capable of "following dozens of professional sports teams, shifting effortlessly from phone to IM (instant messaging) to email in communicating with friends, probing and telescoping through immense virtual worlds [and] adapting and trouble shooting new media technologies without flinching" (2005, p. 144). Arguing that culture is becoming more cognitively complex and demanding, he suggests that a number of today's video games, television shows, and movies require a depth of participation that stimulate neural development and challenge participants to plan and problem solve. Therapists will take note that these latter frontal lobe skills are the essence of cognitive and social development.

POPULAR CULTURE INTERVENTION

As was noted above, popular culture intervention is neither a treatment modality nor theory specific. Instead, it relies on the therapist's ability to extend preexisting therapeutic paradigms and techniques to include the powerful and relevant narratives and metaphors present in comic books, movies, songs, television, video games, literature, and the cyber-world. It is important at this point to differentiate between popular culture interventions and other forms of intervention.

The intervention most closely aligned to popular culture intervention in the literature is what has been termed *cinematherapy,* which according to Dermer and Hutchins is "a specific therapeutic technique that involves selecting commercial films for clients to view individually or with others for therapeutic gain" (2000, p. 164). These particular authors note that movies are particularly useful in psychotherapy with individuals and families because of their universal appeal, ease of integration into a broad range of therapeutic modalities, and applicability to diverse populations. Adding that films allow clients to connect with the characters at an emotional, behavioral, and cognitive level, Dermer and Hutchins, in concert with others before them (Berg-Cross, Jennings, & Baruch, 1990; Christie & McGrath, 1987; Hesley & Hesley, 1988), offer guidelines for utilizing movies in family therapy. Relatedly, Ashcraft, working in the area of sex education with teens, noted that "movies challenge dominant representations of adolescent masculinities and femininities and provide resources for engaging teens in important discourses for sexuality" (2003, p. 38).

It is important to note, however, that cinematherapy does not have an empirical track record to speak of, and is not as simple as asking clients to watch two movies and call you in the morning. Utilizing plotlines and characters in movies (and television shows by association) requires that the therapist be familiar with the films, and that careful consideration be given both to the film's potential impact on the client, and to the client's ability to effectively process the experience.

Another recognized form of treatment that makes use of popular culture is bibliotherapy, which is defined as "the use of written materials or computer programs, or the listening/viewing of audio/videotapes for the purpose of gaining understanding or solving problems relevant to a person's developmental or therapeutic needs" (Marrs, 1995, p. 846). Unlike cinematherapy, which relies on the use of materials that are not designed to be therapeutic per se, bibliotherapy makes use of reading and experiential homework assignments to clients of materials from credible self-help publications. Also unlike cinematherapy, bibliotherapy has received considerable empirical attention in the literature including meta-analytic outcomes studies assessing its effectiveness in the treatment of depression, sexual dysfunction, anxiety, and other minor disorders (Gregory, Canning, Lee, & Wise, 2004; Marrs, 1995; van Lankveld, 1998).

As a popular culture intervention; however, bibliotherapy as discussed in our context, is not the use of self-help books, but of popular literature to engage clients in therapeutic discussions. Just as movies and television shows highlight important discourse on a wide range of issues, so books, comic books, and the emergence and popularity of graphic novels[3] provide the opportunity for clients and clinicians to discuss a wide range of topics of potential therapeutic import. Beres, for example "wondered what range of discourse had been available to the abused women who learned to romanticize or minimize abuse" (2002, p. 432). She explored abused women's engagement with romance novels and concluded that "popular cultural texts are part of clients' imaginative lives, and by discussing favorite texts with our clients, we will be given a glimpse into their imaginative lives" (p. 444). Along similar lines, I have found that superhero comic books can be a valuable means of addressing complex issues with children, teenagers, and adults, including religion, racism, and sexuality (Rubin, 2006).

Another form of popular culture intervention involves the use of music in psychotherapy and counseling. Unlike cinematherapy and bibliotherapy, however, music therapy is an established therapeutic discipline with an extensive history and a broad empirical foundation of support. Interested readers are directed to the American Music Therapy Association (http://www.musictherapy.org) as well as to comprehensive literature reviews and meta-analytic studies of the efficacy of music therapy (Darrow, 2004; Gold, Voracek, & Wigram, 2004; Koger, Chapin, & Brotons, 1999; Wigram, Pedersen, & Bonde, 2000; Wigram, Saperston, & West, 1995). Suffice it to say for our purposes that as a therapeutic resource, music is ubiquitous, particularly with the advent of MTV, the Internet, file sharing, and the iPod, and as such provides endless lyrics for therapeutic dialogue and rhythms for physical and emotional expression (Rosenblum, Daniolos, Kass, & Martin, 1999).

As for the other forms of popular culture represented in this book, including video games and board games, the Internet, and both professional and amateur athletics, I will leave it to the talented team of clinicians that follow to demonstrate their clinical applicability with clients of all ages. By way of this overview of popular culture and the concept of popular culture intervention, I hope to have introduced you to a world of clinical possibilities in the everyday world of the popular.

Part I, entitled "Literature," focuses on the use of several powerful and popular literary stories in play therapy and counseling. In chapter 1, "Metaphors, Analogies, and Myths, Oh My!: Therapeutic Journeys Along the Yellow Brick Road" Lisa Saldaña argues that the story of the Wizard of Oz contains powerful metaphors that have resonated with generations of American children, and continue to do so long into adulthood. Why this story is so powerful, as well as how the characters are used in the therapeutic work of children, adolescents, and adults, is then examined through case discussion including artwork, family counseling, and sand tray therapy. In chapter 2, "Harry Potter and the Prisoner Within: Helping Children With Traumatic Loss," William McNulty observes that children have been able to identify with the trials and tribulations that Harry Potter, an orphan, experiences both at home and at school as he moves through a journey of self-exploration and growth. His chapter focuses on a client's traumatic early loss of parents, and how he used the Harry Potter story to heal. In chapter 3, entitled "Calvin and Hobbes to the Rescue!: The Therapeutic Uses of Comic Strips and Cartoons," Laura Sullivan describes the treatment of a 6-year-old with nighttime fears and sleeping problems who, like she, admired the famous cartoon pair.

Part II, entitled "Music," offers creative insights into the way popular music can be channeled therapeutically. Chapter 4, "The Healing Power of Music," by Nancy Davis and Beth Pickard, demonstrates how to bring music into the therapeutic relationship as a vehicle of change with children, adolescents, and adults with issues such as grief/loss, anxiety, depression, and PTSD. Chapter 5, by Thelma Duffey, entitled "Using Music and *A Musical Chronology* as a Life Review With the Aging," introduces the Musical Chronology as an intervention that can be used with clients working through issues of grief, loss, and other life challenges and transitions.

Part III, entitled "Movies," explores a number of creative ways to incorporate film into counseling and psychotherapy. Chapter 6, "Milieu Multiplex: Using Movies in the Treatment of Adolescents With Sexual

Behavior Problems," by Karen Robertie, Ryan Weidenbenner, Leya Barrett, and Robert Poole, explores the many ways the themes and characters of popular movies have been incorporated into the treatment of inpatient adolescent sex offenders including the use of scriptwriting and movie-making as therapeutic tools. Chapter 7, by Dora Finamore, entitled "*Little Miss Sunshine* and Positive Psychology as a Vehicle for Change in Adolescent Depression," explores the film from both an individual and family perspective, as a vehicle for treating adolescent depression in a school-based group therapy program. In chapter 8, by Linda B. Hunter, entitled "Movie Metaphors in Miniature: Children's Use of Popular Hero and Shadow Figures in Sandplay," Disney movie heroes and their evil counterparts battle, find and use their voices, protect, risk, challenge, rescue, solve problems and save the world—all under the child's control as s/he directs the healing action in the therapeutic sandbox with miniatures drawn from popular movies.

Part IV, entitled "Video and Board Games," demonstrates creative ways in which clinicians bring this popular venue of entertainment into the playroom. Chapter 9, by Deidre Skigen, "Taking the Sand Tray High Tech: Using The Sims as a Therapeutic Tool in the Treatment of Adolescents," demonstrates how the popular and powerful online interactive video game, The Sims, can be utilized as a therapeutic tool in the treatment of adolescents dealing with divorce and adjustment to stepfamilies. Chapter 10, by George Enfield and Melonie Grosser, entitled "Picking Up Coins: The Use of Video Games in the Treatment of Adolescent Social Problems," combines theory and practice to demonstrate use of video games as a bridge for working with boys to increase emotional expression, conflict resolution, confidence, and positive social interactions. Chapter 11, "Passing Go in the Game of Life: Board Games in Therapeutic Play," by Harry Livesay, presents an overview of a variety of popular board games (Life, Scooby Doo, Candy Land) and their therapeutic application.

Part V, entitled "Television," positions the reader in front of the small screen for a discussion of the therapeutic role of several popular TV shows. Chapter 12, by Lawrence C. Rubin, entitled "Big Heroes on the Small Screen: Naruto and the Struggle Within," demonstrates the effectiveness of bringing anime into the therapeutic playroom for children and teens coping with anger and disruptive family circumstances. Chapter 13, "Marcia, Marcia, Marcia: The Use and Impact of Television Themes, Characters, and Images in Psychotherapy," by Loretta Gallo-Lopez, explores the case of a 6-year-old cancer patient within the context of her identification with fictional television icon Marcia Brady of the *Brady Bunch*. Chapter 14, by Thelma Duffey and Heather Trepal, "The Sopranos and a Client's Hope for Justice," utilizes the infamous cable television series in order to help clients come to terms with unfair treatment, challenging life circumstances, and other significant struggles around issues of fairness, ambiguity, and resolve.

Part VI, entitled "Sports," addresses the ways in which amateur and professional athletics and athletes can play an active role in clinical practice. Chapter 15, "Using the Popularity of Sports Culture in Psychotherapy," by Jan M. Burte, illustrates that the sports subculture meets the criteria for a legitimate culture and that by utilizing sports celebrities and sports metaphors in the clinical engagement of both youths and adults, significant psychotherapeutic gains can be achieved. Chapter 16, "Sports Metaphors and Stories in Counseling With Children," by David A. Crenshaw and Gregory B. Barker, utilizes sports metaphors, stories, characters, and analogies to address a variety of clinical issues with children, teens, and young adults.

Part VII, entitled "Innovations in the Use of Popular Culture," takes us into unique and unexpected clinical applications of popular culture. Chapter 17, by Alan M. Schwitzer, Kelly E. MacDonald, and Pamela Dickinson, entitled "Using Pop Culture Characters in Clinical Training and Supervision," draws on characters of popular culture for use in clinical training and supervision to help develop case conceptualization, diagnosis, and treatment planning skills. As illustrations, the chapter addresses addictive disorder of Gollum from *Lord of the Rings*, and the sexual identity questions of E. Lynn Harris's Basil Henderson. Chapter 18, entitled "The Therapeutic Use of Popular Electronic Media With Today's Teenagers," by Scott Riviere, explores the use of popular forms of electronic media including My Space™, e-mail, e-postcards (Postsecret. com), and PowerPoint™ presentations by adolescents to communicate feelings, work out relationships and family issues, and strengthen identity as well as resolve difficult emotional challenges.

NOTES

1. See http://www.billboard.com for its weekly listing of the 100 top-selling songs, artists, and albums.
2. See McLuhan, M. (1960), Classroom without walls, in E. Carpenter and M. McLuhan (Eds.), *Explorations in communication: An anthology*, p. 3 (Boston: Beacon Press).
3. A graphic novel is a type of comic book, usually with a lengthy and complex story line similar to those of novels, and often aimed at mature audiences. The term also encompasses comic short story anthologies, and in some cases bound collections of previously published comic books. For more information, see http://en.wikipedia.org/wiki/Graphic_novelok series.

REFERENCES

Ashcraft, C. (2003). Adolescent ambiguities in *American Pie:* Popular culture as a resource for sex education. *Youth & Society, 35*(1), 37–70.

Beres, L. (2002). Negotiating images: Popular culture, imagination, and hope in clinical social work practice. *Affilia, 17*(4), 429–447.

Berg-Cross, L., Jennings, P., & Baruch, R. (1990). Cinematherapy: Theory and application. *Psychotherapy in Private Practice, 8*(1), 135–156.

Browne, R. (2006). Popular culture: Notes toward a definition. In H. Hinds, Jr., M. Motz, & A. Nelson (Eds.), *Popular culture theory and methodology: A basic introduction* (pp. 9–46). Madison, WI: University of Wisconsin Popular Press.

Cawelti, J. (2001). The concept of formula in the study of popular culture literature. In C. Harrington & D. Bielby (Eds.), *Popular culture: Production and consumption* (pp. 203–209). Malden, MA: Blackwell.

Christie, M., & McGrath, M. (1987). Taking up the challenge: Film as a therapeutic metaphor and action ritual. *Australian and New Zealand Journal of Family Therapy, 8*(4), 193–199.

Darrow, A. (Ed.). (2004). *Introduction to approaches in music therapy.* Silver Spring, MD: The American Music Therapy Association.

Dermer, S., & Hutchins, J. (2000). Utilizing movies in family therapy: Applications for individuals, couples and families. *The American Journal of Family Therapy, 28*(2), 163–180.

Fishwick, M. (2002). *Popular culture in a new age.* Binghamton, NY: The Haworth Press.

Gold, C., Voracek, M., & Wigram, T. (2004). Effects of music therapy for children and adolescents with psychopathology: A meta-analysis. *Journal of Child Psychology and Psychiatry, 45*(6), 1054–1063.

Gregory, R., Canning, S. S., Lee, T., & Wise, J. (2004). Cognitive bibliotherapy for depression: A meta-analysis. *Professional Psychology: Research and Practice, 35*(3), 275–280.

Harrington, C. L., & Bielby, D. D. (2001). Constructing the popular: Cultural production and consumption. In C. L. Harrington & D. D. Bielby (Eds.), *Popular culture: Production and consumption* (pp. 1–15). Malden, MA: Blackwell.

Hesley, J. W., & Hesley, J. G. (1988). *Rent two films and let's talk in the morning: Using popular movies in psychotherapy.* New York: Wiley.

Johnson, S. (2005). *Everything bad is good for you: Why popular culture is making us smarter.* London: Penguin.

Kaiser Family Foundation. (2001). *Talking with kids about tough issues: A national survey of parents and kids.* Retrieved June 13, 2007, from http://www.kff.org/kaiserpolls/3107-index.cfm

Kidd, D. (2007). Harry Potter and the functions of popular culture. *The Journal of Popular Culture, 40*(1), 69–89.

Koger, S., Chapin, K., & Brotons, M. (1999). Is music therapy an effective intervention for dementia? A meta-analytic review of literature. *Journal of Music Therapy, 36*(1), 2–15.

Marrs, R. (1995). A meta-analysis of bibliotherapy studies. *American Journal of Community Psychology, 23*(6), 843–870.

Mattingly, C. (2006). Pocahontas goes to the clinic: Popular culture as lingua franca in a cultural borderland. *American Anthropologist, 108*(3), 494–501.

Miller, T., & McHoul, A. (1998). *Popular culture and everyday life.* Thousand Oaks, CA: Sage.

Neal, A. (1995). Cultural fragmentation in the 21st century. In R. Browne and M. Fishwick (Eds.), *Preview 2001+: Popular culture studies in the future* (pp. 111–125). Bowling Green, OH: Bowling Green State University Popular Press.

Nye, R. (1971). Notes for an introduction to a discussion of popular culture. *Journal of Popular Culture, 4*(4), 1031–1038.

Rosenblum, D., Daniolos, P., Kass, N., & Martin, A. (1999). Adolescents and popular culture. *The Psychoanalytic Study of the Child, 54,* 319–338.

Rubin, L. (Ed.). (2006). *Using superheroes in counseling and play therapy.* New York: Springer Publishing.

Taffel, R. (2005). *Breaking through to teens: A new psychotherapy for the new adolescence.* Guilford: New York.

van Lankveld, J. (1998). Bibliotherapy in the treatment of sexual dysfunction. *Journal of Consulting and Clinical Psychology, 66*(4), 702–708.

Wigram, T., Pedersen, I., & Bonde, L. (2000). *A comprehensive guide to music therapy: Theory, clinical practice, research and training.* London, England: Jessica Kingsley.

Wigram, T., Saperston, B., & West, R. (1995). *The art and science of music therapy: A handbook.* Langhorne, PA, England: Harwood Academic Publishers/Gordon.

PART I

Literature

CHAPTER 1

Metaphors, Analogies, and Myths, Oh My!

Therapeutic Journeys Along the Yellow Brick Road

Lisa Saldaña

A young girl, feeling alone and vulnerable, stands in a grey and overcast farm yard. Dark clouds hang in the background as she wistfully imagines a place "where there isn't any trouble." Yet, this place—as she tells her small furry companion—would not be a place you could get to by any normal means, for it's located "behind the moon" and "beyond the rain." Little does she know that she is about to be hurled over the rainbow, to experiences and relationships that will help her discover that you can't run away from your fears, and whatever it is you seek, it's always right there within you.

THE WONDERFUL WIZARD OF OZ: AN AMERICAN FAIRY TALE

For over 100 years, *The Wonderful Wizard of Oz* "has given faithful service to the Young in Heart; and Time has been powerless to put its kindly philosophy out of fashion."[1] At the dawn of the 20th century, *The Wonderful Wizard of Oz* was published in the United States (Baum, 1900). Often considered the first American fairy tale (Library of Congress, 2000), this beloved children's story has been the basis for a series of over 30 Oz books, and has generated toys, memorabilia, numerous television and stage productions, and of course, one of the most beloved movies of all times: Metro-Goldwyn-Meyer's 1939 musical (LeRoy, 1939).

Today, *The Wizard of Oz* continues to resonate within American culture. The adventures of Dorothy and her faithful companions live on, from kitschy Halloween costumes—complete with ruby slippers and a toy Toto in a basket—to books and articles examining the significance of the tale (Bausch, 1999; Green, 1998; Mills &Crowley, 1986; Morena, 1998; Murphy, 1996; Rushdie, 1992; Schreiber, 1974). What is it about this story that its power is undiminished by time? Why do the story's characters make appearances in the therapeutic work of children, adolescents, and adults?

We Must Be Over the Rainbow!: Fairy Tales and the Realm of the Unconscious

Much has been written of the meaning of fairy tales and their relationship to the unconscious (Roheim, 1953, 1982; Luthi, 1976, 1987; Shapiro & Katz, 1978; Schreiber, 1974; Schwartz, 1956; Von Franz, 1982). Freud (1913) noted that some people may remember their favorite fairy tales in place of real childhood memories. Bettelheim (1976) studied the therapeutic power of fairy tales and their ability to provide guidance and support, assisting children in understanding and coping with the difficulties of life. Children can identify with the main characters of fairy tales, who are often children like themselves, coping with challenges that mirror real situations. The personal, social, and familial conflicts in these tales, as well as the methods by which the characters handle and learn from them, may provide models of coping. As Bettelheim noted,

> Fairy tales carry important messages to the conscious, the preconscious, and the unconscious mind, on whatever level is functioning at the time. By dealing with universal human problems, particularly those which preoccupy the child's mind, these stories speak to his budding ego and encourage its development, while at the same time relieving the preconscious and unconscious pressures. (p. 6)

Fairy tales, when read through a Jungian framework, are examples of the collective unconscious at work. Whenever we work with symbols, whether images on the movie screen, characters in books, or figures in the sand tray, we are tapping into unconscious materials: the repressed or forgotten memories and feelings of our personal unconscious—which are not in our awareness, but might be brought to the fore—and the collective unconscious (Jung, 1964, 1980, 1981). If you look at the elements found in these tales, they correspond to universal symbols, such as Mother,

Father, Hero, Wise Old Man, Great Mother, Child, and Trickster. These archetypes are believed to be the structural components of the collective unconscious—images and symbols found in every culture, in every age.

Whatever the reason, traditional stories, including myths, fables, allegories, fairy tales, and religious writings, are passed from generation to generation because they speak to the conscious and unconscious needs of the people who hear or read them. When a story manages to stay alive and relevant through time, as has *The Wonderful Wizard of Oz,* there is a universality that resonates. As we hear the tale, we identify with characters and situations; we feel, often on a purely unconscious level, that we're hearing *our* story. We may know that these tales of magical places, wicked stepmothers, animals who talk, and children who defeat evil giants aren't real, but we feel and experience them as *true.* Stories that do not connect and resonate within their listeners wither and die.

We're Off to See the Wizard: Metaphors on the Silver Screen

Baum recognized the power of fairy tales. In the introduction to *The Wonderful Wizard of Oz,* he wrote that "Folk lore, legends, myths, and fairy tales have followed childhood through the ages," and that he wanted to create a story "in which the wonderment and joy are retained and the heart-aches and nightmares are left out" (1900, introduction). In Dorothy, Baum provided a protagonist with whom American children could identify: a young girl on a farm in the middle of the United States. Surrounded by hardships, Dorothy and her family struggle to survive on the harsh plains of Kansas. When she finds herself thrown into a strange and alien world, she faces challenges with a calm optimism, courage, and faith.

While Baum's modern fairy tale was a success, selling thousands of copies and propelling its creators to fame and fortune, the story still had not achieved its full power in popular culture. Over the years, different versions of Dorothy's story have been presented on the stage and screen, but it was the 1939 movie that placed Dorothy and Oz firmly into American (and world) consciousness. When the movie debuted on television in 1956, it initiated an annual tradition that became an event for many families. When I discuss the movie in my metaphors workshop, I often share childhood memories of my own excitement at its approach each year. Invariably, the participants will recall their own families' *Wizard of Oz* rituals and share them with the group. In 1980, the video version was released to the public, and every household with a TV and VCR had access to its message. Lines and scenes from the movie have become part of our culture. We immediately recognize the phrases "Follow the yellow brick road," "I'll get you, my pretty," and "We're off to see the Wizard";

we understand what is meant when someone shakes a head and sighs that "we're not in Kansas anymore," or admonishes us to "pay no attention to the man behind the curtain." And of course, everyone knows "there's no place like home."

A Caveat of a Different Color

Since the more powerful images in most people's minds—and therefore in my therapy room—tend to be from the movie, this chapter will focus on those. You may wish to read (or reread) the original book, since there were significant changes made for the film. In the movie, Dorothy's adventures are only a dream, and the only real danger the Wicked Witch of the West. In the book, Dorothy really does travel by cyclone to the Lands of Oz, where she and her companions explore its many realms, meet its various inhabitants, and face and overcome many dangerous challenges before Dorothy finally returns to Kansas. In the movie, Dorothy kills the Witch incidentally to saving the Scarecrow, but in the book, she's a much more empowered young girl, killing the Witch in an angry response to her trickery, and then rescuing her friends.

The book also gives much more depth to the characters and provides the reader with opportunities to think about life's lessons. For example, the characters debate which is more important, the heart—"for brains do not make one happy"—or the brain—"a fool would not know what to do with a heart if he had one" (Baum, 1900, p. 73). Through their numerous adventures, we see again and again how each character embodies that which they seek. The Cowardly Lion acknowledges his fear, and then bravely protects his friends. We read of the Tin Man's gentle care and compassion for every living creature, because he believes that people's hearts provide guidance and prevent them from hurting others, "but I have no heart, so I must be very careful" (p. 86).

In creating the movie, the story's central themes were retained. These include the beliefs that if we trust in ourselves and look within, we find what we seek: ". . . if I ever go looking for my heart's desire again, I won't look any further than my own backyard. Because if it isn't there, I never really lost it to begin with"; and of course, "there's no place like home!" (LeRoy, 1939).

FOLLOW THE YELLOW BRICK ROAD: THE THEME OF THE HERO'S JOURNEY

Like most of the modern stories that have captured our imaginations and now dwell in the popular culture, *The Wonderful Wizard of Oz* is a modern manifestation of what Joseph Campbell identified as "The Hero's Journey" (Campbell, 1968). This theme is not new. It is the outline of every major religious story, of fairy tales, myths, and legends, and is found throughout history and across cultures. Mythology "is psychology misread as biography, history, and cosmology" (p. 256).

There are three phases to The Hero's Journey—Departure, Initiation, and Return—and within these phases are many steps. The Hero receives the call to adventure, in which he is "drawn into a relationship with forces that are not rightly understood" (Campbell, 1968, p. 51) and, like Dorothy, finds himself in "a place of strangely fluid and polymorphous beings, unimaginable torments, superhuman deeds, and impossible delight" (p. 58).

As he begins the Journey, The Hero encounters a mentor or protector who provides guidance. Along the way, allies may join the quest. These companions are an integral part of the story, providing support for The Hero, while coping with their own challenges and limitations. Allies provide assistance, but it is The Hero who must ultimately complete the quest.

As The Hero moves forward, he overcomes obstacles and faces challenges that could destroy him or his companions. By facing and overcoming these challenges, he gains insight, and reemerges with new abilities or a new awareness. At the end of the Journey, The Hero returns "to the kingdom of humanity" (Campbell, 1968, p. 193), where he shares the knowledge he's gained with others.

As Campbell reflected in a series of interviews with journalist Bill Moyers (Campbell & Moyers, 1991), myth and metaphor allow us to connect with our inner self. We react to certain metaphors because our inner world—"the world of your requirements and your energies and your structures and your possibilities" (p. 68)—meets the outer world in a story that resonates within us. These stories work on two levels: the surface level, where we see or read the story, and the deeper, unconscious level, where we identify with characters or situations.

You've Always Had the Power to Go Back to Kansas: The Client's Journey in Treatment

In many ways, The Hero's Journey is a metaphor that mirrors the process and progress of therapy. The core themes in these stories tend to be that of searching. The Hero searches for the true or correct path, his or her place in the world, meaningful relationships, and/or an understanding of his or her world. Clients often come to therapy searching for these same things. Working in therapy, our clients face challenges—often significant ones. We are the guide, providing support, safety, and protection within the therapeutic relationship. We do not provide the answers, only the support our clients need to find the answers themselves. Our clients may have allies in their lives who can assist them in facing their challenges, or we may help them identify allies. Within this support, they are able to face whatever brought them into treatment, overcome their challenges, develop an awareness and understanding of themselves, and share their knowledge with others.

I COULD THINK OF THINGS I NEVER THUNK BEFORE: PSYCHOTHERAPY AND METAPHORS

Metaphor and its use have been woven into psychology since its beginning. Freud's concept of dreams as the "royal road" to understanding the unconscious depended upon the associations made to the allegories and metaphors presented in our dreams. Even Skinner's reinforcement and extinguishing of behaviors are metaphors. Lakoff and Johnson (2003) state that "the essence of metaphor is understanding and experiencing one kind of thing in terms of another" (p. 5). Metaphors relate two objects or concepts that we would not normally connect with each other in such a way that we perceive and intuit a new thing. For example, we create new images when we connect emotions and energy (Desire burned. Anger consumed her. Love warmed his heart.); emotions and place (She went over the edge. He's in La-La-Land.); and concepts with living things (That idea died. Her legacy will live on. His responsibilities beat him down.), or objects (His theory didn't fit. That idea was solid.).

Metaphors in therapy also relate two objects or concepts that we would not normally connect with each other, to provide a new understanding. As Atwood & Levine (1991) note, metaphors "allow clients to perceive a different reality around their problems while still remaining in touch with the problems" (p. 202). As you will see when one client connects her dilemma to the Cowardly Lion, while another connects aggression to the same character, the new understanding is unique to the client's perception of the symbols.

Well, That's You All Over: Matching Client and Metaphor

Research suggests that metaphors are effective in therapy because they speak to the right side of the brain, rather than to the areas of the left hemisphere (Atwood & Levine, 1991; Mills & Crowley, 1986; Sharp, Smith, & Cole, 2002). The left hemisphere contains those logical, analytic areas of the brain that focus on details, and where language is understood at the surface or literal meaning. The right side of the brain can see the big picture and thinks holistically; it contains the creative, imaginative areas, where hidden meaning and humor are understood. By working in metaphor, we may bypass defense mechanisms and speak directly to the areas that are more adaptable and open to change.

There are different types of metaphors people use. In therapy, we are typically working with verbal, behavioral, physical, and physiological metaphors (Bayne & Thompson, 2000). Paying attention to the metaphors our clients use may provide us with insights into their experience and view of the world, and give us strategies to therapeutically use, clarify, and extend those metaphors (Angus & Korman, 2002; Angus & Rennie, 1989; Strong, 1989). A woman who says that she and her partner are "going in different directions" or her relationship is "at a dead end," may view relationships as progressions or journeys. If, on the other hand, she talks about their love as "dying," "growing" or "taking wing," she may see relationships as alive, developing, and living. By matching our response to the metaphor, we speak the client's language and communicate that we understand our client's view of the world. I know that I've missed the meaning when my response to a metaphor doesn't move the discussion forward. For example, when a client told me that he'd "hit a wall at work," my response reflected the concept that he felt he had been moving forward, and now feels blocked. I knew I had stayed within his metaphoric concept when he responded with an affirmation, and built on my response, providing more information: "Yeah, one minute I felt like I knew where I was going in the company, and the next minute, I'm stuck. And I don't know where to go." As the discussion continued, we both gained knowledge and insight about the issue. I know when my response doesn't match my client's perception: I usually get an "uh huh," or maybe an uncertain "um, yeah," or a "no, that's not it."

We can provide metaphors to our clients, but the metaphors they bring into the room are often more powerful, having the most meaning to them, because they come from their own psyche, worldview, and experience. When working with young children in play therapy, the session is often pure metaphor. Because children often lack the verbal and cognitive skills needed to verbalize the issues that bring them to treatment, they use toys and games or create artwork and stories that have meaning to them. Whether working with adults or children, I have found that if I stay within the client's metaphor and frame of reference, therapy is, as one child declared, "Magic!" As Cattanach (2002) notes, "Complex life events cannot always be understood through talking about what happened in reality talk, because the full impact can only be described and contained through metaphor, imagery, myth, and story, or sometimes, play without words" (p. 8).

Toto—I've a Feeling We're Not in Kansas Anymore: The Use of Physical Metaphors in the Playroom

My office is filled with symbols: toys, puppets, and games. My office-mate is a sandplay therapist, so we also have shelves filled with miniatures that represent the cosmos: realistic and fantastical people and animals; plants, trees, and natural elements; religious figures from around the world; buildings, furniture, vehicles, and so forth. While many people think of these therapeutic tools as only being used in play therapy with children, I have found the symbols to be amazingly helpful in working with clients of all ages, and especially helpful with adolescents and adults who have difficulty "finding the words" in my office. By inviting the client to look at the symbols, and find something that represents the person, problem, or issue he or she struggles to articulate, we may examine the symbol and discuss it, rather than what it represents. Using their own metaphors, clients are able to externalize their issues, concerns, and problems, making it easier to discuss and examine them. As Freeman, Epston, and Lobovits (1997) noted, talking about issues and problems in this one-step removed way allows the client safety and distance when working on difficult situations.

When working with angry, desperate, or frustrated couples and families, I often use metaphorical techniques. The distance and safety noted above frequently allow the clients to relate differently and discuss issues in a way that is different and more helpful than their typical communication patterns of fighting, blaming, avoiding, or arguing. This is demonstrated below in the session with Jessica and Mike.

Much has been written about the components of metaphorical stories (Davis, 1990; Gardner, 1971; Kottman, 1995; Mills & Crowley, 1986; Norton & Norton, 1997). Interestingly, they often mirror the format of myths and The Hero's Journey. Sometimes the story is an original one, created by the client and/or therapist in the course of treatment. Sometimes, like *The Wizard of Oz*, it's a movie or a story that the client has identified on some level as having the power to help them. Often, as in play therapy with children, the metaphorical story is a combination of the movies or television shows they have seen and their own imaginative therapeutic process. As you will see demonstrated in the story of Jeremy, metaphorical stories allow the child to personalize or individualize the story's narrative, in order to communicate his understanding of the problem and find the solutions or develop more effective coping skills. These stories feature a character the client relates to who must face challenges, and solve or cope with problems. There are a guide and allies who support and assist him in this endeavor. These characters express thoughts, feelings, and ideas that resonate within the client, although he may not be able to articulate this connection. As in real life, the answers don't come easily and the protagonist often struggles to overcome the challenge or problem and find answers. The other characters can help when needed, but the main character is the leader who makes decisions. The story typically ends with the main character talking about what he went through and what he learned.

YOU'RE OUT OF THE WOODS, YOU'RE OUT OF THE DARK, YOU'RE OUT OF THE NIGHT: *THE WIZARD OF OZ* METAPHORS

To Oz!: The Universality of Oz Symbols

There are as many ways to look at the symbols contained within the *Wizard of Oz* movie as there are people who study them (Bausch, 1999; Green, 1998; Morena, 1998; Murphy, 1996; Schreiber, 1974). There are simple connections: The three companions from Oz might be seen as representing something as simple as animal, vegetable, and mineral. There are complex connections that may be made: Dorothy's four companions may represent the four functions of the psyche, which Jung identified as thinking, feeling, intuition, and sensation (Ekstrom, 2004; Jung, 1981).

Toto may represent loyalty and commitment. Dorothy's adventures begin with her desire to protect her only friend, and he bravely guides the others to her rescue. Toto is at Dorothy's side throughout her adventures. He might represent intuition and insight: it is this faithful little dog who reveals the powerlessness of the supposedly great and powerful Wizard of Oz, and ensures that Dorothy completes the journey of self-discovery when he jumps from the gondola of the hot air balloon.

Dorothy meets the Scarecrow, who hasn't got a brain, when he's immobilized on a pole. He might represent dependence/independence, standing on our own two feet, feeling stuck, competence/incompetence, feeling capable/incapable. Throughout the movie, the Scarecrow longs for a brain, while demonstrating wisdom as the characters face their challenges—"Of course, I don't know, but I think it'll get darker before it gets lighter" (LeRoy, 1939)—and finding solutions to problems.

The Tin Man, who longs for a heart, obviously has one. If not, he would not be the sensitive, emotional character who cries easily, and cares enough about Dorothy to risk the wrath of the Witch to rescue her. When Dorothy discovered and rescued him in the forest, he was frozen or paralyzed. Might he represent fears of being unlovable, our desire to love and be loved, or the idea that connecting with others can free us and allow us to explore life?

We meet the Cowardly Lion as we enter the darkest parts of the forest, a fearful place where dwell "lions and tigers and bears! Oh my!" The Lion believes he lacks courage. He fails to recognize that bravery isn't about not feeling afraid, but in acting even when you are, something he does throughout their journey. He may represent fear of the unknown, uncertainty, doing the right thing in the face of fear, false bravado, or defense mechanisms.

As the characters venture closer to danger, they travel through the Haunted Forest. In the view of psychoanalytic symbolism, forests represent "the place in which inner darkness is confronted and worked through; where uncertainty is resolved about who one is; and where one begins to understand who one wants to be" (Bettelheim, 1976, p. 93).

I tend to view the movie as a metaphor of the human condition. Is there anyone who hasn't longed for a different life? Who at some point hasn't felt that life would be easier or they would be happier if they "only had" the right job or the right car or the right . . . ? That they would be complete if they "only had" the right relationship? As Dorothy sings about "over the rainbow," we all understand her longing. As her companions seek that which they believe will make them whole, we walk in their footsteps.

Dorothy and her allies seek the Wizard of Oz because they believe that only he can give them what they seek. I see him representing the tendency to look for an external solution to problems, rather than recognizing that, like Dorothy and her companions eventually do, we have the knowledge or resources we seek, if we just look within. Dorothy spent much of the movie avoiding the person who frightened and threatened her most: the Wicked Witch. Yet, in order to obtain her heart's desire, she was forced to seek and confront the Witch. When Dorothy faced her biggest fear, when she killed the Witch by throwing water to save her friend, the Witch dissolved. When we face our fears, they lose their power.

I'm Melting! Melting! Using Metaphors to Change Dynamics and Decrease Resistance

When families come to therapy, they typically have a lot of history and emotion attached to their situation. They have usually tried many different ways to solve their problems, and have done and said things that may have hurt each other and caused anger and resentment. By the time they are sitting across from me, it may be very difficult for them to communicate without these intense negative feelings interfering. Metaphors can shift the dynamics by allowing them to focus on a symbol, rather than on each other, and by allowing a discussion of their own feelings and reactions in the here-and-now rather than of past events or interactions. As noted above, a very simple intervention I use is the invitation to use the objects in the room to help me see the problem or issue.

When working with more than one person, I usually start by noting the strengths in their relationship and their history of attempts to cope or solve the problem. I acknowledge how difficult it is for the couple or family to discuss the issue. Lastly, I recognize that this stressful situation has resulted in strong emotions and reactions entering the room when the topic arises. Then I explain that I would like to try something a little different. If they are agreeable, I invite them to use symbols in the room to represent the issue or problem. My wording varies, depending upon the situation; however, it generally follows the lines of: "Look around the room, and see if you can find something that represents (the issue, problem, relationship, challenge, or person). Once you find something, bring it over and place it in the sand tray." I have also used, "Look around the room. If I asked you to find [your boss, your marriage, your job, the issue problem, or challenge] and place it in my hand, what would you choose?" As they work, I am able to observe their verbal and nonverbal interactions, which often provides information not seen when families are sitting and talking to the therapist. When they are finished making their choices, we discuss the objects.

CASE STUDIES

If I Were King of the Forest: The Cowardly Lion and Jeremy

"Jeremy" was 7 years old when he began therapy with me. An only child, his mother had adopted him from foster care. He was doing well at home, but was getting into trouble at school for fighting with other children. His teacher and mother were at a loss. They both described him as sweet and funny with younger children, but withdrawn and aggressive toward peers. His mother had enrolled him in karate, hoping that this would teach him discipline and channel his energy in a more appropriate way, but he continued to get in trouble and had made no friends.

After a first session of getting to know the room, the expectations of therapy, and me, Jeremy came back the next week and went straight to the *Wizard of Oz* miniatures on the shelf. He identified each character and told me about the movie. Picking up the Cowardly Lion, he placed him in the sand tray. He added a combination of other animals and people—although none from the movie—and created a forest for their environment. That day, the Cowardly Lion spent the session growling, snarling, and chasing the other characters, who ran and hid from him. They were afraid of him, and he was in control. He would verbalize that the others were chicken and they weren't going to mess with him. As I watched, I verbally reflected the Lion's feelings of power, as well as the other characters' fear and desire to get away from him. When I wondered aloud if there was anyone in the forest who wasn't afraid of the Lion, Jeremy told me emphatically, "He don't want no friends!"

In the next session, Jeremy once again created scenarios using the Cowardly Lion figure, but this time, as the session progressed, he had some of the other characters stand up to him and fight back. The Lion became frustrated and angry, often destroying the others. Again, I would reflect the Lion's feelings, as well as the others', but I also observed that the Lion was living in the forest all alone, while the other characters seemed to have friendships. They had a community that lived together and often created alliances that stood up to him together. This observation prompted Jeremy to tell me about the Lion's difficult life and his loneliness. He had grown up all alone in a cave in the forest, and the other animals had never accepted him, because he was a lion and they weren't. Everyone was mean to him; he'd even been beaten up and shot at. But the Lion was smart and he had learned to survive. We spent the remainder of the session talking about the Lion's many fears. He was very afraid of people in general, afraid of trying to make friends, and afraid that if he made friends, they would hurt him. By the end of the session, Jeremy and I had decided that Lion's hard life certainly justified being afraid, and that he was being mean and loud because he was feeling very scared and vulnerable. He wanted to be nice and have friends, but he was afraid he'd be hurt again, so he kept everyone away by being so scary.

Before starting the fourth session, Jeremy's mother reported far fewer problems at school. In this session, Lion (through Jeremy) and I discussed Lion's positive attributes. Lion recognized that he was funny, athletic, and smart. He was able to identify Glinda and the Tin Man as two people who knew the real Lion, and might be able to assist him. He brought Glinda and Tin Man to the sand tray, and assigned their roles to me. These friends agreed that Lion really could be nice, once you got to know him. They suggested that he would need to convince everyone else in the forest, since they were now quite afraid of him. The three characters talked about things he might try in order to make friends. They discussed choosing friends carefully, because sometimes friend-making could be tricky. Together, Lion and his allies found out about the others living in the forest, and what they might have in common with Lion.

For the next few sessions, Lion tried making friends with various characters. Sometimes it worked out, sometimes it didn't. Lion struggled with fears of taking risks, feelings of rejection, sadness, and anger, and learning new strategies for connecting with the other denizens of the forest. At the same time, I was receiving reports that Jeremy was becoming a part of the classroom. He was interacting better, and was no longer fighting. By the last session, Lion had made a few friends, and although they sometimes had difficulties and arguments, Lion was no longer aggressive. When there was conflict, Lion was more likely to go find Glinda or Tin Man and talk about how angry or hurt he was. In our last session, Glinda, Tin Man, and Lion celebrated Lion's accomplishments. While acknowledging that there would still be times when he was afraid or when it was hard to make friends, we also identified the new tools and skills he had developed to help him.

When we ended treatment, Jeremy hadn't made any close friends, but he was no longer fighting, and had peers he talked to and played with at school and karate class. His mother and teacher reported that he was much more likely to seek assistance from others, and could seek adults to help him negotiate the challenges of peer relationships.

Jeremy recognized and identified with the Cowardly Lion's false bravado covering his fear. Someone else, on the other hand, might pick the same character for a very different connection. One adult client, who was struggling with a major life-changing decision, was invited to look around the room, and choose a symbol to represent her dilemma. She chose the Cowardly Lion. When asked to tell me about the Cowardly Lion, she identified the scene in the movie where Dorothy's friends plan her rescue:

Cowardly Lion:	I may not come out alive, but I'm going in there. There's only one thing I want you fellows to do.
Scarecrow and Tin Man:	What's that?
Cowardly Lion:	Talk me out of it. (LeRoy, 1939)

In choosing and talking about the Cowardly Lion, she was able to identify and verbalize that she was avoiding making the decision by constantly asking friends and family their opinions on her options. She realized that she hoped they would convince her to make the easiest decision, although she knew it wasn't the right decision. The Cowardly Lion demonstrated his courage in doing what needed to be done, even though he was terrified of what he faced, just as my client recognized she needed to do.

Now I Know I've Got a Heart, 'Cause It's Breaking: Mike and Jessica

"Mike" and "Jessica" married young when Jessica became pregnant with their oldest daughter. Because of an illness in her family, Jessica had bounced around relatives' homes before they married. Together 18 years, Mike was now a successful business owner and Jessica was able to stay home with their children, who ranged in age from 8 to 16. They agreed that their relationship had had its ups and downs, but had been strong and relatively happy until 2 years ago, when they started fighting about money and Jessica's excessive spending. Mike worked long hours, and when the children were in school, Jessica went shopping. Mike felt that she was "wasting [his] hard earned money on things she [didn't] need." Jessica agreed that she spent a great deal of money on shoes and clothing, but she had no other activities besides the house and children. She felt that they were very well off and could afford her purchases. The situation had escalated recently when Mike cancelled her credit cards, and would now only give her an allowance. When they came into therapy, they were sleeping in separate rooms and talking about divorce. In their first session, it was challenging to obtain information as they focused on their anger and hurt, but we were able to identify loving feelings and a level of commitment to each other and their children, as well as a number of positive aspects of their lives together.

When they came into the second session, Jessica noted the *Wizard of Oz* figures on the shelf, and mentioned that she loved the movie, and enjoyed watching it with their children. Mike agreed that it was a family favorite. Recognizing a possible invitation to use these characters, I asked them if they were willing to try something a little different. When they responded positively, I invited them to look at the characters from the movie. "Which one do you think is the most like you? And which do you think is the most like your spouse? Think about it for a minute, and when you decide, go and get them and place them in the sand tray." Jessica was the first to get up. She placed Dorothy and the Tin Man next to each other in the sand. As she did so, I observed that Mike seemed disturbed by her choices. As she walked back to the couch, he went to the shelves and removed the Cowardly Lion. Setting the Lion on the other side of Dorothy, he said he had also chosen Dorothy to represent his wife. The three of us studied the trio for a moment, and then I asked if either of them wanted to comment or ask any questions. When Mike said he did, I asked that they listen respectfully to each other.

Mike told us that he had chosen the Cowardly Lion for himself, because "I'm afraid around my wife." He clarified that he wasn't afraid of her, but of her very emotional reactions. He knew that there were times he needed to address issues at home before they "grew and became bigger problems," but that when he did so, she would "overreact." Sometimes she would cry and accuse him of not loving or understanding her. He then felt guilty, because she was already so unhappy. He described feeling powerless in the face of her pain. At other times, her reaction was angry, resulting in loud arguments that upset the children, and again, he felt responsible for her distress, as well as hurt and angry himself. Because of her reaction, he said he would often avoid an issue until it grew to a point that it had to be addressed, and by then, he acknowledged that he was usually frustrated and angry.

He referred to the scene in the movie when Dorothy sings "Over the Rainbow," as he explained why he had chosen Dorothy to represent his wife. He saw Dorothy as yearning and unhappy; wanting to "escape her home and family." He described his wife in the same way: "She's just so unhappy." He acknowledged her "tough life" and that she was always a little sad, but lately seemed more so. He saw her as wanting to escape "from us, from her family" and he was hurt and worried by this. He described his wife as feeling as though she was missing something. He ventured a theory that her spending was an attempt to make herself happy with "stuff," and wondered aloud if he avoided discussing her spending because he thought she needed to shop in order to be happy.

Jessica listened quietly as Mike spoke, tears in her eyes. When he finished, she described her choice of Dorothy for herself for very similar reasons. She described Dorothy's desperate desire to go home, and connected that to her own feelings as a child. She described Dorothy when we meet her at the beginning of the movie, as she seeks help from her family, but is rebuffed: "No one listened to her. She was so sad and all alone." Looking at Mike, she reassured him that she didn't want to escape him or their children, that she loved them very much; they were her home. She pointed to the tray and explained her choice of Tin Man for Mike. She described a man who she remembered as warm and loving with her. She knew he was still that way inside, because she saw it with their children and his family, but with her, he had become distant and cold. He was no longer the physically affectionate, cuddly man she needed. She didn't know how to get back inside the hard exterior that covered his soft heart. Mike asked if he could speak. When Jessica nodded, he said he had no idea she felt that way. When he had seen her choice, he thought it was because she saw him "as heartless," and he was afraid she didn't love him anymore.

As the session progressed, they were able to talk about their relationship. The issue of money and spending were forgotten as they began to realize that Mike's avoidance of upsetting Jessica had been interpreted by her as withdrawal and abandonment. With his support, she was also able to acknowledge her feelings of sadness and loneliness because of his long work hours and the children being in school. In the course of the session, Jessica recognized the need to resume therapy with her individual therapist and Mike made a commitment to be home early at least three nights a week. As they were leaving the office, Jessica mentioned that when she looked at the three characters in the sand, she was struck by the image of the Lion, Dorothy, and the Tin Man. She noted that Dorothy was "caught between love (pointing to the Tin Man) and fear (the Cowardly Lion)," but that she could also be seen as "being supported by love and courage." We met for two more sessions, and they were able to use this new understanding of each other's feelings to reconnect and make changes in their interactions.

Somewhere, Over the Rainbow, Skies Are Blue: Dorothy and Maria

"Maria" was battling anxiety, depression, and alcohol abuse when she was referred to me by her psychiatrist. An incredibly creative and artistic young woman, she struggled to talk about what had brought her into my office. As we talked, I noticed that her eyes were drawn to the wall of sand tray miniatures, and after a little while, she asked me about them. I explained that sometimes people find they can use the miniatures to discuss hard issues. I offered an invitation to take any miniatures that caught her eye, and place them in the sand tray. Maria readily agreed, and began to thoughtfully select miniatures and place them in the sand. The first figure she chose was Dorothy. She placed her in the center of the tray, and slowly placed an object at each point of the tray: a dove at the top, a figurine of a Madonna on the left, a crystal heart on the right, and a treasure chest at the bottom of the tray. Then she added four raised sand barriers between Dorothy and the objects. When she finished, I asked if there was anything she'd like to share about her sand tray.

She went first to Dorothy, and picked her up. She told me that she had been drawn to the figure because she looked like a happy little girl. She noted that sometimes she felt like a little girl, although not a happy one. She cradled her in her hand for a moment, and then set her back down in the center. She talked about feeling small and vulnerable and very unhappy. Then she explained the meaning of the other objects. They represented the things she sought: a loving relationship (crystal heart); to feel a spiritual reconnection (the Madonna); a better paying, less stressful job (the treasure chest); and to feel at peace with herself (the dove). The walls of sand, she explained, represented the barriers to having those things; between Dorothy and the heart was her distrust of relationships. Between Dorothy and the Madonna was her anger at God. Between Dorothy and the treasure chest was her fear of leaving her job and being poor and losing her home. Between Dorothy and the dove were her feelings of fear and lack of security.

When she was done explaining this, I asked her if there was anything in the room that might be able to overcome any of the barriers. She stared at the shelves for a while, and then chose a set of praying hands. Using her hand, she wiped out the barrier between Dorothy and the dove, and placed the hands in its place. After a moment of studying the tray, she moved the Madonna next to the dove. She stepped back and told me that when she was a child, she had always felt calm and at peace in church. Never taking her eyes off the tray, she said that it was the one of the few places she felt safe. I wondered aloud if there might be a place like that in her life now. Maria responded that there wasn't, and she thought she ought to find one. We ended the session with her making a commitment to finding and visiting a church or similar place where she could feel that sense of peace and safety. Before ending the session, she looked at the tray and asked me if the girl was Dorothy, from *The Wizard of Oz*. Assured that she was correct, Maria left.

Maria opened our next session by telling me that on her way home from our previous meeting, she had rented *The Wizard of Oz*. She had never seen the whole movie, she said. That evening, as she sat in her apartment and followed the yellow brick road with Dorothy and friends, she was surprised at her strong emotional reaction to the movie. She began to write about it in her journal, and realized that Dorothy couldn't get have gotten back home by herself. The following day, she had gone to a 12-step meeting and found a sponsor.

She cried as she quietly described her feelings of connection to Dorothy and her journey through Oz. She told me that her childhood had been one of emotional and verbal abuse and neglect, and, like Dorothy, she had longed to find home, a place of safety and security. A talented artist, she had received scholarships to a number of prestigious schools, and had fled her family as soon as she graduated from high school. Finding herself far from home, in a strange place with no friends, she found the lonely nights terrifying. She focused on her art to keep busy, but often used drugs and alcohol to calm her fears and escape the pain and loneliness.

She asked to work in the tray, and once more placed Dorothy at its center. Finding each of the other characters, she placed them around Dorothy. The Wicked Witch was identified as her past. She told me that she knew she needed to confront the Witch, but she just wasn't ready. She placed the Witch at the bottom of the tray. She picked up the Scarecrow, Tin Man, and Cowardly Lion. At first, she set them in front of Dorothy, saying that she needed friends to help protect her from the past. She went back to the shelves and looked at them for a moment, then walked back and moved the friends so they were standing behind Dorothy. When she did this, she said that she needed friends to "have [her] back" and support her, not get in the way of what she needed to face. Walking back to the shelves, Maria began adding symbols to the tray, placing animals, religious figures, people, monsters, and other objects in a spiral that began at Dorothy's feet and ended at the Wicked Witch. She worked quietly for the remainder of the session, telling me only that this represented her own yellow brick road.

When she was done, she asked for a photo of the tray, which she placed in her journal. During the next nine months of therapy, Maria used sand trays, drawing, and journal writing to record her journey. She bought a copy of the movie, and would often bring in new Oz insights or thoughts about possible meanings in the film. Every so often in therapy, she would take the photo of the sand tray out of her journal. Placing Dorothy in the sand, she would recreate the image, with Dorothy moving forward along the spiraling symbols, closer to the Wicked Witch. Sometimes she would discard, add, or substitute old symbols for new, each time explaining what they meant or why she made the transformation. A symbol representing a past lover was discarded, as she realized she didn't need to revisit that relationship. A symbol of anger was removed and replaced with a symbol of forgiveness as she reconnected with an older sibling. A symbol of death changed to a radiant crystal when she forgave herself for choices she had made and regretted.

As Maria and Dorothy moved forward, she found support, sobriety, and peace. As sometimes happens, there were times she would take a step backward, but each time, she accessed the support system she was slowly building and trusting. It became obvious that bit by bit she was confronting her past, and finding what she sought in her life. In our last session, Maria placed Dorothy directly facing the Wicked Witch and said, "You have no power here! Be gone, before somebody drops a house on you, too!"

CONCLUSION

I first began to study the power of metaphors and the therapeutic qualities of the metaphorical story in 1994, when I was working with children in the foster care system. That summer, all my clients in all my sessions were utilizing the story of a new movie: *The Lion King* (Allers & Minkoff, 1994). This is a film whose story and symbols powerfully resonate with the issues and feelings of children removed from their homes and carrying feelings of guilt and loss. This prompted me to examine the stories I loved as a child, and I realized that all of them had powerful, positive messages. It was then that I realized two things: first, that my love of movies and books such as *The Wizard of Oz* was directly connected to the messages I took from their powerful metaphors. Every time I watched Dorothy and her companions accept their challenges, face their fears, and learn their lessons, I was being told that we all struggle, but that with courage to face my fears, relationships to support and sustain me, and trust in my own inner resources, I would find what I sought. I was in therapy!

My other realization is of how wise Georg Groddeck was when he said that "if psychology was taught through the [movies], literature and books people already know (rather than special textbooks) it would be grasped far more readily by the average individual" (cited in Chetwyn, 1998, p. xi).

And now, to Oz!

NOTE

1. Fade-in introductory on-screen text at the beginning of the 1939 movie.

REFERENCES

Allers, R., & Minkoff, R. (Directors). (1994). *The lion king.* [Motion picture]. United States: Walt Disney Studios.

Angus, L., & Korman, Y. (2002). Conflict, coherence, and change in brief psychotherapy: A metaphor theme analysis. In S. R. Fussell (Ed.), *The verbal communication of emotions: Interdisciplinary perspectives* (pp. 151–166). Mahwah, NJ: Lawrence Erlbaum.

Angus, L., & Rennie, D. (1989, Fall). Envisioning the representational world: The client's experience of metaphoric expression in psychotherapy. *Psychotherapy, 26*(3), 372–379.

Atwood, J., & Levine, L. (1991, June 1). Ax murderers, dragons, spiders, and webs: Therapeutic metaphors in couple therapy. *Contemporary Family Therapy, 13*(3), 201–217.

Baum, L. F. (1900). *The wonderful wizard of Oz.* New York: Harper Collins.

Bausch, W. J. (1999). *The yellow brick road: A storyteller's approach to the spiritual journey.* Mystic, CT: Twenty-Third Publications.

Bayne, R., & Thompson, K. (2000). Counselor response to client's metaphors: An evaluation and refinement of Strong's model. *Counseling Psychology Quarterly, 13*(1), 37–49.

Bettelheim, B. (1976). *The uses of enchantment: The meaning and importance of fairy tales.* New York: Knopf.

Campbell, J. (1968). *The hero with a thousand faces.* Princeton, NJ: Princeton University Press.

Campbell, J., & Moyers, B. (1991). *The power of myth.* New York: Anchor Books.

Cattanach, A. (Ed.). (2002). *The story so far: Play therapy narratives.* London: Jessica Kingsley.

Chetwyn, T. (1998). *Dictionary of symbols.* London: Thorsons.

Davis, N. (1990). *Once upon a time: Therapeutic stories.* Oxen Hill, Maryland: Psychological Associates.

Ekstrom, S. R. (2004). The mind beyond our immediate awareness: Freudian, Jungian, and cognitive models of the unconscious [Electronic version]. *Journal of Analytical Psychology, 49,* 657–682.

Freeman, J. C., Epston, D., & Lobovits, D. (1997). *Playful approaches to serious problems: Narrative therapy with children and their families.* New York: Norton.

Freud, S. (1913). The occurrence in dreams of material from fairy tales. In J. Strachey (Ed. & Trans.), *The standard edition of the complete psychological works of Sigmund Freud* (Vol. 12, pp. 279–288). London: Hogarth Press, 1958.

Gardner, R. (1971). *Therapeutic communication with children: The mutual storytelling technique.* Northvale, NJ: Jason Aronson.

Green, J. (1998). *The zen of Oz: Ten spiritual lessons from over the rainbow.* Los Angeles: Renaissance Books.

Jung, C. G. (1964). *Man and his symbols.* Garden City, NY: Doubleday.

Jung, C. G. (1980). *The archetypes and the collective unconscious.* Princeton, NJ: Princeton University Press.

Jung, C. G. (1981). *The structure and dynamics of the psyche* (R. Hull, Trans.). Princeton, NJ: Princeton University Press.

Kottman, T. (1995). *Partners in play: An Adlerian approach to play therapy.* New York: American Counseling Association.

Lakoff, G., & Johnson, M. (2003). *Metaphors we live by.* Chicago: University of Chicago Press.

LeRoy, M. (Director). (1939). *The wizard of Oz* [Motion picture]. United States: MGM.

Library of Congress. (2000). To please a child. In *The Wizard of Oz: An American fairy tale.* Retrieved April 26, 2007, from http://www.loc.gov/exhibits/oz/

Luthi, M. (1976). *Once upon a time: On the nature of fairy tales.* Bloomington: Indiana University Press.

Luthi, M. (1987). *The fairy tale as art form and portrait of man.* Bloomington: Indiana University Press.

Mills, J. C., & Crowley, R. J. (1986). *Therapeutic metaphors for children and the child within.* New York: Bruner/Mazel.

Morena, G. D. (1998). *The wisdom of Oz.* San Diego: Inner Connections Press.

Murphy, M. J. (1996, Winter). *The Wizard of Oz* as cultural narrative and conceptual model for psychotherapy. *Psychotherapy, 33*(4), 531–538.

Norton, C. C., & Norton, B. E. (1997). *Reaching children through play therapy: An experiential approach.* Denver: The Publishing Cooperative.

Roheim, G. (1953). Fairy tale and dream. In R. S. Eissler, A. Freud, H. Hartmann, & K. Ernst (Eds.), *The psychoanalytic study of the child* (pp. 394–403). New York: International Universities Press.

Roheim, G. (1992). *Fire in the dragon and other psychoanalytic essays on folklore.* Princeton, NJ: Princeton University Press

Rushdie, S. (1992). *The Wizard of Oz.* London: BFI.

Schreiber, S. (1974). A filmed fairy tale as a screen memory. In R. S. Eissler, A. Freud, M. Kris, & A. Solnit (Eds.), *The psychoanalytic study of the child* (pp. 389–410). New Haven: Yale University Press.

Schwartz, K. E. (1956). A psychoanalytic study of the fairy tale. *American Journal of Psychotherapy, 10,* 740–762.

Shapiro, R., & Katz, C. L. (1978). Fairy tales, splitting and development. *Contemporary Psychoanalysis, 14*(4), 591–602.

Sharp, C., Smith, J. V., & Cole, A. (2002). Cinematherapy: Metaphorically promoting therapeutic change [Electronic version]. *Counseling Psychology Quarterly, 15*(3), 269–276.

Strong, T. (1989). Metaphors and client change in counseling. *International Journal for the Advancement of Counseling, 12,* 203–213.

Von Franz, M. L. (1982). *Interpretation of fairy tales.* Texas: Spring Publications.

CHAPTER 2

Harry Potter and the Prisoner Within

Helping Children With Traumatic Loss

William McNulty

Your mother died to save you. If there is one thing Voldemort cannot understand, it is love. He didn't realize that love as powerful as your mother's for you leaves its own mark. Not a scar, no visible sign . . . to have been loved so deeply, even though the person who loved us is gone, will give us some protection forever. It is in your very skin. (Rowling, 1997, p. 317)

The *Harry Potter* series (Rowling 1997, 1998, 1999, 2000, 2003, 2005, 2007) has sold over 325 million copies and has been translated into 65 different languages worldwide (Fierman, 2007). These staggering statistics reflect just how popular and far-reaching the book series is with its worldwide readers. In working clinically with children, I have come to realize that the story lines of the *Harry Potter* books have been and continue to be effective vehicles for helping children change and grow. The themes that weave through the series have a universal appeal that speaks to children, adolescents, and adults alike. The success and appeal of *Harry Potter* has been attributed to the fact that it speaks to people in a universal language that transcends gender, age, and ethnic borders (Lake, 2003). In an age in which video games and online entertainment appear to be more appealing to a generation that has shown an increasingly shorter attention span, these books have created a buzz and a following that is likened to the often frenzied followers of a musical icon or movie star.

The series has been credited with starting a resurgence among children in reading; an accomplishment that has not been seen since Louis Carroll's *Alice* or Berry's *Peter Pan* (Billone, 2004). Not only are these books a pop culture phenomenon, but I am also suggesting that they have contributed to the healing of many children in therapy.

It all begins with a boy named Harry who, at 1 year old, tragically and violently loses his parents to the evil Lord Voldemort and miraculously survives the same attack. He is taken in by Petunia and Vernon Dursley, his maternal aunt and her husband. His 10 years with these nonmagical beings, or Muggle surrogate parents, are filled with emotional abuse and neglect. On his 11th birthday, Harry finds out that he is a wizard and has been accepted into a special school of witchcraft and wizardry called Hogwarts, where he will spend the majority of the next 7 years learning about his powers and the world of magic. Along the way, he learns about himself, his past, and his future and this knowledge guides him along his journey toward becoming a whole person. These books present powerful metaphors through which readers can learn about themselves, overcome adversity, and transcend a sense of helplessness when confronted with seemingly insoluble dilemmas (Frenkel, 2000). The sections to follow will address the popularity of *Harry Potter* as a therapeutic vehicle.

BIBLIOTHERAPY

Bibliotherapy entails the therapeutic use of literature (Hellwig, 1988). Most therapeutic techniques that utilize stories are designed to elicit fantasies that transport the reader to a parallel situation in which they can process their own circumstances from the safety of intellectual and emotional distance. This process of client engagement in bibliotherapy has been described by Huxtable (1982), Davidson (1983), and Pardeck and Pardeck (1984). The latter authors identify three distinct stages in the development and progression of the client's use of bibliotherapy, which are identification and projection, abreaction and catharsis, and insight and integration. The client should be the one who chooses a story that "speaks" to him or her on some level, whether it is conscious or unconscious. The particular story that the child chooses to utilize becomes therapeutic if that choice is in response to a particular life challenge he or she is experiencing. Utilizing the story to address these challenges helps the child overcome feeling alone, embarrassed, ashamed, or resistant (Chan, 1993). Hellwig (1988) also described important stages that transpire within bibliotherapy. Identification occurs when a child sees himself or herself like a character or characters within a particular story. With this identification, there is also projection, during which the child is asked to think about the action of the story and various motives of the actions of the characters in the story. This can be seen as positive in that the child may realize that he or she is not alone with this problem. The child interprets the plot of the story and the therapist attempts to apply the child's interpretation to the problem at hand. The child's identification with the character will often lead to identification with the character's emotional state, which in turn can lead to emotional release. The therapeutic benefit comes with emotional release that accompanies identification with the main character. Insight is acquired as the child becomes able to recognize himself or herself in the characters. The child can begin to integrate the coping strategies learned from the characters in the story and employ them in his or her own situations.

The use of stories as a therapeutic tool has been valuable in my practice with young children. Often, I allow the child to choose which story to bring to the sessions for the purpose of growth and development. The scope of problems that the clients present within sessions is as varied as the clients themselves. Some typical issues that clients have addressed through bibliotherapy include anger, adoption, relational difficulties, and loss. In my work, use of the Harry Potter themes and metaphors has been useful in addressing a number of issues; however I will focus this chapter on loss. With this in mind, in the next section we will discuss the broad genre of fairy tale and fantasy, within which *Harry Potter* resides.

UNDERSTANDING THE USE OF
FAIRY TALES AND FANTASY

Fairy tales are rich cultural communications that contain insights into culture and highlight universal psychological dilemmas (Tisdell, 2002). Therapeutically, they offer children struggling with a variety of issues a vehicle with which to explore and master certain developmental tasks, reduce anxiety, and resolve conflicts. These stories are typically set at an appropriate developmental and emotional level that lends them to insight and understanding. Even though they may be set in a different time, place, and culture, there is a universality to them that speaks to children on many levels. Three theorists who have written extensively on the use and meaning of fairy tales are psychoanalyst Bruno Bettelheim, Jungian Marie Louis Von Franz, and historian Joseph Campbell. The next sections will explore their understanding of these stories and give practical examples from the *Harry Potter* story.

Bettelheim

Bruno Bettelheim was an Austrian-born psychoanalyst who wrote *The Use of Enchantment* (1975), which evaluated fairy tales through a psychoanalytic lens. He believed that man's greatest ongoing and lifetime challenge was to find meaning in life. As children grow, they develop an increased understanding of themselves that helps them to navigate their interpersonal worlds (Noctor, 2006). Bettelheim believed that by dealing with universal human problems, fairy tales speak to the developing ego, and in so doing encourage its development and the developing child's ability to control impulses and solve problems.

For Bettelheim, the fairy tale spoke to the difficulties children experience while growing up in a way that they can emotionally and psychologically identify with. An active imagination is the primary way through which children work through their problems. The child intuitively identifies with the characters of the fairy tale, and understands the latent message as it applies to his or her own life. Through engagement with the characters and action of the fairy tale, the child/reader is moved to rethink his or her own circumstances in order to generate a solution to a real-life crisis he or she is experiencing. To the extent that the story speaks directly to the child's unconscious and provides an outlet and vehicle for resolution of conflicts, it is therapeutic.

Von Franz

Marie-Louise Von Franz was a student of Jung who focused much of her writings on specific aspects of fairy tales, and specifically how they expressed Jungian archetypal patterns and the relationship between the individual and collective unconscious (Jung, 1981). According to Von Franz (1996), every fairy tale is a relatively closed system with complete psychological meaning expressed in a series of embedded symbolic elements including pictures and events. When interpreting a specific fairy tale, the therapist must take into account the emotional experience of the reader. Von Franz (1996) believed that interpretation is highly subjective because readers tend to interpret fairy tales or fantasy stories within the framework of their own experiences, worldviews, and personality type (thinking, feeling, sensing, and intuitive). With the guiding hand of the therapist, fairy tales could take on unique and significant psychological importance for the reader, moving him along the quest to better understand the most important archetype of all, the self.

Campbell

Based upon Jung's idea that archetypes are the underlying structure of all myths, Joseph Campbell (1956) formulated his concept of the *monomyth*. He saw the monomyth as an origin story retold across cultures from the beginning of recorded history. The basic elements within the story are universal and timeless. Campbell saw the role of the hero as the symbol of the self and the adventure a symbol of life (Indick, 2004). The monomyth is divided into three basic stages including *The Departure, Initiation, and Return*. The Departure signifies that destiny has summoned the hero and transferred his spiritual center of gravity from society to the unknown zone. The Initiation is the stage of the journey in which hero enters into the darkness, experiences trials with the aid of a supernatural helper and gains the reward of overcoming the trials. In the final stage, the Return, Campbell articulates three possible scenarios. After attaining enlightenment, the hero can refuse the return and remain in the realm of the gods or go to another place to exist. The hero can choose to return to make humanity better and thus save the world. Finally, the hero can reintegrate into the world of humanity because he is needed.

The *Harry Potter* series also fits well into the framework of the monomyth. We see that Harry is called to adventure each time that he is summoned to Hogwarts. The original calling comes in the form of an acceptance letter delivered by multiple owls. With these invitation letters ignored through the interference of his Uncle Vernon, Harry's acceptance letter is personally delivered by Rubeus Hagrid, the keeper of the keys and groundskeeper of Hogwarts. In subsequent years, he is summoned back to the school by a letter. Harry is transitioned from the nonmagical Muggle world to the magical realm of wizards and witches, Hogwarts School of Witchcraft and Wizardry. Harry enters the darkness in each of his 7 years at Hogwarts by fighting Lord Voldemort, his followers the Death Eaters, and various magical creatures. Along his journey, he is aided by his professors, Sirius Black (his godfather), Dumbledore, and best friends Ron Weasley and Hermione Granger. After the death of his godfather, Sirius, and headmaster Dumbledore, he returns to the wizarding world with the knowledge of how to destroy Voldemort by first decimating the Horcruxes, pieces of Voldemort's soul. This leads to his final and victorious confrontation with Voldemort, his own redemption, and the salvation of the world of wizards.

Taken together, the formulations of fairy tales by Bettelheim, Von Franz, and Campbell provide useful frameworks for understanding the potentially therapeutic value of the Harry Potter tales. Within *Harry Potter*, there are several classical Jungian archetypes who battle against and come to the aid of each other in the unfolding collective unconscious realm that is Hogwarts. These include the shadow (Lord Voldemort), the hero (protagonist, Harry Potter), the wise one (Albus Dumbledore), and the great mother (Lily Potter).

THE *HARRY POTTER* STORY AND THERAPY

Psychoanalyst Selma Fraiberg (1959) described the world of a child as being a magical, unstable, and often frightening place. As the young client gropes his or her way toward reason, he or she must wrestle with dangerous creatures of his or her imagination as well as the very real dangers of the outer world. This statement parallels Harry's struggles as the child searches for meaning within his or her own existence. Harry's experiences in the Muggle and wizarding worlds are metaphors for the client's experience in therapy. For Arehart-Treichel (2002), Harry has experienced overwhelming life experiences beginning with the murder of his parents and followed by the subsequent abuse at the hand of his aunt and uncle, the Dursleys. He leaves this abusive situation and excitedly enters the holding environment of Hogwarts, much like a client entering therapy who is anxious about what lies ahead. The therapist can be seen as a parental figure who supports and offers guidance to the client, much like Headmaster Professor Dumbledore and Housemaster Professor McGonagall guide and support Harry throughout his stay at Hogwarts. In treatment, clients uncover/discover aspects of themselves and work on resolving issues that they struggle with in their lives, just as Harry, who must search within himself as he battles the evil Lord Voldemort. As Harry confronts challenges, obstacles, and victories, so too do clients experience magical moments of growth and understanding by facing their own dark forces in treatment (Mulholland, 2006).

Harry Potter and Loss

"He couldn't remember his parents at all. His Aunt and Uncle never spoke of them and he was forbidden to ask questions. No photos of them. When he was younger he had dreams of some unknown relations coming to take him away . . . this is the same quote as referenced at the end of the sentence. The one memory that he did have was a blinding flash of green light and a burning pain in his forehead" (Rowling, 1997, p. 30). Freud (1909/1970) described what he called "family romance" in which the child becomes dissatisfied with his home and parents and fantasizes that someday his real parents will rescue him from his miserable conditions. The child invents a fairy tale in which he is secretly of noble origin, and may even be marked out as a hero who is destined to save the world (Blum, 1983). This fits in with Harry's story in that he is living with a family that is not his own. He wishes for his real relatives to take him away like in dreams that he has had while at the Dursleys'. What happens is that he is transported into a world of magic where these things actually do come true. He is deemed "The Boy Who Lived" and, later on in the story, "The Chosen One."

Menes (1971) described the mourner as one who experiences emotional pain, loss of interest in the outside world, as well as the capacity to love until the work of mourning is complete. The most important therapeutic task is for the child to loosen ties to their deceased parents with the assistance of caring and loving family (Furman, 1986) and eventually reinvest this energy in new relationships (Silverman, Nickerman, & Warden, 1992). In this context, Hook (2006) describes Harry's task as that of rising like a phoenix out of the ashes of his grief to become a stronger and more complete person.

Harry Potter and the Theme of Resilience

Throughout my work with clients who have experienced loss, the one theme that appears to be common and that they share with the character of Harry Potter is resilience. Even though they have experienced a trauma and developed a variety of psychological, emotional, and behavioral symptoms, these children have survived. The term resilience can be defined as the ability to recover from illness, change, or misfortune (Hook, 2006). Research has suggested that children who display certain characteristics including a positive view of self, attribution of their adversity to an external rather than internal source, and a sense of humor help them to better cope with stressors and adversity (Provenzano & Heyman, 2006). In Harry's case, his parents were murdered and a near fatal attempt was made on his life by Voldemort. Harry Potter is clearly resilient; he is optimistic, good-natured, intelligent, and resourceful and is surrounded for the most part by caring and supportive friends and mentors. While he struggles with demons, both internal and external, he does survive and even more so, thrives and matures. The clinician's task is to identify and harness these curative elements in order to assist clients in surviving their own losses and tragedies. Within the next section of the chapter, I will discuss particular elements within the Harry Potter tale that I have found to be therapeutically useful.

THERAPEUTIC ELEMENTS OF *HARRY POTTER*

The Scar and the Connection to Voldemort

"It was this scar that made Harry so particularly unusual, even for a wizard. This scar was the only hint of Harry's very mysterious past. At the age of 1 year old, Harry had somehow survived a curse from the greatest dark sorcerer of all time. His parents died in the attack, but Harry had escaped with his lightening scar" (Rowling, 1998, p. 4). This passage from the first *Harry Potter* book establishes the foundation for his quest and his many struggles. The fierce attack at the hands of Voldemort leaves a lightning-bolt-shaped scar on his forehead, and a metaphoric scar on his psyche that results in intrusive memories and dreams. It is later explained that this very same scar serves as a transmitter of Voldemort's feelings and actions; a lightening rod of sorts, for evil. This connection has both a positive and a negative impact on Harry's life, offering the opportunity for learning about various aspects of himself, both light and dark. On a positive note, the scar provides Harry access into Voldemort's comings and goings, helping him to combat the evil lord's rise to power. From the negative side, the scar provides Voldemort access to Harry's mind, in which he can implant deceptive images, one of which led to the death of his godfather, Sirius Black.

In treatment, I have used the metaphoric symbolism of the scar in order to help children and teens discuss their own scars, which have resulted from specific traumas in their lives. This opens the door to discussing nightmares and haunting and painful memories.

The Mirror of Erised

Over Christmas holiday during his first year at Hogwarts, Harry has a chance encounter with the Mirror of Erised while exploring the castle under his father's cloak of invisibility. As Harry looked into the mirror, he saw a woman with green eyes like his own and a man whose glasses and untidy hair were also strangely familiar. These images, along with subsequent others, were actually those of his own lost family, which he was seeing for the first time in his life.

Over the course of the next few days, he visited the mirror several times, and on the last day was joined by Dumbledore, who explained its power and purpose. He said "the happiest man on earth would be able to use the Mirror of Erised like a normal mirror; that is, he would be able to see himself exactly as he is. . . . It shows us nothing more or less than our deepest, most desperate desire of our hearts. The mirror will give us neither knowledge nor truth. Men have wasted away before it, entranced by what they have seen or been driven mad, not knowing what it shows is real or even possible" (Rowling, 1997, p. 213). Inscribed above the mirror is the saying "Erised Stra Ehru Oyt Ube Cafru Oyt On Wohsi"; when read in reverse it says "I Show Not Your Face But Your Heart's Desire."

In therapy, I have found the analogy of the mirror useful by asking clients familiar with the story to use it in order to bring to life wishes and dreams related to deceased loved ones' persons. Some clients think about what they would say to the deceased person or pose questions they would ask to the person they have lost. Thus, the mirror is seen as a projective fantasy device, which by virtue of being removed from reality, allows for a safer level of engagement with painful thoughts and feelings.

Dementors and Patronuses

In *The Prisoner of Azkaban* (Rowling, 1999), the Dementors were described to Harry by Professor Remus Lupin, the Defense Against the Dark Arts teacher, in the following manner. "Dementors are among the foulest creatures that walk the earth. They infest the darkest, filthiest places. They glory in decay and despair, they drain peace, hope, and happiness out of the air around them. Even Muggles feel their presence, though they can't see them. Get too near a Dementor and every good feeling, every happy memories will be sucked out of you. If it can, the Dementor will feed on you long enough to reduce you to something like itself . . . soulless and evil. You'll be left with nothing but the worst experiences of your life" (Rowling, 1999, p. 187). When Harry first came into contact with a Dementor, he was forced to relive his memory of the night that his parents were killed. Harry's re-experience of the trauma involved not only memories but also the physical sensations of spine-chilling coldness, labored breathing, and the palpable sensation of drowning; not unlike the experience of clients remembering and reliving a traumatic event

The way to defend oneself against the damaging effects of a Dementor is to conjure a spell called the patronus. A patronus is defined as a positive force, a summoning of the very things that Dementors feed upon but cannot feel, including hope, happiness, and the desire to survive. Each patronus is unique to the wizard who conjures it. To conjure a patronus, the wizard must recall his or her happiest possible memory. Harry's patronus took the form of a stag, which was identical to the one chosen by his father, who parenthetically was an Animagus, a wizard who can transform at will into an animal. Harry's father chose a stag. By choosing the same patronus, Harry introjected his father in a healing way.

Similarly, clients enter therapy to learn skills that will assist them in combating overwhelming anxiety and to work through feelings, thoughts, and memories associated with trauma and loss. Relating the client's experiences to that of Harry Potter can assist the therapist in drawing upon positive experiences from the client's life as part of the healing process

Bogarts

Another dark creature Harry encountered in his travels was the Bogart, described as a shape-shifter who could take the form of whatever it thinks will be most frightening. Harry first encountered this creature while in the Defense Against the Dark Arts class, where he learned that concentration, humor, the close company of companions, and transforming fear into a laughable form were the best protections. This set of protective maneuvers was called the Riddikulus spell. In the wizarding world, each witch and wizard learns how to cast spells such as the Riddikulus by dueling with each other. The various spells are categorized to include those that are either proactive, unforgivable, or defensive. The unforgivable spells include the Imperius curse, which allows the person who cast it to possess another person, the Cruciatus curse, which tortures the other person, and the Avada Kedavra curse, which immediately kills the person without telltale signs. As a note of interest, Harry has been the only known person to survive the Avada Kedavra curse performed by Voldemort. Harry also gained recognition by casting a disarming and nonlethal spell called Expelliarmus, rather than relying upon some of the darker incantations.

From a therapeutic perspective, clients often enter therapy with fears and anxiety related to losses they have experienced or those they anticipate. Utilizing the metaphor of the Bogart can assist them in exploring the shape that their Bogart would take and what they could think of to repel them. Through my work, I have encountered several children who have relied upon fantasy spell casting, which in turn has facilitated exploration and expression of painful feelings.

CASE STUDIES

Brian

Presenting Problem

Brian, a 7-year-old White male, was referred for treatment by his biological mother, who had concerns related to his aggressive behavior at home and at school. His mother described him as a caring person who had a very loving side to him. At the same time, she felt that he had been displaying more of an out-of-control and angry side to him with the members of the family. This aggression had been manifest in hitting, kicking, and breaking objects such as toys and furniture. He had also been displaying crying spells and expressing feelings of sadness, which he had described to his mother as "big missing feelings." According to his teachers, Brian was a good student, whose work had recently suffered because of behavior difficulties including inattention to details, instigating and distracting peers, unprovoked aggression, and lack of focus.

Background Information

Brian was the second of three children to parents who were married at the time of his birth. He was delivered full term without any complications. His older sister was diagnosed as having mood disorder and was receiving psychotherapy and medication management prior to Brian being identified as needing treatment. Brian's younger brother appeared to be relatively well adjusted. Brian was described by his mother as an "easy" baby who attained all developmental milestones within normal limits. At around age three, he suffered the traumatic loss of his biological father from a stroke, which was compounded by the extreme emotional reactions of his immediate and extended family members. Before the death, Brian was reportedly well behaved both at home and school. In the month following the loss, Brian's behavior began to slowly deteriorate to the point that his mother was having difficulty controlling his negative behavior and emotional outbursts. In school, he was fighting with peers over toys, having difficulty following directions, stealing small items from the classroom, and expressing worries over numerous seemingly unrelated issues.

Assessment and Treatment Plan

The lens through which I assess and formulate my treatment of children and their families is psychodynamic; and I often rely upon a nondirective style for interacting with young clients in the playroom. The most important aspect of my treatment is the relationship I develop with the client. The goals are to increase self-awareness and help resolve conflicts as their true feelings are brought into awareness and dealt with in a safe way. Brian was a child who had no reported family history of any major mental illness, violence, or neglect. He was seen by the adults in his life as being a normal boy for his age until the sudden death of his father. After that time, he exhibited symptoms of aggression, intermittent episodes of crying, feelings of sadness, difficulty getting along with peers, and emotional outbursts that necessitated adult intervention. These symptoms became disruptive and problematic at home and at school. He was subsequently diagnosed with Adjustment Disorder with Mixed Disturbance of Emotions and Conduct. As part of the diagnostic evaluation, he was seen by a psychiatrist who recommended individual therapy to address the issues related to the loss of his father. As further part of the evaluation process, a parent interview, family observation, individual play, and psychiatric assessment were conducted. It was decided that individual therapy would focus on the behavioral issues related to bereavement and that his mother would attend parent counseling in order to learn more effective ways of helping her son.

Treatment: Beginning Phase

In the beginning of the treatment, Brian was very difficult to engage. He spent the first few sessions without acknowledging my existence. He would engage in solitary and silent play, with his back turned to me. I believed that a nondirective approach would be effective in allowing Brian to have enough space to explore the room while at the same time developing a sense of safety. I spent much of the time in the first few sessions reflecting the actions of his play. Eventually, Brian and I developed a working therapeutic alliance. His early play involved fantasy themes of soldiers fighting, police and criminals, and Harry Potter. These play scenarios typically involved taking on the role of the powerful character while I was relegated to the role of the enemy or bad guy. During these scenarios, Brian guided my play but typically reprimanded and punished me with incarceration. During duels, Brian often took the role of Harry Potter and deprived me of victory by casting spells. I reflected his feelings related to entering treatment, which included anger, anxiety, and sadness. He was able to engage in discussions about his feelings but was not yet ready to discuss issues related to the death of his father.

Middle Phase

After a few months in treatment, Brian was ready to play out and eventually discuss the issue of loss. He continued to engage in fantasy play and was also introduced to sandplay. Many of his early sand trays contained many mythical creatures and large predatory fighting animals that battled each other. These creatures often protected large treasures that were buried in the sand and were typically threatened by outside and unseen forces that were eventually defeated.

Brian's fantasy activities shifted from playing out various themes of conflict to focusing on exploration of the Harry Potter story. He set up scenarios in which he took on the role of Harry, while I played various other characters including Ron, Hermione, Hagrid, Dumbledore, and Voldemort. In these situations, Brian had Harry engage in searches for certain magical items that would eventually aid him in his journey and at school. He also allowed me to introduce certain exercises through which he could explore his loss. These included drawing out what he would like to see if he had come into contact with the Mirror of Erised. He was able to discuss the pain he experienced from not saying goodbye to his father, and asked questions of him.

Final Phase

As Brian progressed through therapy, he continued to engage in fantasy play and sandplay. His behavior at home and in school improved significantly with few reports of difficulties. His fantasy play continued to involve adventures with Harry and his friends. However, there were more adventures involving Dumbledore and Harry. As Dumbledore, Brian would counsel Harry on what spells he needed in order to protect himself from his enemies. I also introduced the idea of Dementors and protection from them in the form of the Patronus charm. His painful memories, nightmares, and fears were explored through the metaphor of the Dementors. He was able to develop his own Patronus, which protected him from the fears and worries associated with the loss of his father. In one of his final sessions, his play involved a scenario in which he as Harry was able to graduate from Hogwarts and live on his own.

Reflections

Brian had experienced the trauma of loss at an early age, which paralleled Harry's loss of both parents at the hands of Voldemort. Both Brian and Harry were called to their adventure of self-discovery; Brian by his mother and Harry by Dumbledore in the form of an invitation to attend Hogwarts School of Witchcraft and Wizardry. The school became a metaphor for the holding environment of therapy. As Harry learned to rely on friends, Brian sought the assistance of his therapist.

In his fantasy play and subsequent artwork, Brian was able to work through and make sense of his losses. Early on, he utilized spells as a way to keep me at a safe and comfortable distance until he was able to begin to trust and develop a working relationship. As he expanded his Harry Potter play, Brian began to more safely explore feelings associated with his tragedy. By taking on the role of Harry, with whom he shared parental loss, Brian was able to work through the confusing loss-related feelings he had experienced. In the end Brian, like Harry, was able to utilize his relationships and integrate the knowledge that he had learned about himself in order to release his prisoner within.

Andre

Presenting Problem

Andre was a 6-year-old African American male referred for treatment by his school counselor, who had concerns related to behavioral changes that had taken place over the past few months. The counselor related that in the beginning of the year Andre was a good student who had some problems adjusting to a full-day program. After this initial rocky transition, Andre was able to make and maintain friendships and engage in age-appropriate positive behaviors. Prior to entering treatment, Andre had begun to be irritable with peers and teachers, was withdrawn, preferred to play by himself, and would sometimes cry during the day. His mother described him as a loving child but voiced concerns about not "being himself lately." The changes at home included him having bad dreams, not being able to sleep all the way through the night, and regressive behavior such as bed-wetting, clinging to his mother, and baby talk. The mother was looking for individual therapy and parent counseling to better understand and help her son.

Background Information

Andre was the only child of a full-term but unplanned pregnancy; his parents were never married and ended their relationship prior to his birth. He had very limited and sporadic subsequent contact with his father. Andre's father had a history of depression, substance abuse, and trouble with the law, which included time spent in jail for crimes related to drug possession and distribution, theft, and assault. His mother had grown up in a family where there was physical violence, and as a result, she experimented with drugs and alcohol. She had also experienced sporadic depression but had never sought treatment.

Andre's mother stated that he had no significant behavioral problems until his uncle, who lived with the family, was killed by an unknown assailant in the community during a mugging. His uncle was described as the one consistent male figure in his life and "like a father figure." This traumatic event was compounded by the emotional and financial upheaval that it caused his immediate family. Following his uncle's death, Andre regressed behaviorally and emotionally, had difficulty sleeping through the night, and experienced night terrors.

Assessment and Treatment Plan

Information related to the case was gathered through interviews with his mother and school counselor, review of relevant medical and school records, family observation data, and individual play assessment. After the loss of his uncle, Andre was displaying regressive symptoms consistent with a diagnosis of Adjustment Disorder with Mixed Disturbance of Emotions and Conduct, which was later corroborated by the medical director of the clinic. Treatment was to focus on helping Andre cope with the loss of his uncle and to be able to return to a prior level of functioning.

Treatment: Beginning Phase

During the first few sessions of treatment, Andre needed his mother to accompany him. During this time, he played only with his mother but tolerated my observational role. He constructed buildings with blocks and drove cars around them. After several sessions, Andre spontaneously decided that he wanted to come to the playroom without his mother. Throughout this phase, he was restless and had difficulty focusing on play activities for more than a few minutes at a time; however he grew more visibly comfortable with me and seemed to be developing trust.

Around this time, he and his mother were reading the *Harry Potter* stories together as a bedtime ritual, which she observed had a relaxing effect on him. Andre began to introduce the theme of *Harry Potter* into the play room through his drawings and the recounting of parts of the story.

Middle Phase

About 6 months into the treatment, Andre's behavior began to change at school and at home. There was observed improvement in his interactions with peers, and his mother was reporting that he was behaving in a more age-appropriate way at home. He more readily engaged in fantasy play, with particular emphasis on Harry Potter. He took on the identity of various characters and played out themes of being lost, punished, and reaching out for help. During this time, I introduced the theme of Bogarts. Andre role played a Bogart changing shape into things he feared the most, including seeing his uncle at the funeral, being alone, and being blamed for his uncle's death by his mother. All of these themes were then openly discussed in our meetings. Over the course of this play, Andre took on an aggressive role and punished his various enemies for breaking the rules, one of which was his uncle for dying and leaving him.

Final Phase

In the final phase of treatment, Andre continued to work through his angry feelings related to the loss of his uncle as well as toward other family members. He played the role of professors who would punish various students for breaking the school rules. At first he was sadistic in his punishment and would not allow the student (myself) to speak. He became more benevolent, shifting his play to allow students (myself included) to speak. Toward the end of the treatment, he was able to express his sadness and guilt associated with the loss. He was also was able to talk about his own metaphoric scar, relating it to the experience that Harry had endured. Andre explained that just like Harry, his connection to the pain was necessary to grow and change. He intuitively observed that his scar had transformed from an external to an internal symbol of his loss and that he could be sad while also remembering his uncle in a more positive way. At the end of therapy, Andre was sleeping better, had no episodes of regressive behavior at home or at school, and was getting along better with peers.

Reflections

Andre experienced loss, and like Harry, his life was drastically and dramatically changed. The containing space of the playroom was much like Hogwarts and his mother's intuitive use of the *Harry Potter* story to calm him provided a vehicle for emotional containment, identification, and healing. Through this identification and subsequent expansion and exploration of the story, Andre was able to develop an understanding of what his uncle's loss meant to him and how it changed his life. Through his play, Andre was able to explore the theme of guilt and the associated feelings of sadness and anger related to his loss. Andre and Harry were fellow travelers along a similar path, and like Harry he was able to be free of the haunting effect of his uncle's ghost in order to move on with his life and become "The Boy Who Lived."

FINAL REFLECTIONS

"Happiness can be found, even in the darkest of times, if one only remembers to turn on the light" (Cuaron, 2004). The story of Harry Potter has connected with the hearts and minds of countless children and adults who have read the series and seen the films over the past 10 years. As a fan I have been able to utilize the stories therapeutically. I believe that the themes of courage to face life's greatest fears, the strong bonds of friendship we form, and the love from those whom we hold most dear transcend word and image to reflect the journeys that we guide our clients through, as well as those that we pass through in our own lives.

REFERENCES

Arehart-Treichel, J. (2002). Analyst discovers lessons in Harry Potter's ordeal. *Psychiatric News, 37*(5), 33.

Bettelheim, B. (1975). *The use of enchantment: The meaning and importance of fairy tales.* New York: Vintage Books.

Billone, A. (2004). The boy who lived: From Carroll's Alice and Barrie's Peter Pan to Rowling's Harry Potter. *Children's Literature, 32,* 178–202.

Blum, H. P. (1983). Splitting of the ego and its relation to parent loss. *Journal of the American Psychoanalytic Association, 31,* 301–324.

Campbell, J. (1956). *The hero with a thousand faces*. New York: Meridian Press.

Chan, D. W. (1993). Stories and storytelling in teaching and child psychotherapy. *Primary Education, 3*(2), 27–31.

Cuaron, A. (Director). (2004). *Harry Potter and the prisoner of Azkaban* [Motion picture]. United Kingdom: Warner Brothers.

Davidson, M. (1983). Classroom bibliotherapy: Why and how. *Reading World, 23*(2), 103–107.

Fierman, D. (2007, August 3). Harry Potter and the last hurrah. *Entertainment Weekly*, 19–23.

Fraiberg, S. H. (1959). *The magic years: Understanding and handling the problems of early childhood*. New York: Fireside.

Frenkel, R. S. (2000). Harry Potter, psychoanalysis, and hope. *Dallas Psychoanalytic Institute-Institute News, 11*, 2.

Freud, S. (1909/1970). Family romances. In J. Strachey (Ed.), *Sigmund Freud: On sexuality* (pp. 217–227). Harmondworth: Penguin.

Furman, E. (1986). On trauma: When is the death of a parent traumatic? *The Psychoanalytic Study of the Child, 41*, 191–208.

Hellwig, D. L. (1988). Bibliotherapy: The use of children's literature as a therapeutic tool. *Association for Play Therapy Newsletter, 7*(1), 1–4.

Hook, M. (2006). What Harry and Fawkes have in common. In N. Mulholland (Ed.), *The psychology of Harry Potter: An unauthorized examination of the boy who lived* (pp. 91–104). Dallas, Texas: Benbella Books.

Huxtable, M. (1982). Using books to help children. *Social Work Education, 5*(1), 53–65.

Indick, W. (2004). Classical heroes in modern movies: Mythological patterns of the superhero. *Journal of Media Psychology, 9*, 1–13.

Jung, C. G. (1981). *The structure and dynamics of the psyche* (R. C. F. Hull, Trans.). Princeton, NJ: Princeton University Press. (Original work published in 1960).

Lake, S. (2003). Object relations in Harry Potter. *Journal of the American Academy of Psychoanalysis and Dynamic Psychiatry, 31*(3), 509–520.

Menes, J. B. (1971). Children's reactions to the death of a parent: A review of the psychoanalytic literature. *Journal of the American Psychoanalytic Association, 19*, 697–719.

Mulholland, N. (2006). Using psychological treatment with Harry. In N. Mulholland (Ed.), *The psychology of Harry Potter: An unauthorized examination of the boy who lived* (pp. 265–282). Dallas, TX: Benbella Books.

Noctor, C. (2006). Putting Harry Potter on the couch. *Clinical Child Psychology and Psychiatry, 11*(4), 579–589.

Pardeck, J., & Pardeck, J. (1984). An overview of the bibliotherapeutic treatment approach: Implication for the clinical social work practice. *Family Therapy, 11*(3), 241–252.

Provenzano, D. M., & Heyman, R. E. (2006);. Harry Potter and the resilience to adversity. In N. Mulholland (Ed.), *The psychology of Harry Potter: An unauthorized examination of the boy who lived* (pp. 105–119). Dallas, TX: Benbella Books.

Rowling, J. K. (1997). *Harry Potter and the philosopher's stone*. London: Bloomsbury.

Rowling, J. K. (1998). *Harry Potter and the chamber of secrets*. London: Bloomsbury.

Rowling, J. K. (1999). *Harry Potter and the prisoner of Azkaban*. London: Bloomsbury.

Rowling, J. K. (2000). *Harry Potter and the goblet of fire*. New York: Scholastic.

Rowling, J. K. (2003). *Harry Potter and the order of the phoenix*. New York: Scholastic.

Rowling, J. K. (2005). *Harry Potter and the half-blood prince*. New York: Scholastic.

Rowling, J. K. (2007). *Harry Potter and the deathly hallows*. New York: Scholastic.

Silverman, P. R., Nickman, S., & Warden, J. W. (1992). Detachment revisited: The child's reconstruction of a dead parent. *American Journal of Orthopsychiatry, 62*(4), 494–503.

Tisdell, T. M. (2002). Harry Potter and the world of internal objects: An object relations analysis. *Dissertation Abstracts International* (UMI No. 3051885), 1–97.

Von Franz, M. L. (1996). *The interpretation of fairy tales*. Boston: Shambhala.

CHAPTER 3

Calvin and Hobbes to the Rescue!

The Therapeutic Uses of Comic Strips and Cartoons

Laura Sullivan

HUMOR IN WORK, LIFE, AND PSYCHOTHERAPY

Humor is a natural part of humanity. Laughing comes as naturally as breathing. There is nothing more contagious than a baby's laugh, and we delight in hearing babies' unsuppressed giggles. Humor relieves stress and allows us to tolerate one another.

Laughing comes from sharing human experience. When we laugh, it is within a shared moment, present or past, within the context of relationship. Humor is connective when it is shared (and not at someone's expense) and can be an important part of rapport and of strengthening a relationship, whether that relationship is between therapist and client, family members, or with oneself.

Humor heals. As therapists we feel hope when we hear the laugh of a client who had previously lost her way to humor in life. Humor and other forms of play are becoming an increasingly recognized and researched area of physical and mental health (Bhosai, Miwa, & Hilber, 2007).

Humor has been shown to increase immune functioning, decrease cortisol, increase endorphins, lower blood pressure, and enhance respiration (Berk, cited in Howard, 2006). Howard also noted that when problem-solving tests are preceded by laugher outcomes are higher. Newman (cited in Howard, 2006) demonstrated that subjects taught to use humorous monologues while narrating a distressing video had lower blood pressure and skin temperature than subjects using nonhumorous monologues.

Rx Laughter, a not-for-profit research, education, and treatment organization in collaboration with the National Cancer Institute of Thailand, and Yale University School of Public Health, has researched the relationship between exposure to humorous content and the well-being of cancer patients. The researchers measured patient self-reports of pain, anxiety, the ability to fall asleep, comfort levels, and satisfaction, with care before and after humor treatment as the independent variable. Results of the study suggested that in contrast with a control group, patients who received 2 hours of humor videos each day reported statistically significant improvements on all dependent measures. Qualitatively, the hospital staff reported that the humor treatment group became much more pleasant toward the staff and that this pleasantness in turn increased staff morale (Bhosai, Miwa, & Hilber, 2007). These results point to the relationally connective nature of humor. The researchers suggest humor as an inexpensive, noninvasive form of treatment with universal applicability.

Humor has long been considered to be a higher order defense mechanism (Vaillant, 1977). Vaillant (1977) identified four levels of defense mechanisms including: level 1 *psychotic* (psychotic denial, delusional projection), level 2 *immature* (fantasy, projection, passive aggression, acting out), level 3 *neurotic* (intellectualization, reaction formation, dissociation, displacement, repression), and level 4 *mature* (humor, sublimation, suppression, altruism, anticipation). For Vaillant, humor was among the most adaptive, healthy defenses, and as such, coping mechanisms. He states, "Humor is one of the truly elegant defenses in the human repertoire. Few would deny that the capacity for humor, like hope, is one of mankind's most potent antidotes for the woes of Pandora's box" (1977, p. 116). For Vaillant, humor also serves a connective function that draws people together and is the essence of humanity.

Humor is playful creativity itself, reducing stress in the process, in turn enhancing creative expression. Businesses are recognizing the merits of humor and playfulness in developing a creative work environment and increasing productivity. Anne Tryba of the Disney Imagineers has this to say about the Disney work environment:

> Without the ability to laugh at one's errors, and at oneself, it is hard to allow others the luxury of making mistakes. A sense of humor is one of the most important tools we have when it comes to maintaining an atmosphere of creativity. This sense of lightness and humor as a "company culture" comes from "the top down," and is recognized as a way of fostering a safe haven within our campus. Imagineering works hard to keep humor reverberating through its halls. (The Imagineers, 2003, p. 131)

David Kelly, CEO and founder of *Ideo,* a design firm receiving multiple awards for creative innovation of a wide range of products including cameras, toothpaste tubes, small household appliances, and phones, sanctions play on company time to increase creativity. In the documentary film *The Promise of Play* (Brown & Kennard, 2000), Kelly stated, "Play is fundamental to the whole process of coming up with good ideas. Serious goes in a conventional direction. Playful allows you to say something unexpected and that's liable to lead to some new direction." In that same film, David Webster, an *Ideo* design engineer, asserted that when a design team is playful while working they are able to remove "a lot of psychological barriers inhibiting the flow of ideas."

Not only can humor free us to be creative in the workplace, but it can be utilized by therapists in their efforts to effect change. Steven Sultanoff (2003) outlines a theoretical model for implementing humor in psychotherapy. He cautions that in order to apply humor effectively, "it is crucial for the clinician to understand the nature of humor as experienced by the client" (p. 113). Understanding a particular client's sense of humor can be the key to helping them better express their pain and distress as well as connect with the clinician.

Sultanoff believes that intentional use of humor in psychotherapy has the potential to influence change in emotion, behavior, cognition, and physiology. He has observed that humor reduces ratings of stress and anxiety, increases energy and the pursuit of connections with others, assists in correcting cognitions, and has been linked to biochemical changes including higher levels of antibodies and lower stress hormones.

Sultanoff (pp. 125–126) recommends a set of guidelines for using humor during both assessment and treatment. These include recommendations such as:

- Plan appropriate humor for use in therapy.
- Be willing to risk using humor as a therapeutic tool.
- Assess the client's personal style of humor and receptivity to humorous interventions.
- Select humor that is genuine and congruent with the clinician as a person.
- Be capable of self-monitoring motivation for using humor.
- Be prepared to respond to the client's reaction to the humorous intervention.

Importantly, employing humor in psychotherapy does not mean that we are not serious with our clients, because as skilled clinicians realize, jokes, sarcasm, and inappropriate use of humor may signify countertransference. Due to the highly evocative nature of the therapeutic interaction, clinicians experience and acknowledge a wide range of emotional states with clients. Simply, humor can provide alternative perspectives and potential solutions that may otherwise be clinically unavailable.

HUMOR AND LITERATURE AS TRANSITIONAL PHENOMENA

D. W. Winnicott (2005) recognized the continual "oscillation between the inner and outer worlds" (p. xii) in the psychological growth of humans. He described things, people, and places that anchor us during developmental struggles and the integration of new experiences as transitional objects. Transitional objects serve in effect as screens (much like movie screens) or containers where one projects emotional intensity while new experiences and psychological challenges are integrated into the psyche. In common parlance, a transitional object is the teddy bear, blanket, or thumb that helps a child tolerate separation from a beloved caretaker—the primary focus of attachment, according to object relations theory. Winnicott, however, did not limit his description and the importance of transitional objects to blankets and teddy bears.

Although Winnicott recognized that use of transitional objects begins in infancy as early as 4 months, he believed that their use changes shape over time as developmental challenges are met at which time the meaning of the objects becomes diffused (2005). Transitional objects can be anything that serves this projective and integrative function. Winnicott described that when integration is healthy, the object is not repressed, mourned, or forgotten, but integrated throughout the psychic field where the object loses meaning. When the attempt at integration is unhealthy the focus on the object can develop into fetishes, addictions, or obsessional rituals.

Winnicott also introduced the term *transitional state* to designate an "intermediate area of *experiencing,* to which inner reality and external life both contribute" (p. 3). And he defined the concept of *transitional phenomenon* to designate the psychological activity "between primary creative activity and projection of what has already been introjected" (p. 2). For Winnicott, a transitional phenomenon is an experience that may bridge dissonance in experiences, for example, between dream states and wakeful alertness.

Winnicott gave the example of an older child singing songs to prepare for sleep. The child in his example is in a transitional state between the experiences of daytime activity and the quiet of nighttime, soon to be followed by sleep and dreaming. As children often experience anxiety when faced with the quiet of nighttime, the words and melody of the songs are the transitional objects that provide the self-soothing to ease the cognitive and emotional transition from shared social wakefulness to the isolation of sleep.

Literary characters and their stories have served as transitional objects throughout history. Winnie-the-Pooh is a classic example of such a character who has served as both a plaything and transitional object for generations. Winnie the Pooh was A. A. Milne's son's transitional object, and no doubt the adventures of this remarkable stuffed bear have served as transitional experiences as well.

Stuffed Poohs serve as transitional objects for many children in many countries. Since Milne's introduction of Pooh, first published in 1926 when his son Christopher Robin was 6 years old, his stories have been translated into 21 languages. Christopher Robin, Milne's only child, loved visiting the bears at the zoo and was given a stuffed bear from Harrod's when he was just 1 year old (Milne, 1994). Christopher Robin later collected a stuffed pig, donkey, rabbit, tiger, and kangaroos that became characters for the stories his father wrote for and about him.

In his introduction, Milne gives a sampling of how one of the characters serves as a transitional object for Christopher Robin during a stressful moment at school. "Piglet is so small that he slips into a pocket, where it is very comfortable to feel him when you are not quite sure whether twice seven is twelve or twenty-two" (Milne, 1994, introduction).

The stuffed versions of Pooh and his friends are not the only transitional objects. The stories themselves serve as transitional objects. Milne wrote his son into the stories and Christopher Robin's reflections and questions are sprinkled into the books, thus providing Christopher Robin a narrative serving to contain emotional states and sort life experiences for psychological processing and integration of meaning. As child therapists understand, children place anxiety or other emotional states on characters for purposes of modulation, whether those characters are in stories, or are toys such as dolls, puppets, or figures of superheroes. Likewise, an adult may contain a difficult emotional state by repeating a favorite phrase or poem such as the Serenity Prayer.

"Piglet sidled up to Pooh from behind. 'Pooh!' he whispered. 'Yes, Piglet?' 'Nothing,' said Piglet, taking Pooh's paw. 'I just wanted to be sure of you'" (Milne, 1994, p. 284). This excerpt about Pooh and his friend Piglet speaks to the comfort a tangible object can provide. Transitional objects provide a "sureness of" when internal emotional life is unsure. This "sureness of" contributes to the internalization that takes place as we integrate relationships as part of our psychological foundation and personal identity.

Humor can also serve as transitional phenomena and laughter as a transitional state as one moves into emotional, cognitive, physiological, and behavioral change. Bringing humor to pain without offense can ease the intensity of emotion. Similarly, humorous characters can assist in the internal integration of meaning as transitional phenomena. The humor serves as a transitional object.

COMIC STRIPS IN PSYCHOTHERAPY

Blessed are we who can laugh at ourselves for we shall never cease to be amused.

—unknown

Comic strips lie at the intersection of humor and literature, and as such carry great potential to bypass defenses and serve as transitional objects and experiences in their own right. I believe they accomplish this by providing a lighthearted venue for the experience of challenging, and often trying and distressing, life situations. Upon seeing our struggles in a comic strip form, as might nervous parents reading *Baby Blues*™, a self-effacing teen reading *Charlie Brown*™, or an imaginative child traveling with *Calvin and Hobbes*™, the reader quickly recognizes that (s)he is not alone. This instant association, identification, and camaraderie provide us the opportunity to take a step back from ourselves and gain a sense of perspective, appreciation, and context. Vicariously experiencing a perilous adventure through the mazes of adolescence or the confusion of childhood with a favorite comic figure can provide a transitional space for security, problem-solving, and connection. If no one in my life understands what I am going through, at least good old Charlie Brown or Calvin and Hobbes do!

American comics evolved into a source of social commentary and entertainment following the introduction of mass production and distribution of illustrated magazines during the 19th century. Although the roots of cartooning can arguably be traced back to Egyptian hieroglyphics and even prehistoric cave paintings, the 18th and 19th century European use of satirical prints was the direct antecedent to the American comics (Walker, 2002). The American Sunday funnies appeared during the latter part of the 19th century thanks to the developments of color printing, national syndication, and the Sunday edition of the newspaper, which challenged blue laws (Walker, 2002). Since then, humor, in the form of comic strips (the Sunday funnies) has found its way into public consciousness with the proliferation of electronic media, which has given us instant access to our favorite characters through movies, television shows, and contemporary digital venues.

Brian Walker (2002), professional cartoonist, cartoon editor, and founder of the National Cartoon Museum, notes that "comics cover the scope of human experience" (p. 14), and that "The funnies have endured primarily because comic characters have a universal, timeless appeal. Their daily appearances make them familiar to millions. Their triumphs make them heroic. Their struggles make them seem human. Cartoonists create friends for their readers" (p. 15).

As a form of short story, comics have very limited time and space in which to develop the character's dilemma, and therefore must get to the point. Dramatic, colorful, and dynamic imagery, in conjunction with staccato text, along of course with serialization, all help us to get to know our favorite characters quickly and deeply. In order for the reader to get into—get involved emotionally with—a particular character, artists and authors must bring these diminutive protagonists quickly to our attention by immersing them in plotlines, stories, and adventures with which readers can readily identify. With the aid of humor, each cartoon panel or strip provides a quick and painless opportunity to learn about and laugh at life's incongruencies and inconsistencies.

Comic strips are one form of many types of humor available for therapeutic use. Robert Mankoff, cartoonist and cartoon editor of *The New Yorker,* says, "Everything I need to know about creativity I learned from cartoons and cartooning" (Mankoff, 2002, inside cover). Whether favorite comics are brought to therapy by clients, introduced by therapists, or created in the therapy room, they have the potential to address seriousness with levity. The experience of sharing a comic strip with a client, listening as a client reads a favorite, or witnessing a client's comic creation serves as a transitional phenomenon, bridging the gap between life outside and within the safe confines of the therapeutic space.

Comics may be instructional in capacity, such as when illustrating and normalizing gender differences for a couple in treatment through *For Better or Worse*™; narrative, such as when helping a client through mid-life developmental challenges through *Rose Is Rose*™; or containing, such as when offering humor as an outlet for childhood fears and impulses through *Calvin and Hobbes.*™

NIGHTTIME FEARS IN CHILDREN

This overview is offered as a prelude to the case application section, where Adam, a young client struggling with nighttime fears, was assisted by the therapeutic use of cartoon characters—in particular *Calvin and Hobbes.*

Nighttime can be a scary time for children. When the activity of the day winds down and the room becomes quiet and dark, loneliness and fear of being alone in the world often set in. Nighttime can be a truly existential challenge for children. Once past the rapprochement stage, when a child fully understands her physical separateness, darkness and aloneness allow doubts about one's realness and security. This early stage of development is prone to intrusions of images and perceptions that a child may feel threaten to devour her.

In his developmental review, James Fowler (1981) identifies the stage of ages 2 to around 6 or 7 as the *Intuitive-Projective* stage. His review integrates aspects of cognitive, moral, and psychosocial development. Fowler describes an individual's thinking in the *Intuitive-Projective* as "fluid and magical." Lacking in "deductive and inductive logic; it has an episodic flavor in which associations follow one another according to imaginative processes not yet constrained by stable logical operations" (p. 123). During this phase where "reality and fantasy interpenetrate" children are influenced by images and feelings. Fowler notes that the danger of this stage is that the child's imagination can be overwritten with "unrestrained images of terror and destruction" (p. 134).

These unrestrained images often appear at night. Research suggests that younger children experience more frequent passive victimization with less action and mastery in their dreams than do older children and adults (Siegel, 2005). The fluid and magical thought processes also lend themselves to less reality-based dreams. According to Siegel (2005), the young child's dreams have less reality anchors with fewer speaking characters than dreams of the older child.

Levin and Hurvich (1995) found a significant positive relationship between the frequency of nightmares and persons' experiences of annihilation anxiety. They note that prior to an "optimally delineated self" (p. 248) the ego is unable to provide psychic security protecting from fears of danger, helplessness, separation, abandonment, bodily injury, and annihilation of the self.

Cartoons may be one of many helpful treatments in the amelioration of night fears. Cartoon characters can add another presence that provide a container for projected fears and act as third-person observer to strengthen the ego through humor-based mastery of those fears.

CASE STUDIES

Following are some comic favorites that have made their way into my therapy room. These are of course only a few of the endless possibilities. This section begins with two short vignettes of women who brought comics to therapy as a way of communicating concerns relevant to their presenting problems. This section then describes a longer case study of a child with night fears where a common enjoyment of a comic strip between myself and the client became integrated into the treatment process. The section ends with a case where cartoons were created by client and therapist in session.

Kathryn and *Ziggy*™

Ziggy, the unlucky but loveable cartoon character, came into being in 1969 through the pen of Tom Wilson. *Ziggy* became a comic strip in 1971, and later became the work of Tom's son, Tom Wilson II, in 1987 (Universal Press Syndicate, n.d.). Ziggy, a rather nondescript male character save his stout frame, bald head, and big nose, has the luck of Murphy, and the fresh optimism of spring. Ziggy is frequently seen pondering life, at the park, out shopping or eating, at home with his pets, or at his psychiatrist's office.

Kathryn, a mid-adult mother of two, and a longtime fan of *Ziggy*, began bringing Ziggy cartoons early in her therapy to entertain and connect with her therapist. A Ziggy panel was a lighthearted way to begin a session, and a way for Kathryn to ease the awkwardness of knowing she would be talking about herself.

Ziggy was the proverbial grist for the mill. Kathryn loved Ziggy because she identified with him. Like Ziggy, Kathryn often found herself in naïve wonder about how unusual circumstances were a staple in her life. Kathryn could express in a humorous way her fears that her therapist might see her as Ziggy's psychiatrist saw him: as an uninteresting patient of quasi importance.

Discussion of Ziggy's relationship with his psychiatrist opened therapeutic conversation around the belief that she was fundamentally flawed. Reflection on Ziggy gave her an observer's point of view about culpability in events in her own life. Rather than seeing herself as the cause of the actions of others through the lens of Ziggy's passive foibles, she began to see when she was an unknowing recipient of others' projective behaviors. This reflection prompted a shift toward her ability to sidestep exaggerated guilt and frantic attempts to fix others' feelings toward her. She began developing greater confidence in herself and in her ability to build stable friendships while breaking away from her former detrimental relationships. Kathryn evolved from seeing herself as Ziggy's hapless peer to a mentor who could offer him (and herself) valuable insights for living.

Elise and the Peanuts™

In 1950, Charles Schultz gave us his world of *Peanuts* (Schultz, 1999, 2004) featuring the loveable round-headed boy, Charlie Brown, and his unique dog Snoopy (whose alter ego is known as The Red Baron). The

Peanuts cast includes Charlie's best friend Linus, and Linus's famous transitional object, his blanket; Linus's older sister, Lucy; Charlie's little sister, Sally; school chums Peppermint Patty and Marcie; the pianist Schroeder; Franklin; and Snoopy's bird friend, Woodstock. Schultz began *Peanuts* as a comic strip and continued the series as one, but also developed the stories into animated cartoons, providing generations such holiday classics as *A Charlie Brown Christmas* (Melendez, 1965), and *It's the Great Pumpkin, Charlie Brown* (Melendez, 1966). For just shy of 50 years, Schultz wrote and illustrated the *Peanuts* gang until he retired in December of 1999 just 2 months before his death.

Elise, a poised and professional woman, continued during trying times in life to hope for understanding and support from her mother. As an intelligent and independent middle-aged woman, Elise intellectually understood not to expect such a radical change from her mother. Emotionally, she longed for the comfort. She did not find maternal comfort from the woman who brought her into the world, but she did nurture her longing with the world of *Peanuts*.

A perennial challenge for Charlie Brown, as most fans know, is to succeed in kicking the football that his friend Lucy offers to hold for him. The spunky little girl repeatedly convinces Charlie that she will firmly hold the ball in place for him to punt. Each time, whether premeditated or on impulse, Lucy pulls the football away just as Charlie's foot is ready to meet the ball.

Charlie builds his reserve by telling himself "No, I am not falling for this trick again. Absolutely not! Lucy says she'll hold the football, but I don't believe her" (Shultz, 2004). But he then softens as he considers actually standing up to the persistent Lucy. "But maybe she's changed. The odds have got to be in my favor now. Look at her face. That's a face I can trust." Lucy looks down at him from above as once again he lies flat on his back on the ground, and tells him, "I admire you, Charlie Brown. You have such faith in human nature."

When Elise expressed her repeated dashed hopes in relationship to her mother, a friend asked, "How long will you play Charlie Brown to her, Lucy?" This instantly gave Elise a different perspective. It also gave her recognition that she had some choice in the matter.

Elise felt a kinship with Charlie Brown as she was continually seduced by false signs from her mother that she might deliver the coveted compassion, just as Charlie was seduced by Lucy's promises not to yank the football out from under his eager kick. Both Elise and Charlie were disappointed and sore from repeated falls.

Through identification with the cartoon, Elise could master the vulnerability by holding both the experiences of Charlie Brown and Lucy. She could simultaneously be yanker and yanked without harm to anyone.

The clarity of Charlie's dilemma, and continued investment in hope of a different outcome, brought Elise to awareness that she was allowing another's inability too much say-so in defining her security and happiness.

Charlie may spend eternity falling prey to Lucy's empty promises. Elise, however, learned to accept her relationship with her mother as it was—without expectation. Her acceptance has improved her relationship with her mother. The two women can converse without tension about unmet hopes.

Elise keeps a *Peanuts* pop-up book prominently displayed among her tasteful grownup décor as a symbol of her mastery over this particular vulnerability and a reminder to refrain from accepting offers to kick a football. Elise looks to other female relationships for camaraderie and reflective listening.

Adam and Calvin™

In the comic series *Calvin and Hobbes,* which debuted in 1985, Bill Watterson's character Calvin is a young energetic boy who spends most of his time exploring the world through his highly active imagination. His partner in imagination is Hobbes, his stuffed tiger. When in the presence of anyone but Calvin, Hobbes remains an expressionless stuffed animal. When Calvin and Hobbes are alone, Hobbes exhibits not only a full range of living tiger behavior, but of human behavior as well.

Hobbes may be one of the most developed transitional objects in popular culture. Hobbes is the traditional transitional object in that he comforts Calvin at night and through separation from his parents. But Hobbes assists Calvin through many transitioning psychological states. In Calvin's world, Hobbes embodies every human emotion and serves many roles such as playmate/companion, coadventurer, conscience, antagonist, foil, and comfort.

Hobbes and Calvin have philosophical discussions about the meaning of school and the meaning of parents. They contemplate life as they sled across snow-covered hillsides, hold clubhouse meetings, engineer replicating machines, play ball, fight like siblings, and ward off monsters under the bed. They plan sneak attacks on one another with snowballs, and look forward to friendship at the end of the school day where Hobbes is awaiting Calvin in eager anticipation.

Hobbes's presence allows Calvin to feel opposing or intense experiences by temporarily having Hobbes contain part of the emotion. Hobbes encourages, scolds, guides, goads, comforts, and shares disappointments, joys, and guilt. When Calvin needs a temporary place to contain blame after a parental scolding for making too much noise, Hobbes is accused of playing the cymbals. When his father is irritated with him for needing yet another nighttime reassurance, Calvin suggests that it is Hobbes who is requesting another bedtime story.

Because of Calvin's ability to imagine, Hobbes is able to assist Calvin by bolstering—sometimes providing—courage to explore the world, take on challenges, recover from disappointment, and generally move psychologically forward. Without Hobbes the world may seem too scary, lonely, or meaningless to meet challenges necessary to move him along in his development.

Adam's Story

Adam, a 10-year-old boy with dark curly hair and engaging green eyes, came to play therapy due to nightmares he experienced frequently off and on from age four. The nightmares had increased in frequency over the past year, and were occurring almost nightly. His parents had tried everything they knew to do such as comforting him, having a bedtime ritual, and cutting off scary movies and television. Adam usually did not remember his nightmares.

Adam was the oldest of three brothers. A well-behaved boy, he worried about the impulsive and rebellious behavior of his brother 2 years his junior. He exceeded the expectations of parents and teachers with politeness, organizational skills, and responsible behavior.

Adam enjoyed dark or scary movies and television shows such as *The Ghost Whisperer* (Moses, 2005–present) and *Goose Bumps* (Carol, 1995–1998). As a bright, articulate boy, Adam talked easily about his nighttime experiences and almost anything in his life, such as family, friends, school, sports, and video games. He could describe that the supernatural stories themselves were not a problem for him, but that the visuals troubled him as images often crossed his mind during the day. Although his family no longer watched the shows, and for the most part he was in agreement, he admitted to missing the excitement of the shows and the closeness it brought with his father and brothers.

Though we sat in a room full of toys, Adam did not play. During the first several sessions he sat contentedly on the playroom floor intellectualizing the elements of his week. At 10 years old, Adam was poised to better understand cause-and-effect relationships, and in particular, the one between his television viewing choices and his nightmares. Unfortunately for Adam, this understanding did little to alter his experiences. He could not figure out why after discontinuing his viewing, he continued to have nightmares.

One session, Adam asked, seemingly out of the blue, "Do you know Calvin and Hobbes?" As a long-time fan of *Calvin and Hobbes*, I responded enthusiastically (maybe even losing my therapeutic self for a moment while I indulged my own child within). We began to talk about our favorite episodes and the little boy and his stuffed tiger became regular visitors in our sessions. While becoming cognitively more sophisticated, Adam was still influenced by his powerful and unrestrained imagination.

Adam loved the mischievousness of Calvin. He especially enjoyed Calvin's trips into his imagination when he became superheroes Spaceman Spiff or Stupendous Man. He became animated as we recounted Calvin's trips as Spaceman Spiff (a character within a character) to such faraway planets as Gloob and Zorg. Through Calvin's pranks, Adam could explore wishes and fantasies and explore limits that he would not test in his real world.

Each session began with a discussion of a few episodes of *Calvin and Hobbes.* Following our discussions Adam became more spontaneous in the playroom as for the first time he explored the play items and engaged in animated play with action figures.

In our sharing of *Calvin and Hobbes,* we reviewed Calvin's nighttime fears on only three occasions. When we did, we focused on the humor in the characters' expressions, the humor in the arguments that erupted between Calvin and Hobbes, and the manner in which they relied on one another for strength in overcoming the drooling monsters in the closet and under the bed.

Just as Hobbes is a transitional object for Calvin, the comic strip of boy and tiger became a transitional object for Adam. As a cartoon character Calvin did not carry the frightening elements of the graphically real images Adam had viewed on television and in movies. He could play and imagine the antics of Calvin without feeling overriding guilt or psychic consumption. Calvin is a character drawn by, and therefore loved by, an adult. Although Calvin's parents are frequently stressed by his behavior, Calvin is never really in danger of abandonment.

In some respects, Adam was experiencing a collision between developmental stages. Still influenced by lingering images from unrestrained imagination and attempts to impose logic to free himself from their influence, he was unable to process and resolve the experiential fright brought on by dark TV images, complicated by a heightened sense of responsibility and desire to please adults.

Adam and I never discussed whether he saw Hobbes as alive independent of Calvin, or as a stuffed animal alive only in Calvin's imagination. We did not discuss that as a stuffed tiger, Hobbes's words and actions were actually aspects of Calvin himself. Explicit discussion of Hobbes "realness" wasn't necessary to our purposes and might have interfered with the focus of Adam's work. For Adam, images from earlier childhood along with repressed impulses and current images from indiscriminate media viewing interfered with feelings of safety. The images erupted at night and interfered with his sleep.

Calvin's stories contained Adam's fears, desires, and impulses. Through the stories Adam recognized that one could explore imagination, even mischief, and remain loveable, loved, and secure. Acceptance of Calvin in the therapy room allowed Adam to break out of his formalized way of relating to adults as he began to examine, experience, and integrate action, thought, images, and emotion in a more balanced way. Adam's parents contentedly discontinued therapy after several weeks of him sleeping through the night without nightmares. At 2-month and 6-month follow up calls, he was still sleeping peacefully through the night.

Justine

Justine entered the playroom, and I ran through the usual introduction of myself, the playroom, and the structure of the sessions in 9-year-old language. I offered, "You can play or not play, talk or not talk." Her choice?—not talk and not play. Justine sat on the floor about 6 feet from me, turned her back, focused on a children's magazine, and was silent for the entire session. This was a first for me.

True to my word, I allowed the silence despite my discomfort. In self-defense, I picked up blank paper and pencil and began to sketch a cartoonish reflection of the silent girl with her back to me. I sketched her shoulder-length blondish brown hair, the one arm and leg that I could see, her left tennis shoe tucked under her right leg, and the open magazine on her lap.

Time passed relative to my discomfort—slowly. When I broke the silence to announce the end of the hour, she quietly stood and headed to the door. I handed her the sketch. No words were spoken, but she looked at the paper and then looked up at me and smiled. We had connected. Without plan, I had mirrored her in a way that felt nonintrusive to her.

Justine required much in the way of physical, psychological, and emotional space from me. Although it was often difficult to tell when she needed me nearer or distant, I did my best to read her signals. She forgave my misreads and apparently I read well enough that she made progress at home and school by becoming more outgoing. She eventually became more spontaneous in session, and did not forget the drawing from session one.

After many sessions of sandplay, she moved to paper and wanted us to draw together. I followed her lead and together we began to draw cartoonish characters of people and animals.

Together we measured and drew playing-card-sized rectangles across the large lightweight poster board. Within each rectangle we drew cartoons of people, animals, and objects. We talked about our selections and some possible storylines to help cue our imaginations for additional characters.

Colored pencils and markers gave our characters the richness they deserved, and scissors gave them their independence. We now had a deck of cartoons of our own creation and were ready to bring them to life. For several of our following sessions, we included stories from the deck. Each week we began with spreading out the cards and choosing a beginning card. Together we created stories with themes that ranged from helplessness, nurturing, and aggression, to resolution and mastery. The main character of the stories was a girl about Justine's age. Initially, she thrived on the continuity of beginning the session with the cards. Always following her lead, I was ready to observe cues from her indicating whether to begin with the cards or that she was ready to move on. Following stabilization of her mastery themes, she no longer chose the cards and moved on to varied other play activities. She completed her play therapy process shortly after.

It is hard to say whether or not Justine would have developed the cartoon story deck without the introduction of the portrait, but it is safe to say that the projection into the characters and stories was important in developing mastery over her social anxiety. Giving Justine the lead in character and story development allowed her to maximize her growing self-efficacy.

Postscript to Justine

In reflecting back on my cartoon work with Justine, I acknowledge that clients may bring their favorite comics to the therapist as a way of communicating who they are and what they are experiencing. Clients may have developed their own characters outside of therapy or may choose to develop their own within the therapy. Alternatively, the therapist can suggest existing literary characters or cocreate them with the client. Introduction of literary characters may be either client or therapist generated (see Table 3.1).

In the area of creating characters, clients often have written, drawn, or imagined their own. Asking about creative outlets often reveals these

Table 3.1 Guidelines for Creation of Comic Strip Characters

Client	Therapist
Existing and mentioned in session	Existing and suggested by therapist
Existing and brought to session	Existing and brought by therapist
Created outside of session	Ask client about favorite characters
Created within session	Ask client to make up characters
	Suggest a character based on knowledge of the client

characters. Client-generated characters take precedence over therapist-generated ones in order to maximize client self-directed mastery of intra-psychic struggles. In the absence of client-created or chosen characters, the therapist can suggest characters to choose or cocreate character/s with the client.

The therapist can follow up by assigning that the client clip and bring meaningful comic strips to future sessions. The therapist can also bring relevant strips to sessions to add to the therapeutic narrative. Together client and therapist can write additional scenarios for the existing characters to consider new possibilities. For example, we may consider the possibility that Ziggy shops for a new psychiatrist. He may visit several before he finds one who is confirming of Ziggy's worth.

CONCLUSION

The rich variety of available comic strips and cartoons provide the therapeutic relationship with a wealth of potential humorous interventions. Laughing with these friendly interventions serves as a natural antidepressant impacting emotional, psychological, behavioral, and physiological change. The humanity of literary characters lends to instructive, projective, and containing purposes for a range of presenting problems. Well-timed use of comics can lead the therapeutic narrative in creative and productive directions.

REFERENCES

Bhosai, S., Miwa, S., & Hilber, D. (2007). Understanding the effects of humor therapy on patients' self-reports on pain, comfort and anxiety: Humor as a medium for non-invasive pain management. *Rx Laughter*. Retrieved September 22, 2007, from http://www.rxlaughter.org/RxLNCIfinalApril2nd2007.doc

Brown, S. L., & Kennard, D. (Directors). (2000). *The promise of play* [Documentary movie]. United States: Direct Cinema Limited.

Carroll, W. (Producer). (1995–1998). *Goosebumps* [Television series]. Los Angeles: Hyperion Pictures.

Fowler, J. (1981). *Stages of faith: The psychology of human development*. New York: HarperOne.

Howard, P. (2006). *The owner's manual for the brain: Everyday applications from mind-brain research*. Austin: Bard Press.

Imagineers, The. (2003). *The Imagineering way*. New York: Disney Enterprises.

Levin, R., & Hurvich, M. (1995). Nightmares and annihilation anxiety. *Psychoanalytic Psychology, 12*(2), 247–258.

Mankoff, R. (2002). *The naked cartoonist.* New York: Black Dog & Leventhal.

Melendez, B. (Director). (1965). *A Charlie Brown Christmas* [Television movie]. Studio City, CA: CBS Television.

Melendez, B. (Director). (1966). *It's the Great Pumpkin, Charlie Brown* [Television movie]. Studio City, CA: CBS Television.

Milne, A. (1994). *The complete tales of Winnie-the-Pooh.* Boston: Dutton's Children's Books.

Moses, K. (Producer). (2005–pres.). *Ghost whisperer* [Television series]. New York: ABC Studios.

Schultz, C. (1999). *Peanuts: A golden celebration.* New York: HarperCollins Publishers.

Schultz, C. (2004). *Peanuts: A pop-up celebration.* New York: Little Simon.

Siegel, A. (2005). Children's dreams and nightmares: Emerging trends in research. *Dreaming, 15*(3), 147–154.

Sultanoff, S. (2003). Integrating humor into psychotherapy. In C. E. Schaefer (Ed.), *Play therapy with adults* (pp. 107–143). New York: Wiley.

Universal Press Syndicate. *About Tom Wilson.* Retrieved September 18, 2007, from http://wwwamuniveral.com/ups/features/ziggy/bio.htm

Vaillant, G. (1977). *Adaptation to life.* Boston: Little Brown.

Walker, B. (2002). *The comics since 1945.* New York: Harry N. Abrams, Inc.

Winnicott, D. (2005). *Playing and reality.* New York: Routledge Classics. (Original work published 1971, Great Britain: Tavistock Publications).

PART II

Music

CHAPTER 4

The Healing Power of Music

Nancy Davis and Beth Pickard

It [music] gives a soul to the universe, wings to the mind, flight to the imagination, a charm to sadness, gaiety and life to everything.

—*Plato*

Music is the shorthand of emotion.

—*Tolstoy*

The arts are the soul of our existence. Music gives birth to emotion and emotion gives birth to music. Emotion and music are one and the same. We as human beings seek the pleasant beauty of music. "Human existence is defined by the ways we cope with obstacles and problems—music often gives solace during wrenching moments such as funerals, lost loves, and fears" (Cornett, 2006, p. 338).

Music is often used as a coping device. Slaves used (and unfortunately are still using) music to help them endure and control suffering. Many times, music has eased the burden of work and/or oppression. Music is often used to make life better! When faced with health problems, music gives one a more positive attitude and can help put suffering in perspective. With music, things don't seem so bad. Brooks, McCarthy, Ondaatje, and Zakaras (2004) state that many health benefits can be realized from the use of music and, as a therapeutic agent, it can bring about a relaxation response during many types of medical and surgical procedures. He notes that music can contribute to "improved health for a variety of patients . . . premature babies, mentally and physically handicapped . . . and those

---

Beth Pickard and Nancy Davis are mother and daughter.

suffering from . . . depression" (2004, p 12). Health providers often try to tailor match the patient with his favorite type of music. Music can be a magic potion! Almost anyone who has been involved with music for any time at all knows this secret. I (Pickard) have been a music teacher all of my life and have seen music work its magic.

MUSIC IN COUNSELING

Music is widely known to bring about relaxation, creativity, self-discipline, and motivation. Music has impacted lives by facilitating the expression of emotions, an appreciation for diversity, and a deep awareness of self, all of which contribute to the foundations of a healthy culture. Ever since the first drumbeats were heard in primitive lands, music has been known to be a soothing influence. Music alters our perception of time and mood, relaxes us, and gives us energy. Music can even change our state of consciousness in very real ways.

We have all experienced smiling and even laughing with faster musical rhythms in music. Endorphins, natural painkillers, are produced when we feel this pleasure. Listening to music causes changes in blood flow, respiration rate, pulse, blood pressure, and papillary (heart) muscle tone. Music is a type of intelligence, a way of knowing and expressing feelings and ideas (Cornett, 2006). Jensen (2000) speaks of emotional intelligences as being comprised of the ability to identify and label feelings, expressing feelings effectively, understanding and managing feelings, controlling impulses and gratification, reducing stress, and knowing the difference between feelings and actions. Music can contribute to the development of these skills.

Music colors our world. This is very helpful because we are able to maintain a more positive outlook on life by listening to positive, uplifting music. Music seems to soothe tensions. It takes off the rough edges of human interactions. Music just makes the world seem more friendly!

Music has the ability to put one in an altered state. Altered states may be measured by cycles per second of brain activity (Jensen, 2000). When listening to certain types of music an individual may picture faraway places and faraway times. Music seems to bring about a more pleasant state of mind.

However, music can also have a negative effect. Took and Weiss found that students who preferred heavy metal and rap music had a higher incidence of poor school grades, behavior problems, sexual activity, alcohol and drug use, and trouble with the law (1994). Gardstrom (1999) found that most of the students she studied felt that the heavy metal and rap music mirrored their feelings about society and did not, as some believe, cause their behavior. She found that this type of music gave them expression to their feelings and did not necessarily encourage antisocial behaviors. While these findings are contradictory, they mirror the many contradictions inherent in the lives of contemporary adolescents.

Sounds have been found to affect behavior. What we hear may regulate behavior. When autistic children experienced low-volume rhythmic drumbeats, their behavior improved. It seems that body and mind synchronize with the rhythmic drumbeats. Research seems to support the idea that music and specifically the hearing of music affects the body and mind in very positive ways (Jensen, 2000).

Music can be a tool to encourage relaxation and seems to bring about the same effects as soothing words or massage. Music seems to bring about long-term strengthening of the immune system.

Stress is caused by many things in our culture. Our daily lives are often filled with too much noise and confusion. Music can help us tune out the static. It can also make it easier to bear the confusion. Campbell suggests that music masks unpleasant sounds and feelings (2001).

Because music is widely accepted in our culture as a mood elevator, young students may use music as a means of regulating mood in the case of depression. Students who play an instrument have reported more self-confidence. Making music or playing an instrument forces one to create, reflect, bare one's soul, ponder, and react in new ways. I (Davis) found that my own children gained more self-confidence through the playing of musical instruments.

Music affects body and brain. Brain research has shown measurable reasons to prove that the effect of music on our whole body is very real. If we neglect using music, our souls "wither like a malnourished plant in winter" (Jensen, 2000, p. 51). Through the use of music one may lose the sense of time and place. Many times we are lost in our memories or in our hopes and dreams when we listen to certain meaningful pieces of music.

THE MAGIC OF MUSIC

These findings are very supportive of that article I read many years ago. When I (Pickard) taught in the elementary schools, I brought many styles and tempos of music into my music classroom. I encouraged my students to find a peaceful piece of music with a slow tempo and then suggested that they find a special quiet place in their home where they could go when they felt stressed or angry. "Music is a natural pacemaker" (Campbell, 2001, p. 67). Heart rates slow to match the speed of the tempo of the music. A slower heart rate "creates less physical tension and stress, calms the mind, and helps the body heal itself" (Campbell, 2001, p. 67). Listening to a favorite peaceful slow piece of music seemed to slow the students' heart rates and allow them to relax in body and mind. I wanted to give them a tool to handle the stresses they would encounter in the course of their hectic days including academic preparation and social interactions.

Later, when working with university students, I mentioned the fact that music could give them relaxation of body and mind. I gave them an assignment. I asked them to pick a favorite piece of music, no matter what style or tempo, and to play that piece of music for 10 minutes. I asked them to find an ostinata or short repeated rhythm pattern to fit their music. I then asked them to play that ostinata for the 10 minutes while listening to their favorite piece of music. Following this listening time, I asked them to write a couple of paragraphs about their feelings during the time in which they completed their assignment. Many students expressed a sense of peace and the belief that their stresses could be managed. In doing so, they seemed to gain a perspective on their worries and a resource for coping with stress

CASE APPLICATIONS

Music has charms to soothe the savage beast
To soften rocks, or bend a knotted oak.
—William Congreve (1670–1729)

Natalie

Reason for Referral and Presenting Problem

Nightmares, flashbacks, and panic attacks plagued 25-year-old Natalie. She complained of exhaustion, irritability, and insomnia. Her problems were beginning to affect her job performance. Natalie reported that she was having passive suicidal thoughts that frightened her enough to consider therapy.

Background Information

Natalie had never been in therapy. She was a quiet private person who had few confidants. She was very hesitant to open up and share her life with a total stranger. She started by sharing the safe, easy-to-divulge information and it took several months to uncover some of the imprisoned issues from the past that were screaming to be acknowledged. Once released, healing could commence.

To the outside world, Natalie's childhood appeared ordinary. She grew up in a household with both biological parents and two younger siblings. Her father was a self-proclaimed minister of a small congregation and her mother stayed at home to take care of the family. They lived comfortably in a small town where most people knew each other. Her extended family united several times a year and enjoyed their time together. She had become a successful, independent woman with strong family ties. Natalie was initially hard pressed to identify any conflicts or problems in the family.

Natalie excelled in academics. A gifted student, Natalie was the first in her family to attend college. She graduated and quickly got a job at a local newspaper. She had a job that she declared as "one of the greatest joys of my life." Her exhaustion and lack of concentration were affecting her performance. The past was haunting her and threatening to devour her world. As time went on in therapy, Natalie began to share that she often traveled into a nearby metropolitan city and would meet strangers and have sex. After each encounter Natalie would carry extreme guilt accompanied by a tormenting pursuit for answers into the cause for this behavior. She punished herself through self-inflicted injuries. She rightfully worried about contracting sexually transmitted diseases.

Eventually, Natalie revealed that from the ages of 4 to 15 she had been the victim of numerous sexual abuse perpetrators. Her aunt and her uncle had repeatedly abused her as they babysat whenever Natalie's mother ran errands. Other men joined in this sexual abuse, which often involved weapons and threat of violence upon her as well as her family. This was the primary source of her wounding, although other cases of sexual abuse by cousins, strangers, and a traveling minister were also uncovered. Natalie had never shared any of these horrifying events from her life with anyone. She viewed her silence as protecting the family and was unable to see herself as a victim. Natalie perceived her absence of disclosure as consent and the repeated incidences of sexual abuse by perpetrator after perpetrator as punishment for her sins.

Clinical Use of Music in Therapy

Talking in therapy was tremendously difficult for Natalie. Nonverbal techniques proved to release information that words would not. Natalie revealed that she kept journals and would sketch when feelings and thoughts overwhelmed her. Her creativity paired with artistic talent was a tremendous asset in therapy. Tapping these gifts was vital in helping Natalie. Several times, music evolved as a therapeutic intervention for growth and change.

Natalie entered one session and discussed that she really liked the singer KT Tunstall. I asked her to bring in some of her favorite music so that we could "play with it." *Eye to the Telescope* was her favorite album and she chose two songs to share. The first song was *Through the Dark* (Tunstall, 2006), which is about making difficult and painful choices.

Together we listened to the song in silence. I instructed her to "just be" and not try to analyze or think too much. I find that often this becomes somewhat of a sacred time. It is as if the client and I join together on a different level. I explained that I would like for her to express herself through drawing or creating something as we listened to the song for a second time. I asked Natalie to choose how she wanted to express herself on a piece of paper. I offered her crayons, colored pencils, pastels, markers, or chalk. She selected a combination of pastels and chalk. I started the song and let her create. Natalie was so involved in her artwork that I played the song for a third and fourth time as she finished her piece. As she worked, I tried to write down the lyrics to keep myself involved in the activity as well. She indicated that she was finished by putting down the chalk (see Figure 4.1).

I (Davis) typically initiate the dialogue by asking how the experience was for the client. Natalie shared that it had been good for her. She enjoyed it and felt positive about her piece. I then asked how she felt about her picture. She said, "It looks really dark. I didn't want it that dark!" She revealed that the blue (the teardrops) in her picture "looked sad." The red boundaries around the blue (outline of the teardrops) represented "walls of pain." "If the red was not there, the black would get in," Natalie stated. She quietly murmured that "if I'm happy, I stop and think that I shouldn't be so the wall of pain stops me from being happy. The sadness is contained within the pain." Her voice trailed off.

The color yellow (splotches scattered throughout the image) symbolized happiness for her. Yellow was interspersed with the darkness. She noted that the darkness was more intense on the left side of her drawing and the yellow became more obvious as she shifted her gaze from left to right. We had previously discussed the progression on the page from left to right possibly meaning past to present to future. Her voice strengthened as she saw a positive change within her picture and possibly in her life.

The stitches on the page also stood out to her as she analyzed her art. Interestingly, this image was conjured up from the lyrics of the song about pieces of a puzzle. She was trying to make sense of her life piece by piece by pulling together the past and the present.

Natalie factually said that the "chalk sticks to the pastels." I asked, "Is there a way to keep the yellow pure and free from the black?" Natalie replied, "I could choose not to use the chalk." So I reframed and said, "So you're saying that you'd do something different?" She chuckled, "Oh, that was sneaky!" Natalie got it. We then launched into a conversation of how she could do something different in her life to feel something different. Natalie was finding her way through the dark.

A few weeks later Natalie invited KT Tunstall and her tunes back into the session. *Silent Sea* (Tunstall, 2006) was another favorite song, which is about finding oneself after being cast adrift from a secure relationship.

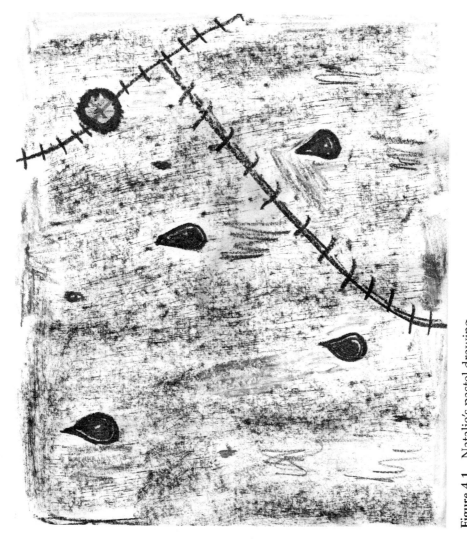

Figure 4.1　Natalie's pastel drawing.

As the music played on my CD player, I asked Natalie to list words or phrases that came to her mind as she listened. During the second listening I requested that Natalie incorporate the written expressions into a picture of what she envisioned during the song. As she worked on her piece, I kept the music flowing as she poured herself onto the paper. As she concluded, she sighed and put the crayons and colored pencils away (see Figure 4.2).

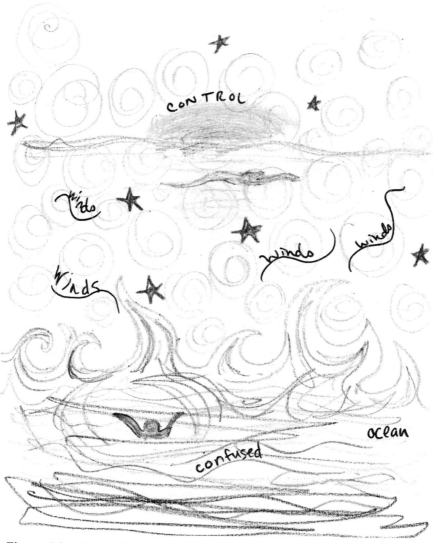

Figure 4.2   Natalie's crayon and pencil drawing.

Natalie explained that in the past the song had a calming effect, but her focus had been on the storm. During this experiential exercise, she altered her focus to the calm and to the warm sun at the top of her page. She had "more pronounced revelations" after her processing. The main phrase of the song about becoming inured to pain permeated her picture from the top of the page to the bottom. She noted that the base of the picture was dark and brooding and included the words confused, ocean, and bruise. The setting sun and the surface of the "silent sea" were near the top of the page. In between the "polar extremes" were the swirling sea and the whimsical breezes she labeled as winds.

There were two people identified in her work. One person was drowning in the black and red murky waters with hands held up for help. The water rose up from darker blue to a frothy hue, showing her journey from "confusion" to "control." The stars were her "remembrance of the past" and "constant reminders of past stuff." We discussed how this is a similar metaphor to "walking beside your abuse" rather than having her past constantly in front of her to stumble upon in her life or shoving her history of abuse behind her to bite her on her backside. The stars were "just there." Beneath the sun was a second person. "She was peaceful and enjoying her swim near the calm surface." Natalie said that she really enjoyed creating the upper half of the picture, which was fanciful and uplifting. She stated that the polar extremes were where she had been and where she wanted to be, which was perfectly summed up in the song lyrics that were about taking control in life. This continued to pave our path toward Natalie finding where she wanted to be. It was often through music and lyrics that this young woman found resolution to the question in her life.

Natalie journaled, "I therapist shopped for awhile. Most of them just expected me to say everything aloud and get it out that way. I just don't do that. But with a picture [or music] I can get everything in and then explain it. If I can't quite find the words, the story is still there. I'm not the best with talking about what I feel but I can draw or paint a picture that says it all. . . . That's why I think that I've meshed so well with my therapist. She works with me in ways that others haven't."

Nathaniel

Reason for Referral and Presenting Problem

Nathaniel, age 15, came to counseling with his paternal grandfather. Nathaniel was having difficulty falling asleep and would then refuse to get up and go to school nearly every morning for the past few months. He had stated that he "wanted to go to sleep and not wake up." The school continually tried to work with the family to help Nathaniel's attendance without success. He was extremely irritable and had even gotten into a physical fight with his grandfather. He often made threats to harm others. His grandfather was concerned that Nathaniel was suicidal. Nathaniel had told him that he had thoughts of stabbing himself with paper clips and pencils. Nathaniel often left the house without his grandfather's knowledge and no one knew exactly where he would go. There had been a history of drug use, but Nathaniel's grandfather could not determine if this was a current problem.

Background Information

Nathaniel lived with both of his biological parents for the first 2 years of his life. During these years, his parents constantly fought, used alcohol, and often sent Nathaniel to spend time away with his paternal grandparents. After the divorce, his father was granted full custody and his mother received visitation. The relationship between his parents remained conflicted and Nathaniel spent more time with his paternal grandparents than with either of his parents. When Nathaniel was 7, the court awarded custody to his paternal grandparents, as both parents were considered incapable of providing a safe environment for their child. Contact with both parents continued on an infrequent basis.

When Nathaniel was 11 years old, his mother died in a car accident. Nathaniel went into a deep depression. He attempted to hang himself "to be with my mother." His grades, which were below average prior to this, dropped to the place where retention was considered. No counseling services were sought during this time. From that point on, Nathaniel's academic performance bordered each year on failing.

Nathaniel's paternal grandmother was a stern, angry woman. According to his grandfather, she had experienced a traumatic brain injury as a young girl and had "never been right." She resented raising her grandson and often provoked Nathaniel. Nathaniel was labeled as a bad kid by his grandfather. His grandmother's mental and physical health declined to the point of admission into a long-term care facility when Nathaniel was 13 years old. His grandparents divorced shortly after her out-of-the-home placement. Nathaniel remained in the custody of his grandfather, who reported no true health concerns with his grandson. However, Nathaniel often complained of physical ailments. Frequent trips to the doctor rarely found any medical basis for his concerns.

During the intake session, Nathaniel did admit that he had smoked marijuana in the past, but he denied that he was doing any drugs at that time. He stated that he had smoked cigarettes since the age of 10. Nathaniel appeared skeptical that he could benefit from counseling. He denied having any problems; however, he agreed to "give it a try."

Clinical Use of Music in Therapy

Nathaniel was resistant in the first therapy session. He mumbled short responses, avoided eye contact, and kept looking at the clock. It quickly became obvious that he did not want to sit around and talk. Over the course of the next few sessions Nathaniel relaxed a bit and talked about the challenges of school, problems with girlfriends, and how much he did not appreciate the rules and boundaries his grandfather had placed on him. He quickly changed subjects whenever his past was approached.

After five sessions Nathaniel shared that his father had given him a guitar. His father had never learned to play the guitar and Nathaniel had expressed interest in it. A friend had helped him learn a few chords and he had been practicing daily. He asked if he could bring his guitar to the next session and I told him that I would look forward to this. The next session, Nathaniel brought his guitar. He strummed a few chords and was obviously pleased with himself. He said that he had started listening to some of his favorite bands and was trying to play along. He proudly held up his hand to show me the blisters he was awarded for his efforts. I watched, listened, and applauded his efforts.

Nathaniel continued to bring his guitar to future sessions, each time gaining more confidence and skill. His blisters turned to calluses that he attributed to mastery of his instrument. He had found other peers were playing guitars and he joined up with them. He reported that they would sit around and have jam sessions. He was somewhat amazed that he could have so much fun and be sober at the same time. He admitted that he had not stopped smoking marijuana, as he had told us in the intake session, but now he was going to try to stay clean.

Nathaniel was soon able to talk and play the guitar at the same time. His selection of music appeared to match his moods as he started to open up about the topics that he had previously avoided. He played Top 40 tunes and reached back in time to play the Beatles. I must admit that when Nathaniel played songs from the 1960s and 1970s, which was pop music in my day, I felt a special connection and understanding. When Nathaniel played recent hits, he educated me on the significance of the music and lyrics. He often knew the history of the artists and was able to relate to some of the trauma that his rock idols had experienced. He began talking about his mother and the relationship that they had prior to her death. He reminisced about the good times and became tearful as he described the events that surrounded her death. Eventually, he shared his experiences from the funeral and the longing he still had for his mother. In other sessions, he would play his guitar and slowly work up to discussing the anger he had at his father. Feelings of abandonment and betrayal came out while his guitar sounded loud and echoed his anguish. His thoughts often stormed through the torment he felt from his grandmother. He recalled all of the name-calling, the pain, and the useless efforts to please her.

Nathaniel's grandfather reported encouraging changes in his grandson's life. He no longer talked of hurting himself, he was actually attending school, his grades were improving, and grandfather and grandson were beginning to talk rather than argue. The transition occurred slowly and with much hard work in therapy. Nathaniel's guitar was able to rise to the occasion and help him explain and explore the past that he had so desperately tried to convince himself was benign. Long after Nathaniel had moved on from counseling sessions, he was able to continue his therapeutic work with his faithful companion, his guitar.

Aubrey

Reason for Referral and Presenting Problem

Aubrey, age 16, was crying out for help, according to her distraught mother, Marissa. Marissa had called to initiate counseling services because Aubrey desperately needed to talk to someone and she believed Aubrey to be in an emergency situation. Aubrey was having problems sleeping, was crying uncontrollably, and had been missing school due to numerous physical complaints. Fears of being kidnapped were preventing her from leaving the house alone. Most communication between Aubrey and her mother ended up in loud and disturbing arguments. Aubrey's doctor had suggested counseling as an option to deal with her physical complaints, and the school recommended counseling due to the extended absences and concern over Aubrey's emotional state.

Background Information

Aubrey's biological parents, Marissa and Derrick, divorced when she was 4 years old. Marissa was granted joint custody and primary physical custody of Aubrey. Aubrey lived alone with her mother from age 4 until age 7, at which time, Marissa remarried. From the beginning, Aubrey had a strained relationship with her stepfather, Mark who was described as being aloof, reserved and noncommunicative with her. Aubrey was accustomed to her mother's full attention and was jealous of the time her mother spent with Mark. When Aubrey was 12, Marissa gave birth to Aubrey's half brother, Andrew. Aubrey's relationship with her stepfather grew even more distant as Mark became a "perfect dad" to his one and only son. The family struggled financially although both parents worked full-time jobs. Often Aubrey was left to care for her little brother in the parents' absence.

Aubrey had been very close to her father and missed him greatly after her parents separated. Initially after the divorce Aubrey and her father, Derrick, maintained contact through consistent visitation. However, Derrick remarried within the year, moved a hundred miles away, and started a new job that took him out of state for long periods of time. Visitation became infrequent and inconsistent. Derrick and his new wife had two other children over the next 3 years. When Aubrey did visit her father, she would return to her mother and complain about her father's lack of attention. Aubrey had begun to refuse visitation with her father. Phone calls with her father were typically ending with Aubrey yelling and hanging up the phone.

Aubrey had no significant medical conditions; however, she went to the family doctor several times a month for various physical complaints ranging from stomach problems to headaches. Aubrey's doctor had referred her to several specialists, ordered countless tests, and eventually labeled Aubrey's problems as psychosomatic. Aubrey had no history of alcohol or drug usage. It was suggested that counseling might help alleviate her physical symptoms.

Academically, Aubrey was on target. Despite the fact that she missed school on average 1–2 days per week, her grades were well above average. Often teachers felt that she was a gifted student. Aubrey's mother reported that it was extremely difficult to convince Aubrey to go to school each morning and each year was getting progressively worse. Once at school, Aubrey often called her mother and cried for her to come and bring her home. Marissa was beginning to experience pressure at work due to the time she had to take away from her job in order to deal with Aubrey.

Socially, Aubrey had a small number of close friends. She had been involved in limited extracurricular activities. She had spent several years on the soccer team, but had not pursued the sport for the last year. She had enjoyed playing the clarinet in band, but stated that she planned on quitting after the semester. She reported an interest in listening to music.

Clinical Use of Music

Several sessions were held with Aubrey who was eventually willing to verbalize her feelings about her family. She confided that she felt "lost." She claimed that she did not feel special to anyone. She reminisced about her memories of her father and how she had been a daddy's girl until he remarried and forgot her. Her mother was "so busy with her own life that she doesn't have time for me." Even though Aubrey was able to let her feelings out in therapy, she did not believe that she could ever share these thoughts and feelings with her family.

Marissa and Aubrey both reported that some improvement was noted after several sessions. Aubrey was able to get to sleep more easily, she was not crying as much, and her school attendance had improved. However, her relationships with her parents remained extremely conflicted.

During the course of one session, Aubrey talked about one of her new favorite songs. We began discussing music and how certain songs affected her moods. I asked Aubrey if there was a song that could help her express how she felt about her parents. Challenged by the task, Aubrey agreed to do some research and bring the song into the next session.

Prior to the next session and unbeknownst to me, Aubrey mustered up courage and sent an e-mail containing the words of a song to her parents. I received a frantic phone call from Marissa claiming that her daughter was suicidal because Aubrey had just sent an e-mail to her and to her father, which led them to fear that Marissa was sending them a veiled suicide threat.

Not knowing exactly what was occurring, I immediately held a session with Aubrey. Aubrey brought in a CD by Beyoncé Knowles. She requested that we play the song *Listen* (Knowles, 2007) which is about trying to find one's voice and the pain of not being heard or understood by someone else. She had printed the lyrics of the song so that I could follow along. These were the same lyrics sent to her parents. After the song, Aubrey said, "That's how I feel." I asked her to listen to the song again, this time writing down words or phrases that captured the essence of her feelings. Aubrey wrote down lyrics that reflected her burgeoning sense of control and freedom. Aubrey said the song made her feel "set free" and "happy because I realize that I need to move on and be myself." The music itself was inspiring and uplifting. She denied that the song held any suicidal meaning for her. Aubrey then agreed to include her mother in the session.

Marissa joined the session and Aubrey was able to explain to her mother that she sent the e-mail because "nobody understands me." Marissa had never heard the song, which was recently from the movie *Dream Girls* (Condon, 2006). I played the song *Listen* for Marissa and then I asked them to listen a second time while writing down phrases and words that stood out to them. They then shared what they wrote. As they opened up to each other, Aubrey was able to express that she was angry at her father for "not acting like a dad" to her. She explained that she felt that her mother "never sees" her because Marissa was always working and when Marissa was home, she was always too busy to notice her. Listening to the song together helped Aubrey convey her thoughts and feelings to her mother and aided her mother in understanding how all the pieces fit together to make Aubrey a very sad, angry girl. This was the therapeutic breakthrough that paved the way toward healing the hurts that were so deep within Aubrey.

circumstances. The therapist may choose to join in on this activity by suggesting therapeutic words, phrases, or lyrics. The lyrics are written down and even possibly sung together as the music is played.

Another version of this technique was developed by Janine Shelby. Shelby revised the words to "Twinkle, Twinkle Little Star" for a client who had been sexually abused. Shelby's lyrics were: "I am safe and I am strong."

DISCUSSION TOPICS

1. What do you hear, see, feel, or experience when you listen to the original music?
2. What do you hear, see, feel, or experience when you listen to your own lyrics to the song?
3. Can you think of a time when you might think, hum, or sing your own lyrics in order to feel or experience something different?
4. What do you think the original artist would think of your personalized lyrics?
5. Imagine that you are the artist singing your lyrics with the band. What would your music video look like?

Exercise 4.2: Mood CDs

OBJECTIVE

jective of this technique is to have the client create a music CD ludes songs that express different feelings such as joy, anger, anxiss, or any feeling identified by the client. Clients will come to that the music they listen to affects how they feel and that in return, can be altered by the music they select at any

MATERIALS

ssigned as homework, the client must have access o legally download or copy songs onto CDs or vention is undertaken in the therapist's office, ess to music and a system to record. In either ds to have the equipment to play the music

the
to
t the

DESCRIPTION

The therapist initiates a discussion of how music can affect our feelings, moods, and perceptions and discovers whether the client has favorite songs, artists, or musical groups. The client is assigned the homework of creating a Mood CD where certain feelings are identified and corresponding songs are selected. Using current technology, the client then produces a CD that eventually includes an entire list of feelings and songs. Downloading the songs into an iPod or MP3 player can produce the same results, but the therapist must have the equipment to play the music in the office.

Ask the client if he or she would share the Mood CD in sessions. Numerous ways of exploring the music could range from creating artwork, using clay, journaling, creating sand trays, experiencing guided imagery, or discussing the songs.

By creating a CD that has all of the chosen music in one location, the client can easily find the music that is desired in times when healing is sought.

Additional steps in the therapeutic process could entail the client creating an album cover for the CD, selecting a title for the CD, and sharing the songs with family members or friends either in or out of session.

DISCUSSION TOPICS

1. How can different music affect your feelings and your mood?
2. What does the music tell you about yourself?
3. Does your mood reflect the lyrics, the rhythm, or the music of each song?
4. Does each song match your mood or does each song change your mood?
5. What do you know about the artists and how do you identify with them?
6. In what situations would you find yourself wanting to listen to each of your different songs?
7. What songs would you have chosen a year ago? Five years ago? How have your tastes in music changed?

REFERENCES

Brooks, A., McCarthy, K., Ondaatje, E., & Zakaras, L. (2004). *Gifts of the muse: Reframing the debate about the benefits of the arts.* Santa Monica, CA: RAND.

Campbell, D. (2001). *The Mozart effect: Tapping the power of music to heal the body, strengthen the mind and unlock the creative spirit.* New York: Harper Collins.

Condon, B. (Producer). (2006). *Dream girls* [Motion picture]. United States: Dreamworks SKG.

Cornett, C. (2006). *Creating meaning through literature and the arts: An integration resource for classroom teachers.* Upper Saddle River, NJ: Merrill Prentice Hall.

Gardstrom, S. C. (1999). Music exposure and criminal behavior: Perceptions of juvenile offenders. *The Journal of Music Therapy, 36,* 207–221.

Knowles, B. (2007). Listen. On *B'Day* [CD]. New York: Colombia Records.

Jensen, E. (2000). *Music with the brain in mind.* Thousand Oaks, CA: Corwin.

Took, K. J., & Weiss, D. S. (1994). The relationship between heavy metal and rap music and adolescent turmoil: Real or artifact? *Adolescence, 29,* 613–621.

Tunstall, KT. (2006). Through the dark. On *Eye to the telescope* [CD]. United Kingdom: Virgin Records.

Tunstall, KT. (2006). Silent sea. On *Eye to the telescope* [CD]. United Kingdom: Virgin Records.

CHAPTER 5

Using Music and
A Musical Chronology
as a Life Review
With the Aging

Thelma Duffey

Sarah is vibrant, energetic, and young at heart. She first attended therapy following a medical scare that reminded her of "how vulnerable we are, particularly as we age" (Sarah, personal communication). Introspective by nature, Sarah sought the help of a therapist who would walk with her through personal challenges related to aging and loss. She wanted to deal authentically with her feelings and to have a realistic perspective on her experiences. She described herself as having been a dreamer much of her life, and lamented on how difficult it had historically been for her to leave the past behind and walk enthusiastically in the present. Now, with so much of the past behind her, she wanted to revisit her experiences with a fresh perspective and walk gratefully in the present, mindful of every opportunity she had. Further, Sarah wished to be free of the second-guessing retrospection that had plagued so much of her life.

Sarah is not alone in this quest. Discussions on the individual's quest for meaning are age-old. Since the beginning of time, people have reflected on what purposes their lives serve, what legacies they leave behind for future generations, and what impact they have had on those around them (Birren & Deutchman, 2005; Cadrin, 2006; Derrickson, 1996; Haight, Schmidt, & Burnside, 2005; Thibault, Ellor, & Netting, 1991; Wong, 2000). No doubt, the meaning-making experience is fundamental to our growth and development as a species. Further, making meaning of our experiences is spiritually, psychologically, and relationally relevant. As a result, the meaning we ascribe to our experiences ultimately impacts the way we behave toward others, our self-perceptions, and our expectations of life. Although these considerations are important at any stage in life, they can be particularly prominent as we approach later life (Butler, 2002; de Vries, Westwood, & Blando, 2005; Erickson, 1963). In this chapter, we will explore how the use of popular music, through a vehicle I developed, entitled *A Musical Chronology and the Emerging Life Song* (Duffey, 2005a, 2005b; Duffey, Lumadue, & Woods, 2001) can help clients like Sarah come to terms with life experiences and discover their meaning and purpose.

Researchers and theorists have long discussed the meaning-making experience. Cassell (1982) suggests that the degree of suffering we experience at the end of life is influenced by the meaning we ascribe to our experiences, and by our ability to connect with the sense that something larger than ourselves exists. Frankl (1992) purported that deriving meaning from our experiences was central to the therapeutic process. Erikson (1963) also contended that, although meaning-making is a course we all undergo throughout our lives, this process is particularly salient in our generative stage of life.

Therapists working with older adults can help their clients discover and document their meaning-making experiences through a life review (Butler, 2001, 2002; Burnside & Haight, 1994; Gibson & Burnside, 2005; Haight, 2007; Prickett, 1998; Soltys & Kunz, 2007). Although most studies on life review have been done with older persons who are homebound or in care facilities or institutions, Arkoff, Meredith, and Dubanski (2004) posit that life review can be helpful for the large portion of older people who are well-functioning and have many years of life remaining. They further state that life review for adults in this group should be proactive, using insights from the past to help create a better present and future. Life reviews can also serve as legacies for loved ones and future generations (Cadrin, 2006).

Popular music, in the form of *A Musical Chronology and the Emerging Life Song*, is one resource that can be used with clients conducting their life reviews. This intervention is founded on the principle that popular music often plays an important role in people's lives, given that "music has long been considered the language of emotion and has historically been a component in the ancient healing rituals of cultures throughout the world" (Duffey et al., 2001, p. 399).

Indeed, popular music has been historically relevant to people of all ages. For example, Christianson and Lindlof (1983) note how music has a significant emotional impact on children. Larson & Kubey (1983) describe how music reflects the range of emotional experiences that adolescents encounter in their daily lives. Eich and Mecalfe (1989), and Terwogt and Van Grinsven (1991) focused on music with adult populations, discovering that music can induce specific emotional states and alter mood. Pricket (1998) states that music can assist older adults who are well with various life tasks such as maintaining an active lifestyle, maintaining or building social contact, and maintaining and building cognitive skills. According to Bright (1997) music serves two primary roles in the lives of older people. First, it evokes emotions, memories, and past connections in a person's life. Second, it can facilitate the enjoyment of shared interests and activities.

A Musical Chronology is supported by research such as Baumgartner's (1992) study, which investigated the relationship between emotions that describe the original experience and those aroused in hearing music that reawakened feelings. Participants reported that listening to a personally important piece of music created powerfully clear recollections of past experiences that frequently appeared with images reminiscent of the original events. Indeed, music provides an avenue for understanding life experiences as it elicits a range of emotions and the listener associates past or present life events with a musical piece (Hays, 2005; Hays & Minichiello, 2005; Karras, 1987; Kenny, 1999). More recently, Cadrin (2006) discusses how popular music can serve as legacy work in palliative care and can be a catalyst for helping clients create meaning at the end of life.

In that vein, Porchet-Munro (1993) described how "music tends to be mythic, symbolic, and archetypal and enables journeys of insight" (p. 39). Insight comes to us at all ages, but is particularly poignant as people grow older. During this time in life, many reflect on their lives: their successes, regrets, accomplishments, and unrequited dreams. Further, as Cadrin (2006) notes, many "seek to make amends for past events that have not been reconciled . . . to gain a larger understanding of . . . life experiences . . . and to share the values and beliefs that have been learned" (p. 114). They do this by reminiscing on their experiences and genuinely assuming responsibility for them. More specifically, *A Musical Chronology* is an intervention that can facilitate clients' access to memories and their emotional responses to life (Duffey, 2005a, 2005b; Duffey et al., 2001). Additionally, it can assist older adults with forming more meaningful connections with loved ones (Duffey, Somody, & Clifford, 2006/2007). This process serves as a musical scrapbook, of sorts, that allows us to revisit our experiences and the meanings we ascribe to them. The process also helps us become more accountable and replace unproductive narratives with healing perspectives (Bortnick, 2005; Duffey, 2005a; Duffey et al., 2001). *A Musical Chronology* is framed within a Narrative Therapy framework.

NARRATIVE THERAPY

Gregory Bateson suggested that it is the attribution of meaning rather than an underlying dysfunction that determines behavior (Bubenzeer, West, & Boughner, 1994; Gladding, 1998; Kurtz, Tandy, & Shields, 1999; White & Epston, 1990). According to Narrative Therapy, our personal stories not only reflect our life experiences, but also create them (O'Hanlon & Beadle, 1994; Parry & Doan, 1994; White & Epston, 1990, 1992). Stories provide us with a way to structure our experiences and make sense of them. They help us put into words the meaning we make of our experiences, and we make choices by taking into account the meaning we attribute to our life events (Freeman, Epston, & Lobovits, 1997). These stories either facilitate or impede the success of our life goals.

White and Epston suggest that we can create an alternative story based on lived experience, even though a dominant story may be imposed by society (Becvar & Becvar, 1996; White & Epston, 1990). Durant (1993) describes how "People are engaged in a constant process of making sense of themselves, their relationships, and what happens to them. This view of self is what determines how people feel and behave" (p. 27). Even though our life narratives are influenced by a number of factors, they generally become autonomous (Hodas, 1994), to the point of shaping our lives (White & Epston, 1992). Narrative therapy deconstructs "taken for granted realities and practices" (White & Epston, 1992, p. 12). The narrative therapist assists clients with separating from their problems, and reauthoring their stories. Zimmerman and Dickerson (2001) state:

> The therapist engages the client in a process of telling another story about themselves in relation to the problem. This is a heroic story of persons standing up to problems that are primarily not of their making and putting them out of their lives (as opposed to a pathological story of the person or family). (p. 420)

Hodas (1994) proposes ways to help clients re-author their lives in ways that promote personal agency. He refers to this as a "therapeutic sharing ritual" between client and therapist. This ritual can be particularly meaningful in our work with aging populations.

A MUSICAL CHRONOLOGY AND THE EMERGING LIFE SONG

A Musical Chronology is an intervention that can facilitate clients' access to their emotional responses to life (Duffey, 2005a, 2005b; Duffey et al., 2001; Duffey et al., 2006/2007). Further, the chronology process provides us with a vehicle for identifying the restrictive narratives (White & Epston, 1992) we form in reaction to life events. As a therapeutic medium, patterns of behavior or emotions can be discovered through the chronology and the clients' personal narratives clarified (Duffey, 2005a, 2005b; Duffey et al., 2001). By participating in the process, clients are led to recognize the effects of their narratives on current relationships and life experiences. Langer (1951) posits that "because the forms of human feelings are more congruent with musical forms than with forms of language, music can reveal the nature of feelings with a detail and truth that language cannot approach" (p. 199). *A Musical Chronology* deconstructs restrictive narratives and facilitates clients' re-authoring of their lives through the use of music consciously selected (Duffey et al., 2001).

Musical Chronology Assumptions

1. Music is a common means for some men and women to connect with their life experiences.
2. Music and lyrics can contribute to clients' creation and maintenance of narratives and stories.
3. If our perceptions are negatively skewed, they create a restrictive narrative that can result in a relationally rigid worldview that impedes the potential for sustained connection and commitment.
4. Music is one vehicle by which we may form, maintain, or alter unproductive perceptions and restrictive relational narratives.

Chronology Objectives

1. To facilitate clients' access to their emotional responses to past relationships.
2. To provide a forum for clients to identify and process relational grief and loss experiences that may create unproductive perceptions and restricted narratives.
3. To help clients recognize the effects of these perceptions and relationship narratives on present relationships.
4. To assist clients to deconstruct restrictive narratives and re-author their lives through the use of music consciously selected and reinforced.

The Chronology Process

A *Musical Chronology* is a four-stage process best facilitated within the context of a comfortable connection between client and therapist, and can be adapted to diverse therapy needs. Below is a framework for its implementation.

Stage I

Counselor and client discuss the viability of using music to revisit past memories and associations. Consistent with most therapeutic processes, the chronology structure can be adapted, and is essentially flexible, depending on the needs of the client and the unfolding of the therapy experience.

Stage II

Clients identify musical selections that have been important to them or that trigger associations to important life events. Clients, with the counselor's help, compile the list of musical selections and arrange the song titles chronologically. This part of the process assists clients in conceptualizing and mentally organizing their experiences. Clients and counselors find the lyrics for the songs they choose to include in their chronology. Clients are often surprised to discover patterns with respect to language, and messages that color and inform their experiences and expectations. Clients and counselors compile a CD or audiotape.

Stage III

Clients play the music and discuss their thoughts, memories, and associations. This leads to a revisiting of historical events while listening to the music. In this stage, music is used to evoke feelings, thoughts, and memories.

Stage IV

Client and counselor listen for relational themes and restrictive narratives or unproductive perceptions that impede connection or deepened relationships. Client and counselor work collaboratively to facilitate clients' awareness of any restrictive relational narratives and to create the possibility of alternate perspectives. Clients find and play a song that represents their beliefs, values, and convictions. They often select songs for their loved ones—songs that represent their shared experiences, their feelings toward them, or their hopes for their futures.

A Musical Chronology can be used to create a lyrical biography, of sorts, and clients can actually narrate the selection and record their messages on the CD. These messages, along with the musical chronology, not only serve to help clients put to words the meaningful events in their lives; they can also serve as an auditory legacy for their friends and families, and for generations to come.

CASE DISCUSSION: SARAH

Sarah conducted a life review as part of therapy following a medical scare. The musical chronology process was particularly salient for Sarah because of her lifelong interest in music and her current interest in creating a coherent life context. She hoped this context would provide her with a productive "lessons learned" perspective on her life events and a meaningful roadmap for her future.

Although Sarah reported experiencing many blessings and a full, rich life, she has also felt haunted by ghosts from the past. And now, at this point in life, she didn't want to give these previous hurts and experiences any more time or energy. Still, she described a need to make meaning of her experiences, to honor them, and to let go of those that no longer served her life purpose. Further, she wanted to clarify her thoughts, beliefs, and values in such a way that she could communicate them to her children and other loved ones. Sarah wanted the people she loved—the people who loved her—to know the parts of her she deemed most significant while they still had time together. Also, she wanted her loved ones to be left with these parts when she was no longer here. Toward that end, we worked together as she conducted a life review.

When asked, Sarah described her children as the greatest accomplishments in her life. She is proud of them and profoundly enjoys their time together. Sarah is also grateful for her relationship with her parents. She sees them to be wonderful people and acknowledges how familial challenges had ultimately brought her closer to them, an experience for which she is immensely thankful. Sarah also sees herself as a good friend and appreciates the friendships she sustains. Additionally, Sarah is proud that she established a career doing something she loved, being a sole proprietor of a local bookstore, where she had the opportunity to inspire people to love books as she always has.

On the flip side, Sarah describes her greatest liability as her attachment to hurts from the past, with her greatest wish being to free herself from these attachments. She describes herself as a deep feeler, albeit a person entrenched in her perspective. This characteristic can make it difficult for her to let go, even when she knows that to do so would be in her best interest. Sarah feels limited by these patterns of thought and behavior. Although she has gained considerable insight into her patterns throughout the years and in previous therapy experiences, she now seeks a more experiential process—one that will help her create new meaning from her experiences. Her hope is that as she attributes meaning to these experiences, she can embrace them for the value they have had in her life, and then release them as experiences that have served their purpose. Because Sarah is aware of her past-focused perspective and the restrictive narratives these create for her, she has taken great care in organizing her musical chronology.

Sarah's Process

Sarah was excited at the prospect of compiling music that had been important to her and invested in the process enthusiastically. She had long been a music lover, and described how music had been her friend ever since she was a child. In fact, some of her earliest recollections involve sitting on the floor next to the stereo speakers in her family home, playing her favorite records over and over. She explained how music, more than half a century later, still moves her. And now, as part of the chronology process, Sarah is bringing out old records to create a musical landscape of her life experiences. The music serves as a catalyst in her therapy, as Sarah describes her life and places it in a context she can understand.

In the initial part of the chronology process, Sarah included many songs that reflected lifelong themes of anticipation, hope, yearning, and loss. Beginning with the death of her grandparents, and later, her parents' divorce, these themes were poignant. Later experiences involved her divorce and an unfortunate relationship. Sarah also regretted lost friendships at various points in life.

At the same time, Sarah's music also reflected a number of happy, rewarding times, illustrated by themes of passion, love, and fulfillment. She also recalled the deep friendships that endured across time, the very genuine relationships she has with her children and grandchildren, and the very real love she shares with her parents. In conducting a life review, Sarah began to place her diverse experiences in context.

Sarah's Chronology

Sarah begins her chronology with Carly Simon's (1971) "Anticipation." In describing her life and in listening to this song, Sarah discussed how her children and grandchildren have always been the bright spot in her life. She recalls the time in life when her children were young, and how her family was busy "building, becoming, and doing" (Sarah, personal communication). Although that period is resoundingly powerful for her, she has regrets. According to Sarah, this song reflects how Sarah has characteristically chased her dreams. It also makes her recall her first marriage, and how much she had wanted it to be long-lasting. Although the decision to part was mutual, she recalls the guilt she has felt for being young, immature, stubborn, and shortsighted.

Sarah recalls how difficult it was for her to be in love with the moment; how, despite the great moments before her, she would often look forward to something else; how she would *wait* for more. Sarah no longer wants to wait, and like the song, she wants to see the present as the good old days.

Interestingly, while conducting her chronology, Sarah began to see how her history was filled with many "good old days," complete with good times, bad times, challenges, and triumphs. Sarah describes feeling grateful for them at the same time she regrets that her head and heart carried other preoccupations while she lived those moments. But she no longer wants to live with regret. Now, she has another chance. Today *is* her new day *and* her good old day. Sarah wants it to become second nature for her to recognize her great moments as they occur. The 1970s hit song, "Anticipation" (Simon, 1971), helped her put words to that desire. Further, it helped her communicate this value to her children and loved ones.

Sarah's second song in her chronology, "Happiest Girl in the Whole USA" (Fargo, 1999), was also popularized in her youth. However, in this song, the singer appears to appreciate her good life. Sarah always enjoyed the song, and she enjoyed hearing how happy someone can be in a mutually satisfying relationship. In listing this song in her chronology, Sarah is reminded of the part of her that is genuinely hopeful.

Sarah thinks about how wonderful it is to truly appreciate our blessings. Sarah smiles as she thinks about how happy she is with her life as it is, and how blessed she has been. She is especially grateful that she has discovered how to have a relationship with God. This struggle has been hard-won, regardless of, and perhaps because of, the gains and losses in her life. Happiness to Sarah is directly related to feeling connected in life. There are times when Sarah feels very connected to the people she cares about and to God, but there are other times when she feels disconnected from everyone. During these times, she has historically lamented losses and shattered hopes. More often, Sarah tries to remember that she *is* connected to others, to God, and even to deceased loved ones, even when feelings of loneliness come over her. At the end of the day, she feels more connected because she believes that God exists, and she appreciates that her loved ones are life gifts. When Sarah feels isolated or especially alone, she reminds herself that these feelings are part of the human condition. By remembering the "bigger picture" and the spiritual connection she shares with others, she feels comforted. Recalling the hope she felt as a child, her trust in God, and her expectation that life would be good to her, she uses lyrics sung by Cat Stevens in the form of "Morning has Broken (Farjeon, 1971). This song represents her belief that our lives have meaning; that there is a design to life; and that we are cocreators of this design.

At the same time, she remembers another Cat Stevens song, "Wild World" (1970), popularized in her adolescence. She included the song because it reminded her of her excitement at the idea of new beginnings and her fears of separation and disconnection. These feelings have been age-old themes in her life. According to Sarah, she first recognized them when she was a senior in high school, attending an out-of-town field trip. It was on that trip that she first heard the song. The field trip was exciting on a number of fronts. In addition to participating in leadership activities, Sarah also visited her first shopping mall. She was at the shopping mall when she heard "Wild World" played over the loud speaker.

This song represented both excitement and risk. For one, Sarah describes the excitement she felt at being in another city—at seeing so many stores and so many people. Her boyfriend, a boy she loved and had tremendous respect for, did not participate in this school trip and she missed him. Sarah describes how close they were and how much they depended on one another. Still, Sarah had doubts as to whether they should maintain the relationship after college, and, in hearing Stevens' song, imagined what it would be like for them to part. Sarah was afraid of being out in the world at the same time that she was attracted to the idea. Moreover, she couldn't imagine living life without her boyfriend, and grieved the possibility of that loss. Further, she was in touch with her childlike feelings and concomitant insecurities. Indeed, a number of family deaths and early life separations fueled her fears.

Now, Sarah wants her own grown children and grandchildren to feel confident at the same time that she wants them to be safe. She has always felt fiercely protective of them, and is just now facing her limitations and the reality that she does not have that kind of power. Sarah understands that it is their turn to live life in the world and to make their own life choices. And, she wants to watch them soar with anticipation rather than fear; with great expectations rather than trepidation. Sarah no longer wants her childhood losses or the old Cat Stevens (1970) song, "Wild World," to affect her or her children's expectations of what the world can bring. And like the song, she believes that yes, there is a lot of bad out there. And yes, we do not navigate life without encountering the bad in one context or another. All the same, her hope is to carry hopeful anticipation when they walk the world. They do so with such courage and adventure. She so admires them. And, what of her fears? She doesn't have any expectations that her hardwiring will be drastically changed. She still has fears! The good news is that she also has trust. She trusts her children, she trusts God, and she is trying to trust life.

Sarah's Marriage

Sarah had felt comparable struggles with fear and trust with respect to the ending of her marriage. She and her husband had, for the most part, been good to each other, and their parting was bittersweet. She didn't like the idea of facing the world without him. Still, she was ready to try. Sarah recounts how she did encounter "bad" in a subsequent relationship and wished she had listened to her instincts. These experiences again reminded her of her friendship with her husband and the way an early Carole King (1999) song, popularized by James Taylor, would remind her of him. The song "You've Got a Friend" is among her favorites.

To her surprise, even though she always saw her husband to be the strong one, she saw how she, too, provided him with a helping hand, and how she continued to support him long after the divorce was finalized. These memories comforted her and reminded her of how important it is to treat all people, but especially the people you love most, with consideration. They also reminded her of how important it is to be treated with compassion and respect. She sadly recalls times where this was not the case. At the same time, Sarah is reminded of the value of friendship.

These songs helped Sarah give context to the many experiences and feelings she has thus far encountered. The songs have both validated and challenged her caution. More importantly, they have helped her remember the complexity of life, its joys, and the inevitability of its sorrow. No easy task for Sarah, she wanted to be mindful of her present so she would not take her future for granted. Equally important, she understood the value of an open heart, risk, and the good fortune of good luck as depicted in the song "It Don't Come Easy" (Starr, 1971).

Here Sarah recognized her own power to take her freedom, to choose to see possibilities, and to anticipate the best in them. She also discovered that to do so requires that she regain trust and hope in her heart that at the end of the day, all would be well. She needed to trust that she could and would handle life as it comes—she wasn't destined to lament. She needed to remember how her connections with others and God were sources of rich supply; resources that would sustain her. She also needed to remember how she provided much comfort to others and that her own belief in others inspired them to risk in new and exciting ways. These were all life gifts. And at this time in her life, she was fortunate to recognize them.

This experience was depicted in Carly Simon's (1989) "Let the River Run" from the *Working Girl Soundtrack,* which she included in her chronology. Here, Sarah was able to make meaning of her struggles with perfectionism and self-criticism, and she was able to honor the dreamer within her. For example, when difficult things happened in her life or the lives of her loved ones, she had characteristically blamed herself for not doing better and for not making it work. Sarah came to see how much of a dreamer she was, and how much she had, indeed, risked in her lifetime. She had been an adventurer in her own right without knowing it. As she recalled her many successes, she was humbly grateful. She still struggles when difficult situations transpire. However, she no longer expects that she can control them or fix them. She is beginning to achieve a greater sense of acceptance that life happens in a full tapestry of color. And in so doing, she is beginning to accept herself as a beautiful, albeit imperfect, person in her own right. She selected the legendary song "Amazing Grace" written by John Newton (1779) as her song to "live into." Sarah recognizes her fears but also recognizes the grace that could transform them. She gives context to her experiences in her appreciation for the power of grace. While she acknowledges the dangers, and difficulties, that come with life, she also gives credit to grace for leading her home (Newton, 1779).

CONCLUSION

Like Sarah, clients in therapy seek to make meaning of life experiences in a number of creative ways. Music, as a medium found in popular culture, is rich in possibilities. By using popular music that characterizes important times in people's lives, clients are able to revisit these experiences. And because music evokes memories and the feelings that come with them, clients are able to work with these memories and feelings to give them context. *A Musical Chronology* is one intervention used by therapists toward this end. Here, clients have an opportunity to take stock of their experiences, become more genuinely at peace with them, and perhaps make amends or connect with important others. At the end of the day, when used as a life review, it can serve as a catalyst for some as people learn to accept, or come to peace with, who they are and how they have lived.

REFERENCES

Arkoff, A., Meredith, G.M., & Dubanoski, J.P. (2004). Gains in well-being achieved through retrospective-proactive life review by independent older women. *Journal of Humanistic Psychology, 44,* 204–214.

Baumgartner, H. (1992). Remembrance of things past: Music, autobiographical memory, and emotion. *Advances in Consumer Research, 19,* 613–620.

Beckvar, D.S., & Becvar, R.J. (1996). *Family therapy: A systemic integration.* Boston: Allyn & Bacon.

Birren, J.E., & Deutchman, D.E. (2005). Guided autobiography groups. In B. Haight & F. Gibson (Eds.), *Burnside's working with older adults: Group process and techniques* (4th ed., pp. 191–204). Boston: Jones and Bartlett.

Bortnick, B. (2005). Music and other arts activities in the lives of older adults. In B. Haight & F. Gibson (Eds.), *Burnside's working with older adults: Group process and techniques* (4th ed., pp. 205–222). Boston: Jones and Bartlett.

Bright, R. (1997). *Wholeness in later life.* London: Jessica Kingsley.

Bubenzer, D.L., West, J.D., & Boughner, S.R. (1994). Michael White and the narrative perspective in therapy. *The Family Journal: Counseling and Therapy of Couples and Families, 2,* 71–83.

Burnside, I., & Haight, B.K. (1994). Protocols for reminiscence and life review. *Nurse Practitioner, 19,* 55–61.

Butler, R.N. (2001). The life review. *Journal of Geriatric Psychiatry, 35*(1), 7–10.

Butler, R.N. (2002). Age, death, and life review. In K.J. Doka (Ed.), *Living with grief: Loss in later life.* Hospice Foundation of America. Retrieved August 11, 2007, from http://www.hospicefoundation.org/teleconference/2002/butler.asp

Cadrin, M.L. (2006). Music therapy legacy work in palliative care: Creating meaning at end of life. *Canadian Journal of Music Therapy, XII*(1), 109–137.

Cassell, E.J. (1982). The nature of suffering and the goals of medicine. *New England Journal of Medicine, 306,* 639–645.

Christianson, P.G., & Lindlof, T.R. (1983). The role of the audio media in the lives of children. *Popular Music and Society, 9*(3), 25–40.

Derrickson, B.S. (1996). The spiritual work of the dying: A framework and case studies. *Hospice Journal, 11*(2), 11–30.

de Vries, B., Westwood, M., & Blando, J. (2005). Group work with older adults at the end of life. In B. Haight & F. Gibson (Eds.), *Burnside's working with older adults: Group process and techniques* (4th ed., pp. 247–258). Boston: Jones and Bartlett.

Duffey, T.H. (2005a). A musical chronology and the emerging life song. *Journal of Creativity in Mental Health, 1*(1), 141–147.

Duffey, T.H. (2005b). When the music stops: Releasing the dream. In T. Duffey (Ed.), *Creative interventions in grief and loss therapy: When the music stops, a dream dies* (pp. 1–23). Binghamton, NY: Haworth Press.

Duffey, T.H., Lumadue, C.A., & Woods, S. (2001). A musical chronology and the emerging life song. *The Family Journal: Counseling and Therapy for Couples and Families, 9,* 398–406.

Duffey, T.H., Somody, C., & Clifford, S. (2006/2007). Conversations with my father: Adapting a musical chronology. *Journal of Creativity in Mental Health, 2*(4), 45–63.

Durant, M. (1993). *Residential treatment: A cooperative, competency-based approach to therapy and program design.* New York: Norton.

Eich, E., & Metcalfe, J. (1989). Mood dependent memory for internal versus external events. *Journal of Experimental Psychology: Learning, Memory, and Cognition, 15*, 443–455.

Erikson, E. (1963). *Childhood and society* (2nd ed.). New York: Norton.

Fargo, D. (1999). The happiest girl in the whole U.S.A. On *The happiest girl in the whole U.S.A.* [CD]. Universal Special Products.

Farjeon, E. (1971). Morning has broken [Recorded by Cat Stevens]. On *Teaser and the firecat* [Record]. Santa Monica, CA: A&M Records.

Frankl, V.E. (1992). *Man's search for meaning.* Boston: Beacon Press.

Freeman, J., Epston, D., & Lobovits, D. (1997). *Playful approaches to serious problems: Narrative therapy with children and their families.* New York: Norton.

Gibson, F., & Burnside, I. (2005). Reminiscence group work. In B. Haight & F. Gibson (Eds.), *Burnside's working with older adults: Group process and techniques* (4th ed., pp. 175–190). Boston: Jones and Bartlett.

Gladding, S.T. (1998). *Family therapy: History, theory, and practice.* Upper Saddle River, NJ: Prentice Hall.

Haight, B.K. (2007). The life review: Historical approach. In J.A. Kunz & F.G. Soltys (Eds.), *Transformational reminiscence: Life story work* (pp. 67–84). New York: Springer Publishing Company.

Haight, B., Schmidt, M.G., & Burnside, I. (2005). Demographic and psychosocial aspects of aging. In B. Haight & F. Gibson (Eds.), *Burnside's working with older adults: Group process and techniques* (4th ed., pp. 7–24). Boston: Jones and Bartlett.

Hays, T. (2005). Well-being in later life through music. *Australasian Journal on Ageing, 24*(1), 28–32.

Hays, T., & Minichiello, V. (2005). The meaning of music in the lives of older people: A qualitative study. *Psychology of Music, 33*, 437–451.

Hodas, G.R. (1994). Reversing narratives of failure through music and verse in therapy. *The Family Journal: Counseling and Therapy for Couples and Families, 2*, 199–207.

Karras, B. (Ed.). (1987). *"You bring out the music in me": Music in nursing homes.* Binghamton, NY: Haworth Press.

Kenny, C. (1999). Beyond this point there may be dragons: Developing general theory in music therapy. *Nordic Journal of Music Therapy, 8*, 127–136.

King, C. (1999). You've got a friend. On *Tapestry* [CD]. Sony.

Kurtz, P.D., Tandy, C.C., & Shields, J.P. (1999). Narrative family interventions. In A. C. Kilpatrick & T.P. Holland (Eds.), *Working with families: An integrative model by level of need* (pp. 171–191). Boston: Allyn & Bacon.

Langer, S.K. (1951). *Philosophy in a new key* (2nd ed.). New York: New American Library.

Larson, R., & Kubey, T.R. (1983, Spring). Television and music: Contrasting media in adolescent life. *Youth and Society, 14*, 13–33.

Newton, J. (1779). Amazing grace. *Olney hymns.* London: W. Oliver.

O'Hanlon, B., & Beadle, S. (1994). *A field guide to possibility land: Possibility therapy methods.* Omaha, NE: Possibility Press.

Parry, A., & Doan, R. E. (1994). *Story re-visions: Narrative therapy in the post-modern world.* New York: Guilford Press.

Porchet-Munro, S. (1993). Music therapy perspectives in palliative care education. *Journal of Palliative Care 9*(4), 39–42.

Prickett, C. A. (1998). Music and the special challenges of aging: A new frontier. *International Journal of Music Education, 31,* 25–36.

Simon, C. Anticipation. (1971). On *Anticipation* [CD]. Electra Entertainment.

Simon, C. Let the river run. (1989). On *Working girl: Original soundtrack album* [Record]. Global/Warner.

Soltys, F. G., & Kunz, J. A. (2007). Reminiscence and older adults. In J. A. Kunz & F. G. Soltys (Eds.), *Transformational reminiscence: Life story work* (pp. 41–66). New York: Springer Publishing.

Starr, R. (1971). *It don't come easy* [Record]. United Kingdom: Apple Records.

Stevens, C. (1970). Wild world. On *Tea for the tillerman* [Record]. Santa Monica, CA: A&M Records.

Terwogt, M. M., & Van Grinsven, F. (1991). Musical expression of mood states. *Psychology of Music, 19,* 99–109.

Thibault, J. M., Ellor, J. W., & Netting, F. E. (1991). A conceptual framework for assessing the spiritual functioning and fulfillment of older adults in long term care settings. *Journal of Religious Gerontology 7*(4), 29–45.

White, M., & Epston, D. (1990). *Narrative means to therapeutic ends.* New York: Norton.

White, M., & Epston, D. (1992). *Experience, contradictions, narrative, and imagination.* Delaide, South Australia: Dulwich Centre Publications.

Wong, P. T. P. (2000). Meaning in life and meaning in death in successful aging. In A. Tomer (Ed.), *Death attitudes and the older adult* (pp. 23–36). Philadelphia: Brunner-Routledge.

Zimmerman, L., & Dickerson, V. (2001). Narrative therapy. In R. J. Corsini (Ed.), *Handbook of innovative therapy* (2nd ed., pp. 415–425). New York: Wiley.

PART III

Movies

CHAPTER 6

Milieu Multiplex

*Using Movies in the Treatment
of Adolescents With Sexual
Behavior Problems*

Karen Robertie, Ryan Weidenbenner,
Leya Barrett, and Robert Poole

COMING ATTRACTIONS

The Onarga Academy is a residential facility specializing in the treatment of children who have demonstrated sexually problematic behavior. Program I, "Field of Dreams," works with clients between the ages of 12 and 16 and their families. This particular population is highly diverse, coming from varied locations around the state of Illinois, at the request of both social and legal agencies and with a wide variety of family backgrounds, behavioral problems and emotional problems, abuse histories and legal issues. Common diagnoses include oppositional defiant disorder, conduct disorder, attention deficit hyperactivity disorder, bipolar disorder, adjustment disorder, depressive disorder, and posttraumatic stress disorder. Cognitive, emotional, and social development deficits are quite common. Many clients have also experienced abuse, neglect, abandonment, and loss. They typically need to work through a multitude of difficult family issues; still others will need to learn how to mourn the loss of a family system that they have never known. Many of these clients have been placed in residential treatment as a last resort after failing to make progress in outpatient therapy and/or other residential treatment centers. As a group, they tend to have exceedingly poor self-images, a low sense of self-efficacy, poor frustration tolerance, external locus of control, depression, and often seemingly little internal motivation to change.

In general, our population of children with sexual behavior problems is not antisocial per se (Isaac & Lane, 1990), but do experience behavioral and social problems that are self-reinforcing and typically difficult to extinguish through traditional outpatient cognitive-behavioral means (Kahn, 2001). From a developmental perspective, these children seek immediate gratification despite a pattern of increasing adverse consequences. They have cognitive styles predominated by self-serving distortions that encourage continued abusive behavior, provide a false sense of perceived power and control over others, and facilitate the avoidance of both consequences and self-examination. These distortions in turn ground their worldviews in the need for revenge, anger, and power (Lane, 1997).

The treatment philosophy of the Onarga Academy is based on the introduction of a new cognitive schema grounded in a total milieu approach. This includes introducing and reinforcing beliefs, values, and behavioral patterns that are more heroic in nature: prosocial, empathic, sharing, communicative, honest, and facilitative of healthy gender identity and sexuality. Cognitive behavioral methods are generally considered the best practice when working with this population, since these methods have proven consistent, effective, and efficient in practice (Bengis et al., 1997; Delson, 2003; Erooga & Masson, 1999; Longo & Bays, 1999; Stickrod, Hamer, & Janes 1984). This approach is supplemented with an individualized multimodal intervention that emphasizes the differences between children who have demonstrated sexual behavior problems and their adult counterparts (Longo & Longo, 2003).

Residential treatment centers often make good use of the treatment culture and treatment peer group grounded in social learning and reality theory. Because our particular population often has additional attachment-related problems, we also implement experiential/expressive methods including narrative and art therapy (Bengis et al., 1997; Longo & Longo, 2003). We believe that these latter modalities provide an effective means of reaching clients on a deeper and more emotional level than traditional cognitive-behavioral approaches. Because the treatment team in our "Field of Dreams" (Program I) has programmatic control and full institutional support, we are able to combine intensive individual and milieu techniques, which also incorporate these other cutting-edge experiential approaches (Robertie, Weidenbenner, Barrett, & Poole, 2007). The more tools in our treatment box, the better the chance of making an impactful connection with clients (Kendall, 1991; Liebman, 1986). This multimodal/multitheoretical treatment framework, while initially based upon similar work with adult sexual offenders (Bays & Freeman-Longo,

1989; Bays, Freeman-Longo, & Hildebran, 1990) also recognizes that child offenders have their own unique developmental issues (Longo & Longo, 2003; Longo & Prescott, 2006). One of the experiential treatment methods that Program I has found most useful and productive has been the therapeutic use of movies.

Big Issues on a Little Screen

Movies can generate powerful emotional responses from clients, sometimes reaching beyond their defenses and creating otherwise unavailable opportunities for engagement, insight, and change. Movies can be a useful and effective treatment tool, but like most tools, only when done so with clear therapeutic intention and consideration of the potential (positive and negative) impact on the client(s). This requires far more than simply showing movies to a passive audience, and instead entails careful planning, tailoring the movie to the clinical and developmental needs of the individual clients and the group as a whole, and actively engaging them in discussion and processing both during and after the film. Prior to viewing films, the clients are helped to understand the purpose and place of movies in their treatment. While entertaining, the movies are not presented as entertainment per se, but rather, as a necessary and important component of their treatment.

Some treatment issues, especially those related to abuse, trauma, and family conflict, can be so difficult to approach in treatment that the presentation of evocative movies can result in the release of very powerful and potentially explosive feelings and behavior, requiring considerable therapeutic preparation and support (Klorer, 2000). For the purposes of this chapter, there are two general ratings that we provide: M, for mature themes requiring considerable therapeutic preparation and support, and G, for general viewing, which are much less intense and evocative.

Movies can create a safe therapeutic distance between a client and his or her issues, allowing the processing of very powerful feelings elicited by a character in the story. Movies can also provide for a vicarious emotional experience without actually exposing the client to unnecessary potential risk and/or harm. Movies can therefore provide a viable medium for addressing treatment issues, which if presented during the early stages of intervention might result in resistance and avoidance. There can be almost an inoculation effect provided by a series of vicarious emotional experiences afforded by movies or "reel life," which allow a client to build up the emotional strength, endurance, and capacity to cope with actual treatment issues or "real life." The safe emotional distance provided by a movie can be a holding environment in which the client can develop a sense of safety and control (Nathan & Mirviss, 1998).

Movies can convey the gamut of human emotions and experiences: from rage to sorrow, fear to elation, regret to hope. One has only to observe the clients cringing during an abusive scene in *Radio Flyer* (Donner, 1992) or silently crying during *Antwone Fisher* (Washington, 2002) to realize the potential emotional impact of movies. Clients who often have difficulty identifying and clarifying their own emotions and experiences can, with the aid of movies, begin to make sense of their own lives. Clients can even at times relate to movies and movie characters more readily than they can to other people or even their own lives. They feel that they know and understand these characters and relate to them on a level that they are not yet prepared to do with people in real life.

Watching movies can also provide a shared emotional common ground for a group of clients, and function as a reference point for future social interactions. At a programmatic level, movies can make it easier for the clinicians to determine when all the clients are "on the same page." When using a familiar scene in *The Lion King* (Allers & Minkoff, 1994) as a treatment tool, for instance, staff can be assured that the clients are not only familiar with the subject matter but they can also focus the clients' attention and emotional energy upon a particular message that they are seeking to communicate with a better-than-average chance of the message getting through. After all, the future Lion King, Simba, had difficulty in understanding the advice of the wise baboon Rafiki until the message literally hit him over the head. The clients, as movie audiences so often do, seem to understand the situations and life lessons presented to the movie characters much more readily than do the actual characters in the movie.

Once you have used movies to illustrate various treatment points with a group of clients for a long enough period of time, it begins to become a self-sustaining reaction; the staff and the clients themselves begin to see treatment messages in everyday movies shown for purely recreational purposes. A movie character will say something patently untrue and/or antisocial only to have a number of clients quietly whisper, "Thinking error," and another movie character will say something truly profound or wise and the clients will murmur, "Treatment message," almost in unison. Rather than detract from the pleasurable experience of watching movies, relating the content to treatment concepts actually seems to enhance the viewing experience as well as assuring clients that their favorite movies might well be presented again within a treatment context.

As a therapeutic teaching tool, movies reach clients on both a cognitive and emotional level. Movies can illustrate concepts on both a visual and an auditory level, which is particularly important given the different processing styles of our clients. Movies can provide concrete examples of abstract concepts such as empathy, communication, emotional expression, and relationships. Favorite and impactful dialogue stays with clients, who then utilize the favorite words almost mantra-like in their day-to-day life. Because movies are so multisensory, and typically fast-moving, they provide innumerable opportunities for learning. Movies are often excellent reflections of the perceived social mores and cultural values of the times in which they were made.

Movies can also provide a common basis for understanding a shared language for communicating concepts that are readily understood and remembered by clients. Everyone enjoys talking about a movie they recently watched and enjoyed. The life experiences of our clients have often been far removed from many of the common experiences most people have had while growing up; therefore, their understanding of what constitutes a relatively normal childhood might be decidedly skewed, with considerable gaps in terms of development and learning. Movies can fill in these gaps by providing an approximation of other people's experiences for the clients to utilize as a reference point with which to compare and contrast their own life experiences.

In the same fashion, the life experiences of our clients have often varied widely from those of the clinical and care staff. Movies can provide a common ground for both clients and staff to gain a greater understanding of what the other side has experienced in their own lives, allowing them to walk a mile in others' shoes without actually putting these shoes on.

Movies are also undeniably entertaining, involving, and interesting. Using movies in treatment can make a group seem less like treatment and more like recreation. Movies are also a good way to structure time for a program. One can either show the whole film or just specific sections to highlight treatment points. Clients often already have a naturally occurring interest in movies and basing your group and/or interventions on these movies means meeting the clients where they are. Movies can hold the clients' interest and attention over a prolonged period of time, no small feat in and of itself. Even more miraculously, however, discussion of these same movies tends to borrow a portion of that same interest and attention a long time afterward. Some movies are not only enjoyed by the clients; they are much anticipated, even breathlessly awaited, eagerly talked about and discussed, in the absence of any staff prompting whatsoever. Imagine channeling some of that energy into therapeutic uses!

When using movies as a treatment tool, there is a lot of hardware out there to put in the treatment toolbox. There are often movie posters available, sometimes even sporting the exact lines and/or treatment messages that you are trying to teach the clients. There are often images available in newspapers, magazines, and on the Internet. There are even movie soundtracks for audio memory recall. Program I, the "Field of

Dreams," made extensive use of movie-related materials during an extended series of therapeutic interventions known as Super Hero Week, later Super Hero Month, and eventually Super Hero Summer (Robertie et al., 2007).

In the old days, theaters would feature a single movie option, just like the treatment practices for our client population often featured a single linear treatment path based almost exclusively on one treatment modality (cognitive-behavioral). A moviegoer who did not happen to care for the movie that was playing there was simply out of luck. Nowadays, multiplex theaters offer many more movie options, and treatment practices offer many more options for helping a client deal with his problem issues. In the spirit of the multiplex, this chapter will feature a number of different applications for the use of movies in therapy. Here is what's playing!

THEATER ONE: MOVIES THAT ADDRESS SEXUAL OFFENDING/ABUSIVE BEHAVIOR ISSUES

Many of the movies listed in the trauma section of Exercise 6.1 at the end of this chapter obviously can be used to illustrate sexual offending/abusive behavior issues. Treatment of our clients primarily includes education regarding dysfunctional behavioral patterns and cognitive distortions, seemingly unimportant decisions (SUDs), and thinking errors. It is in these areas where pop culture movies can be truly helpful, as the following movies normalize the fact that cycles of behaviors exist everywhere. *Groundhog Day* (Ramis, 1993) illustrates the theme of repeating one day over and over again, until the protagonist "gets it right." Viewing and processing this movie is an easy way to discuss repetition of behavior (cycles) and how to escape the negative behaviors by replacing them with positive behaviors.

Back to the Future (Zemeckis, 1985) is an example of a movie illustrating seemingly unimportant decisions. In *Back to the Future*, Marty McFly makes a seemingly unimportant decision to save his future father from the path of an oncoming car. This very same action also prevents Marty's future parents from meeting, and sets off a chain of events that could ultimately result in Marty and his siblings ceasing to exist. Viewing and discussing this movie has encouraged clients to look at the events of their lives and the ramifications of their actions. This intervention can become even more experiential by having clients create their own time machine, and then asking them to determine at what point in time would they return, what would they change, and what would be the ramifications?

The flip side of seemingly unimportant decisions is understanding that one's present is the sum of all of one's past experiences. This is succinctly demonstrated in a clip from *13 Going on 30* (Winick, 2004). Jenna Rink, age 13, makes a wish to be 30. Several days after the wish is granted, she decides that she does not like the person that 30-year-old Jenna has become. In an effort to reclaim her 13-year-old self, Jenna retreats to the family home. During this visit, Jenna asks her mother what she would change in her life, if she were granted a "do-over." Jenna's mother thinks for a moment, then admits that she would not change anything, even the unpleasant moments, because all of the moments of her life are what make her who she is today.

Thinking errors, cognitive distortions, lies you tell yourself in order to make your actions defensible, play a significant role in the treatment of our clients. In general, adolescents with sexual behavior problems are masterful in the use of thinking errors. Pop culture movies can assist these adolescents in recognizing and correcting these thinking errors. One of the best pop culture movies to illustrate thinking errors is *Willy Wonka and the Chocolate Factory* (Stuart, 1971). Each one of the children touring the chocolate factory illustrates a different thinking error, as do their family members. Veruca Salt is the best example of Problem with Immediate Gratification and/or Entitlement of any screen diva: "I want it all and I want it now!!"

Possible interventions include:

1. Have clients list the thinking errors uttered by each of the main characters, and then have them list corrective statements for each of the thinking errors.
2. Have clients determine which of the children they are most like and describe how they are like that child.
3. Have clients identify their primary thinking error, and then write an Oompa Loompa-style rhyme about their thinking error.
4. Review the disasters that befall each of the children. Have clients determine what disaster their own thinking errors would create.

If you are looking for movie clips that illustrate thinking errors, one place to begin is *Monty Python and the Holy Grail* (Gilliam & Jones, 1975). While it is unfortunate that large sections of the movie are not appropriate for adolescents with sexual behavior problems, two sections are particularly helpful in demonstrating thinking errors. The Black Knight in the forest, who systematically has his limbs cut off, while loudly proclaiming that nothing is wrong ("It's just a flesh wound!"), and that he will win the fight, epitomizes minimizing and denial and how self-defeating these thinking errors can be. Toward the end of the movie, when the knights reach the horrible monster and see that it is "just a bunny," only to have several of their number murdered by the bunny, demonstrates just how dangerous minimizing can be. It is simple to expand the metaphor of this intervention. After the clips are shown to clients and discussed, a shared language exists. Clients who are minimizing can be redirected with the simple question "Is that 'just a bunny' you are talking about?"

These are just a few examples of how pop culture movies can be used to illustrate thinking errors. Thinking errors abound in popular culture; your use of pop culture movies is only limited by your own imagination!

THEATER TWO: MOVIES THAT INCREASE EMPATHY

Our clients have deficits in experiencing empathy, the capacity to understand and show regard for the feelings of others. In order to engage in sexually problematic behavior a client has to ignore, distort, and/or act in opposition to thoughts, feelings, and rights of others. A crucial element in treatment is assisting clients in developing empathy. The presence and use of empathy in a client acts as an internal barrier helping to protect against or reduce the likelihood of future sexually problematic behavior (Kahn, 2001).

Pop culture movies can assist clients in developing alternative perspectives and movies can generate genuine emotion, caring, and action in clients in ways that other modalities may not. Teaching empathy is challenging and can leave clients experiencing a variety of uncomfortable and distressing emotions. Through movies, clients can relate to and experience empathy in small doses for the characters as well as for themselves and for their own and others' vulnerabilities. Once the client can comfortably experience empathy for himself, he can then begin to practice empathy on a larger scale for others.

One movie that can begin to assist clients in experiencing empathy for themselves in manageable doses is *Freedom Writers* (LaGravenese, 2007). In this movie a teacher and a group of at-risk students explore literature that examines themes of intolerance, including *Anne Frank: The Diary of a Young Girl* (Frank, 1958). The students begin to examine the intolerance they experience in their daily lives and discover ways that the students can succeed despite the many obstacles set before them. The students begin to journal their own diary entries and they are candid and revealing in their writings. Relating to the background and struggles of the students in the movie, clients are able to find elements of themselves in this story. Clients can begin to identify with the powerlessness that is sometimes felt under overwhelming circumstances and the client can find hope in the success that the students in the movie achieve. Another added benefit is that the movie inspires creativity, writing, and healthy expression of thoughts and feelings. Showing this movie is a good introduction to journal writing, allowing clients to see the benefits of the task and to feel empowered to succeed in it despite their writing abilities.

Intervention: Using Foreign Movies to Build Empathy in Clients

Explain to the individual client or the group that he will be watching a foreign movie, where the characters speak in a different language and may or may not have subtitles. The movie *The Way Home* (Lee, 2002) is useful. If possible, view the version without subtitles. Ask the client to determine what the story is about and which emotions each character is experiencing. After the movie, discuss the client's reactions and the story they believe the movie told. Ask the client to explain how they determined which emotions the characters were experiencing. Encourage the clients to focus on the facial expressions, body language, tone of voice, and gestures as indicators to the emotions being experienced. Then assist the client in identifying how they can apply these emotional recognition skills at determining the emotional state of an individual during their interactions with others. These skills should be fairly instinctual, but for clients who have purposely ignored or distorted the feelings of others, these skills are often underdeveloped.

THEATER THREE: MOVIES THAT CAN BE USED TO ADDRESS TRAUMA HISTORIES

A quick look at any movie database is sufficient to demonstrate how many pop culture movies exist with plotlines that include stories of physical abuse, neglect, sexual abuse, and/or other forms of trauma. However, the intensity level of each of these movies could earn them a "Mature Audiences Only" rating. The question then becomes not "Can I use movies and/or movie clips to illustrate the point when I am dealing with trauma issues?" but "How can I use movies/and or movie clips to illustrate the point, without re-traumatizing clients?" We have created interventions using movie clips to lessen the impact. In essence we seek to "inoculate" clients, to dip their feet in the traumatic issues, to build up their reserves, so that the impact is not retraumatizing. A specific example of this is an intervention using two trauma-related movies not listed above, *Good Will Hunting* (Van Sant, 1998) and *Antwone Fisher* (Washington, 2002), and a movie most probably would not expect to see connected with trauma, *The Lion King* (Allers & Minkoff, 1994). The intervention is as follows.

In *The Lion King,* Rafiki (the wise guide) hits Simba (the student) on the head. Simba complains and asks why. Rafiki replies that the incident does not matter, because it is in the past, and hits Simba again. Simba again complains, this time stating that it hurts. Rafiki assures Simba that the past can hurt, and challenges Simba to see that one can either learn from the past, or run from it. Rafiki attempts to hit Simba a third time, and Simba avoids the blow (thus effectively learning from his past). Show this scene to your clients, and discuss. Our clients are easily able to make the connection to the metaphor in the movie and their own traumatic pasts.

Antwone Fisher is the based-on-real-life story of a young sailor who is ordered to see a Navy psychiatrist due to his continued physical altercations with other Navy personnel. Initially, Antwone refuses to talk to the psychiatrist. Over the course of the movie, Antwone allows himself to progressively trust the psychiatrist, and begins to tell the story of his life. Antwone's trauma history includes abandonment by his mother, extreme emotional and physical abuse by his foster parent, sexual abuse by a foster cousin, and witnessing the murder of his friend (the only support person Antwone had in his life). Antwone's healing process follows a typical pattern of moving forward, regressing, moving forward, regressing until the moment when Antwone achieves a feeling of empowerment over his trauma. Antwone demonstrates empowerment in two ways. First, Antwone asks the psychiatrist if he thinks he will "make it." The psychiatrist replies, "I know that you will make it. What do you feel?" Antwone states, "I think in another life or another time, I'd be king." Second, Antwone is able to return to the home of his abusive foster mother and foster cousin and confront them about the abuse they inflicted upon him. The two women deny any wrongdoing; however, Antwone proudly speaks for all trauma survivors when he proclaims, "You couldn't destroy me. I'm still standing. I'm still strong, and I always will be."

Good Will Hunting is the fictional story of a troubled mathematical genius with an explosive temper. A Harvard University professor recognizes Will Hunting's potential, and intervenes on his behalf with the court system after he is jailed for his involvement in a fight. Will is offered parole in exchange for agreeing to attend therapy twice a week, and agreeing to work on mathematics with the professor. Will agrees to the terms, apparently in order to get out of jail; he repeatedly proclaims his belief that he does not need therapy. Toward that end, Will demonstrates his talents for manipulating therapists, identifying their weaknesses and, in an attempt to maintain an emotional distance from the therapists, pushing their buttons.

After successfully alienating five therapists, Will meets his match in the form of therapist Sean McGuire, whom he greets with one of pop culture's best additions to the therapeutic process, "Let's do it; let the healing begin!" When Sean does not immediately allow himself to be manipulated by Will Hunting, Will resorts to a tactic used by Antwone Fisher, and many of our clients: he simply refuses to speak. Eventually, Will loses interest in this tactic, as did Antwone Fisher, and he begins to speak to Sean. Slowly, Will allows himself to trust Sean, and a therapeutic relationship develops. Eventually, Sean and Will discuss Will's history of physical abuse at the hands of his foster father. Will acknowledges the physical and emotional pain, and the subsequent diagnosis of attachment disorder. Will is able to discuss how his trauma history impacts his current life as he talks about fear of abandonment leading him to choose to break up with his girlfriend, instead of risking emotional intimacy. Sean assists Will in healing from his trauma by guiding Will into a cathartic moment: "It's not your fault." Will is able to express long repressed feelings. In true cathartic fashion, this is the point in the movie at which Will's life begins to take a turn for the better.

Shown together, these three clips demonstrate why it is important to discuss trauma issues, validates the difficulty clients may have in discussing these issues (many of our clients identify completely with the initial game playing that both Antwone and Will utilize to attempt to avoid discussing their issues), and offer hope that clients can tell their stories, and can resolve their trauma histories. In addition, both Antwone Fisher and Will Hunting are able to resolve their trauma histories to the extent that they are no longer at the mercy of the aftereffects of their trauma histories. They are able to empower themselves, establish healthy relationships (they both "get the girl"), and take control over their lives. And perhaps most importantly for the adolescents with whom we work, both Antwone and Will establish relationships with females, and live, so to speak, happily ever after. Antwone Fisher has the added benefit of being a true story: the real Antwone Fisher wrote the book upon which the movie was based, and wrote the movie's screenplay. This serves as a stellar example of rewriting one's life script. Interestingly, these three movies can be used to conceptualize the stages of treatment.

THEATER FOUR: MOVIES THAT EXPLORE FAMILY ISSUES

Exploring family issues with our clients is no small feat. On a good day, these clients can be vague and evasive. They would rather attend any other group and discuss any topic other than family issues. Yet, identifying the family dynamics that contributed to the client's development of sexually problematic behavior is crucial. Treatment and family therapy can allow the client and his family to successfully address the specific contributing factors, including their family dynamics, relationships, rules, routines, and functioning. Families often worry that they are going to be blamed for their child's sexually problematic behavior and the parents may feel like failures. Due to the naturally secretive nature of sexually abusive behavior and the sensitivity of this issue, thoughtful care and attention is required when addressing the topic with clients and their families. Few topics are as likely to create as much abject reaction and conflict as family issues. Movies can be a helpful, creative, and thoughtful way to engage clients in the exploration of relevant family issues.

Many of our client's families have significant issues involving family boundaries and roles. However, explaining the concepts of boundaries and roles to clients and their families can be both difficult and confusing. Movies can be helpful in depicting examples of family roles and boundaries and the impact that these concepts have on family functioning. Two particular movies that illustrate these concepts include *My Big Fat Greek Wedding* (Zwick, 2002) and *The Addams Family* (Sonnenfeld, 1991). In *My Big Fat Greek Wedding,* a woman from an emotionally effusive Greek family meets, dates, and weds a man from a reserved traditional Protestant family. The movie focuses on how the couple gracefully and comically navigates the family traditions, cultural beliefs and values, hierarchical system, and family roles of their two vastly different families. While *The Addams Family* is "mysterious and spooky and all together ookey," they demonstrate clearly defined family roles and healthy family dynamics in many aspects. Using movies to address relevant family issues makes it easier for a family to make themselves vulnerable, and movies normalize their particular issues and validate their experience. The movies confirm that the clients and families are not alone.

Often clients and their families do not fit the standard definition of the typical family. Movies that can illustrate the "family of choice" concept are helpful in assisting the client in defining their family. *Ice Age* (Wedge & Saldanha, 2002), reinforces the concept that a family can be composed of members that you choose. In this movie, the most unlikely trio of animals band together for a common goal. Despite their differences and conflicts, the trio finds loyalty, friendship, and ultimately family with one another. For clients who have had chaotic and abusive family experiences, movies can assist in developing a more healthy and normalized point of reference regarding family relationships. Movies can fill in the gaps left by chaotic family experiences, providing clients with an example of what positive, healthy family interactions may look like for them in the future. The movie *Sky High* (Mitchell, 2005) is useful in this regard in that a family of superheroes face challenges and changes while demonstrating healthy family functioning.

With careful selection, a movie will provide clients with a nonthreatening way to begin identifying, discussing, and gaining insight into their own family dynamics. In movies, clients can find the story of themselves and their family. Their personal family dynamics can be normalized as they see their struggles shared by others in the movie.

The movie *Lilo and Stitch* (DeBlois & Sanders, 2002), demonstrates a variety of therapeutic themes that can be explored with clients. Three particular themes that are helpful to expand upon include the ideas that a family can be "small and broken but still good," that you can choose your family, and that even if you were created to cause destruction you have the power to change and make different choices. In the movie, an alien biological experiment, 626, was created for destruction. The creature 626 flees to earth and is adopted by a young girl, Lilo, who believes 626 is a dog. Lilo lives with her sister since her parents have died and her sister is struggling with the responsibility of caring for Lilo. Lilo names her new pet Stitch and decides she is going to teach Stitch how to be good despite his increasingly destructive behavior. Stitch's bad behavior causes trouble for Lilo and her sister, who are then placed in jeopardy of being removed from the home. The movie concludes with Stitch learning the meaning of family and choosing to help rather than hurt others. A recurring motto in the movie is, "*Ohana* means family and family means nobody gets left behind or forgotten."

Intervention

Have the client or group view *Lilo and Stitch*. Depending on the focus of the group or session, provide a list of questions about the movie before or after the viewing. Discuss the client's thoughts, feelings, and reactions to the movie. It is important to determine what the client believes is the moral or treatment message of the movie. This will provide the therapist with an understanding of the client's perspective and the issues he may be most open to exploring with regards to his own family. Ask the client how the movie relates to himself and his family. This response gives the therapist permission to begin addressing those issues acknowledged by the client. Other helpful questions include: Which characters did he most like and dislike? Which characters were most and least similar to him? As a group or session activity, review the family motto of *Ohana* and ask the client to create his own family motto. Provide art supplies, stencils, and other materials to the client to help him make his family motto concrete and reinforce the message. Assist the client in elaborating on how his family motto could be put into practice and how the client would know if his family was following the motto. Alternative methods for exploring family issues in greater depth are collages, sand trays, artwork, and a variety of other therapeutic modalities.

THEATER FIVE: MOVIES THAT ILLUSTRATE TEAM BUILDING, PRIDE, AND COURAGE

Our clients demonstrate tendencies to remain emotionally closed or withdrawn. They often feel alienated from their peers and have little understanding and/or experience with concepts such as teamwork, personal courage, or pride. As therapists and counselors, we are constantly asking clients to give up their old, maladaptive lifestyles, but we also need to replace those old patterns with new healthy ones.

Clients are often reluctant to attempt to make healthy changes in their lives. Clients are fearful of change and view change with a sense of loss for being required to give up on a part of themselves. It then becomes our job to instill a sense of courage or pride in the clients as they progress in treatment—the courage needed to make healthy changes. This can be accomplished through individual therapy efforts, but is often more effective in the group setting. You can motivate an individual within the group or motivate the group as a whole.

There is a wide variety of movies that can be used to illustrate the concept of teamwork. Many sports movies focus on this very concept. These movies also often address a host of secondary issues such as racism and overcoming adversity. The subject matter varies in its appropriateness for your target audience and target issues. Below is a sample intervention demonstrating how to expand the movie's teamwork metaphor focusing on the movie, *The Fantastic Four* (Story, 2005). The intervention helps to demonstrate how teamwork can be demonstrated, along with the potential challenges of being a leader or working as an "individual" on the team. At the end of *The Fantastic Four,* all four members of the team must work together to defeat Dr. Doom. However, throughout the movie, two of the main characters, Johnny Storm and The Thing, have an ongoing feud and often appear at odds with each other. If the members of the team fail to work together, Dr. Doom prevails and the Fantastic Four are defeated. However, The Fantastic Four put their individual differences aside, unite as a team, and defeat evil. These group dynamics exemplify those of many of our clients.

As stated in the introduction, watching movies can be more of a passive process, but the discussion and processing of the film should be an active one. An exercise to demonstrate team unity, as well as its challenges, is provided as follows. Using *The Fantastic Four,* you can show a short clip to set the stage for your teamwork exercise. The scene in the DVD chapter 29 titled ("Doomsday") provides an example of super-hero teamwork. Now, using that as the catalyst for this exercise, divide a group into five clients. Give four of the clients a marker and designate the fifth client as the leader. Set up a large piece of drawing paper onto a wall or easel. Next, assign each client with a marker for a specific skill. For example, one client can only draw vertical lines, one client can only draw horizontal lines, one client can only draw diagonal lines, and one client can only draw squiggly lines. (Note that clients can also be assigned to draw specific shapes to provide variety to the exercise.) Next, assign the leader a type of drawing, such as a house or a creation within their realm of skill level. Now, instruct the designated artists to follow only the EXACT instructions that their leader gives them. They are not to make any moves or draw any other way except for what they have been assigned. Next, the leader instructs each member of his team to step up to the paper, one at a time, and begin drawing their creation. The designated artists are not to make any marks on the paper unless the leader says so. The leader must also tell them exactly where to place their line on the paper. "A little to the left, a little to the right, a little higher, and a little lower" are common and ongoing instructions. This exercise gives the leader a sense of power, and also gives the other members the sense of being a follower, however, with the overall goal of having to work as a team to create their drawing. Then, as the first drawing is completed to the best of their abilities, you switch roles and redo the activity multiple times. Results can be widely varied, based on the leadership skills of the clients and how well the overall team interacts. This allows for discussion of how it feels to be a leader, what challenges were faced, how challenges were overcome, and how it felt to be the member of a team.

The movie *Miracle* (O'Connor, 2004), which details the accomplishments of the 1980 United States Olympic hockey team, is a prime example of both teamwork and pride. The teamwork focus is on how the young Olympians came together as individuals, but learned to be a team. The pride factor is defined in the team defeating one of the powerhouse nations of the time. When clients learn that pride can be a healthy emotion, along with the accolades that typically accompany it, they rarely want to let go of this feeling and it tends to remain with them for long periods of time. A discussion around this particular movie can also incorporate a discussion of "positive" and "criminal" pride. Positive pride involves preparation, prolonged effort, delayed gratification, and the result that a person feels good because others approve of him and his accomplishments. Criminal pride involves entitlement, ability for negative risk taking, criminal thinking, and the result of elevating oneself by putting down others. Several sports movies focus on instilling a sense of positive pride into the audience, and the therapist or counselor can assist in explaining the emotions that the client is feeling during the movie. Once clients understand this distinction, they can better appreciate the therapeutic power of this particular movie.

Another genre that can be utilized to discuss personal and group courage is that of the historical/war movies. Again, designed for a mature audience only, the critically acclaimed movie series *Band of Brothers* (Hanks, 2001) is a good tool for discussing both courage and teamwork. The series chronicles the men of Easy Company during their tour of duty in World War II. Organized into 10 separate one-hour segments, the series is a plethora of situations of personal courage in times of great duress, as well as an ongoing example of a team of soldiers and how they relied on each other for aid, comfort, and survival. It also affords an excellent opportunity to teach clients American history and to instill pride into how they view their country and those who have labored, fought, and died to preserve their freedoms. These short segments are a good source for focused discussions and worksheets on these topics.

THEATER SIX: SPECIAL FEATURE: TREATMENT TOWN!

As therapeutically useful as it can be to show clients movies to illustrate various treatment concepts, it can be even more productive, educational, and fun to make your own movies. In the Treatment Town video intervention, clients create a Treatment Monster, a visual representation of the problem issues that tear down their treatment. These Treatment Monsters first rampage through the miniaturized community of Treatment Town, but the clients then rebuild Treatment Town and defend it against the next attack.

The idea for Treatment Town is based on the classic giant monster movies of Japan. Before the advent of computer-generated imagery, the only real requirement for filming a giant monster rampaging across a city was a variety of miniaturized props, a production assistant in a cheap rubber suit or perhaps a puppet to represent the monster, and the use of forced perspective with a camera to make the destruction appear epic in scale. This creative and extremely low-budget concept created such pop culture icons as Godzilla, Gamera, and Ultra Man, all instant status heroes with young males everywhere. Gamera is, after all, the friend of all children.

The Treatment Town concept is simplicity itself. First, ask the client to construct a miniature community based on the giant monster-plagued city of Tokyo, out of readily available materials such as cardboard, felt, glue, markers, and Styrofoam. When constructing props for Treatment Town, the clients are free to use their imaginations to create anything that might conceivably be miniaturized and included in the town. Examples include cars, telephone lines, stop signs, fences, roads, drive-in theaters, skate parks, subways, swimming pools, and movie stars. This miniature community will be called Treatment Town. By way of inspiration, show clients an assortment of Godzilla videos during both the preproduction and filming stages of the project. All of these movies are rated PG or less and are readily available for rental or purchase. Mystery Science Theater 3000 episodes are particularly useful. Have staff present during these preparations to assist the clients in creating the set.

Direct the clients to identify and create their own personal Treatment Monsters, visual representations of those factors that serve to tear down and destroy their treatment. Examples have previously included Mr. Worry (excessive anxiety about family issues beyond the client's ability to affect) and Fear of Success (self-defeating behaviors designed to keep expectations low). On camera, interview each client individually. Ask each client: "What is the name of your Treatment Monster? How does your Treatment Monster act to destroy your treatment?"

Film each Treatment Monster as it rampages through the Treatment Town accompanied by music. There is actually Godzilla theme music available, but it can be very illuminating to have the clients create their own musical selections. Afterward, ask the client to rebuild Treatment Town. Then interview the client again. Ask each client the following questions: "How long did it take to build Treatment Town? How long to tear Treatment Town down? What could you do to defeat the Treatment Monster?"

Each possible solution to the Treatment Monster issue is then designated as a Nemesis (that which will defeat the Treatment Monster). Film each client with their Treatment Monster again, but in the second take, the Treatment Monster is defeated by the Nemesis before destroying too much of Treatment Town. Each client is filmed in sequence: no rehearsals, no do overs, no repeats, no stopping, no script, no budget, and no talent necessary. Truly a tribute to low-budget film making!

The Treatment Town movies can be shown in-house to an often delighted audience of clients, staff, family, and collateral contacts such as probation officers and social service case workers. With the simple addition of having the clients wear a mask, however, the options for presenting the Treatment Town video in venues beyond the facility, literally taking the show on the road, are vastly expanded. Be aware of any applicable confidential policies before doing this.

The appeal of Treatment Town is not difficult to figure out. Treatment Town targets our client population where they truly live. Our clients already love monsters, movies, and mayhem! Like many other treatment interventions, staff can only expect clients to be as excited, motivated, and involved as the staff members themselves are willing to be. Each year, the production seems to become bigger and better, although the working budget itself never seems to increase beyond a few dollars.

Treatment Town also provides a very powerful treatment metaphor. Our clients are often told what their problem issues are and what they should be doing about these problem issues. Here is a perfect opportunity for a client to identify what he himself perceives as the problem issue holding him back in treatment as well as create a solution to his problem. What does the problem issue look like? How does it act? How does it affect the client? What can the client do about this issue?

This particular intervention also illustrates the resiliency of the human spirit through the construction, destruction, and rebuilding of Treatment Town. This is a very familiar treatment path for many clients. Reminding the clients that it is never too late to make their situations better or worse is very important since the clients themselves are often plagued by all-or-nothing, rigid thinking. Clients also learn to make connections between actions and consequences, delaying the immediate gratification of negative short-term feel-goods for the more sustained satisfaction of positive long-term feel-goods. Above all, the clients learn that any Treatment Monster, no matter how fearsome or destructive, can be defeated.

Treatment Town can also be used as a measure of treatment progress over time. Clients may make incremental progress over a prolonged period of time but these changes are much more salient when reviewed after a significant time period. Treatment Town makes an ideal intervention to coincide with the Halloween holiday season. After the Treatment Town movie is made, it can be periodically reviewed to compare and contrast the client's current functioning, the status of his Treatment Monster, with his previous functioning captured on film.

The Treatment Town movie project utilizes multiple learning modalities: audio, visual, kinesthetic, conceptual, and concrete. The clients are given the opportunity to visualize and then operationalize working through their problem issues before actually implementing these positive changes on a more behavioral level. It is sometimes the simplest treatment messages that actually end up getting through to a client, and interventions don't come any simpler than Treatment Town.

So what are you waiting for? All you need is a camera, a client, and a dream to make your own Treatment Town video! The copyright is free and the budget is certainly affordable to anyone. What you really need to invest in this project is what is most important and difficult to create: time, energy, and enthusiasm. We hope that you enjoyed the shows!

Exercise 6.1

THEATER ONE: MOVIES THAT ADDRESS SEXUAL OFFENDING/ABUSIVE BEHAVIOR ISSUES

Bress, E., & Gruber, J. (Directors). (2004). *Butterfly effect* [Motion picture]. United States: BenderSpink.

Gilliam, T., & Jones, T. (Directors). (1975). *Monty Python and the holy grail* [Motion picture]. UK: Michael White Productions.

Leder, M. (Director). (2000). *Pay it forward* [Motion picture]. United States: Bel Air Entertainment.

Marshall, P. (Director). (1988). *Big* [Motion picture]. United States: Gracie Films.

Kassell, N. (Director). (2005). *The woodsman* [Motion picture]. United States: Dash Films.

Ramis, H. (Director). (1993). *Groundhog day* [Motion picture]. United States: Columbia Pictures.

Stuart, M. (Director). (1971). *Willy Wonka and the chocolate factory* [Motion picture]. United States: David L. Wolper Productions.

Winick, G. (Director). (2004). *13 going on 30* [Motion picture]. United States: Revolution Studio.

Zemeckis, R. (Director). (1985). *Back to the future* [Motion picture]. United States: Amblin Entertainment.

THEATER TWO: MOVIES THAT INCREASE EMPATHY

Anspaugh, D. (Director). (1993). *Rudy* [Motion picture]. United States: TriStar Pictures.

Anspaugh, D. (Director). (1986). *Hoosiers* [Motion pictures]. United States: De Haven Productions.

Atchison, D. (Director). (2006). *Akeelah and the bee* [Motion picture]. United States: Spelling Bee Productions.

Carter, T. (Director). (2005). *Coach Carter* [Motion picture]. United States: Coach Carter Company.

Davis, J. (Director). (2006). *Ant bully* [Motion picture]. United States: Signet Sound Studio.

Docter, P., & Silverman, D. (Directors). (2001). *Monsters Inc.* [Motion picture] United States: Pixar Animation Studios.

Friedlander, L. (Director). (2006). *Take the lead* [Motion picture]. United States: New Line Cinema.

Gonera, S. (2007). (Director). *Pride* [Motion picture]. United States: Cinered Internationale Film Production.

Halstrom, L. (Director). (1993). *What's eating Gilbert Grape* [Motion picture]. United States: J&M Entertainment.

Henson, J. (Director). (1986). *Labyrinth* [Motion picture]. United States: Delphi V Productions.

Johnson, P. (Director). (1995). *Angus* [Motion picture]. United States: Atlas Entertainment.

Mandel, R. (Director). (1992). *School ties* [Motion picture]. United States: Paramount Pictures.

Mayer, M. (Director). (2006). *Flicka* [Motion picture]. United States: Twentieth Century Fox.

Petersen, W. (Director). (1984). *Never ending story* [Motion picture]. United States: Bavana Studios.

Seltzer, D. (Director). (1986). *Lucas* [Motion picture]. United States: Twentieth Century Fox.

Sharpsteen, B. (Director). (1941). *Dumbo* [Motion picture]. United States: Walt Disney Productions.

Tollin, M. (Director). (2003). *Radio* [Motion picture]. United States: Revolution Studios.

Underwood, R. (Director). (1993). *Heart and souls* [Motion pictures]. United States: Alphaville Films.

Wang, W. (Director). (2005). *Because of Winn-Dixie* [Motion picture]. United States: Twentieth Century Fox Film Corporation.

Yakin, B. (Director). (2000). *Remember the Titans* [Motion picture]. United States: Jerry Bruckheimer Films.

THEATER THREE: MOVIES THAT CAN BE USED TO ADDRESS TRAUMA HISTORIES

Allers, R., & Minkoff, B. (Directors). (1994). *The lion king* [Motion picture]. United States: Walt Disney Feature Animation.

Clark, L. (Director). (1995). *Kids* [Motion picture]. United States: Excalibur Films.

Donner, R. (Director). (1992). *Radio flyer* [Motion picture]. United States: Columbia Pictures Corporation.

Eastwood, C. (Director). (2003*). Mystic river* [Motion picture]. United States: Warner Brothers Pictures.

Huston, A. (Director). (1996). *Bastard out of Carolina* [Motion picture]. United States: Showtime Networks.

Jenkins, P. (Director). (2004). *Monster* [Motion picture]. United States/Germany: Media 8 Entertainment.

Kaplan, J. (Director). (1998). *The accused* [Motion picture]. United States/Canada: Paramount Pictures.

Mangold, J. (Director). (2000). *Girl, interrupted* [Motion picture]. United States/Germany: 3 Art Entertainment.

Shyamalan, M. (Director). (1999). *The sixth sense* [Motion picture]. United States: Barry Mendel Productions.

Speilberg, S. (Director). (1985). *The color purple* [Motion picture]. United States: Amblin Entertainment.

Streisand, B. (Director). (1991). *The prince of tides* [Motion picture]. United States: Barwood Films.

Van Sant, G. (Director). (1998). *Good will hunting* [Motion picture]. United States: Be Gentlemen Limited Partnership.

Washington, D. (Director). (2003). *Antwone Fisher* [Motion picture]. United States: Mundy Lane Entertainment.

THEATER FOUR: MOVIES THAT EXPLORE FAMILY ISSUES

Allers, R., & Minkoff, B. (Directors). (1994). *The lion king* [Motion picture]. United States: Walt Disney Feature Animation.

Anderson, S. (Director). (1997). *Meet the Robinsons* [Motion picture]. United States: Walt Disney Feature Animation.

Atchison, D. (Director). (2006). *Akeelah and the bee* [Motion picture]. United States: Spelling Bee Productions.

Bird, B. (Director). (2004). *The Incredibles* [Motion picture]. United States: Walt Disney Pictures.

Dayton, J., & Farris, V. (Directors). (2006). *Little Miss Sunshine* [Motion picture]. United States: Big Beach Films.

DeBlois, D., & Sanders, C. (Directors). (2002). *Lilo and Stitch* [Motion picture]. United States: Walt Disney Feature Animation.

DeVito, D. (Director). (1996). *Matilda* [Motion picture]. United States: Jersey Films.

Dunham, D. (Director). (1993). *Homeward bound* [Motion picture]. United States: Touchwood Pacific Partners.

Dylan, J. (Director). (2005). *Kicking and screaming* [Motion picture]. United States: Universal Pictures.

Gyllenhaal, S. (Director). (1995). *Losing Isaiah* [Motion picture]. United States: Paramount Pictures.

Herskovitz, M. (Director). (1993). *Jack the bear* [Motion picture]. United States: American Filmworks.

Hoen, P. (Director). (2007). *Jump in* [TV]. United States: Disney Channel.

Leder, M. (Director). (2000). *Pay it forward* [Motion picture]. United States: Belair Entertainment.

McNamara, S. (Director). (2004). *Raise your voice* [Motion picture]. United States: Brookwell-McNamara Entertainment.

Mitchell, M. (Director). (2005). *Sky high* [Motion picture]. United States: Max Stronghold Productions.

Noonan, C. (Director). (1995). *Babe* [Motion picture]. United States: Kennedy Miller Productions.

Sharpsteen, B. (Director). (1941). *Dumbo* [Motion picture]. United States: Walt Disney Productions.

Sonnenfeld, B. (Director). (1991). *The Addams family* [Motion pictures]. United States: Orion pictures.

Stanton, A., & Unkrick, L. (Directors). (2003). *Finding Nemo* [Motion picture]. United States: Walt Disney Pictures.

Wang, W. (Director). (2005). *Because of Winn-Dixie* [Motion picture]. United States: Twentieth Century Fox.

Washington, D. (Director). (2002). *Antwone Fisher* [Motion picture]. United States: Mundy Lane Entertainment.

Wedge, C., & Saldanha, C. (Directors). (2002). *Ice age* [Motion picture]. United States: Twentieth Century Fox Animation.

Zwick, J. (Director). (2002). *My big fat Greek wedding* [Motion picture]. United States: Big Wedding.

THEATER FIVE: MOVIES THAT ILLUSTRATE TEAM BUILDING, PRIDE, AND COURAGE

Anspaugh, D. (Director). (1986). *Hoosiers* [Motion picture]. United States: De Haven Productions.

Boaz, Y. (Director). (2000). *Remember the Titans* [Motion picture]. United States: Jerry Bruckheimer Films.

Carter, T. (Director). (2005). *Coach Carter* [Motion picture]. United States: Coach Carter.

Dunham, D. (Director). (1994). *Little giants* [Motion picture]. United States: Warner Brothers Pictures.

Friedlander, L. (Director). (2006). *Take the lead* [Motion picture]. United States: New Line Cinema.

Gartner, J. (Director). (2006). *Glory road* [Motion picture]. United States: Glory Road Productions LLC.

Gonera, S. (Director). (2007). *Pride* [Motion picture]. Germany: Cinered Internationale Filmproduktionsgesellschaft mbH & Co. 1. Beteiligungs KG.

Hanks, T., et al. (Director). (2001). *Band of brothers* [Mini-Series]. United States: DreamWorks SKG.

Herek, S. (Director). (1992). *The Mighty Ducks* [Motion picture]. United States: Avnet/Kerner Productions.

Joanou, P. (Director). (2006). *Gridiron gang* [Motion picture]. United States: Columbia Pictures Industries.

O'Connor, G. (Director). (2004). *Miracle* [Motion picture]. United States: Pop Pop Productions.

Ritchie, M. (Director). (1976). *The bad new bears* [Motion picture]. United States: Paramount Pictures.

Singer, B. (Director). (2000). *X-Men* [Motion picture]. United States: Bad Hat Harry Productions.

Story, T. (Director). (2005). *Fantastic four* [Motion picture]. United States: Twentieth Century-Fox Film Corporation.

Wedge, C. (Director). (2002). *Ice age* [Motion picture]. United States: Twentieth Century Fox Animation.

Zieff, H. (Director). (1989). *The dream team* [Motion picture]. United States: Imagine Entertainment.

REFERENCES

Allers, R., & Minkoff, B. (Directors). (1994). *The lion king* [Motion picture]. United States: Walt Disney Feature Animation.

Bays, L., & Freeman-Longo, R. (1989). *Why did I do it again?: Understanding my cycle of problem behaviors.* Orwell, VT: The Safer Society Press.

Bays, L., Freeman-Longo, R., & Hildebran, D. (1990). *How can I stop?: Breaking my deviant cycle.* Orwell, VT: The Safer Society Press.

Bengis, S., Brown, A., Longo, R., Matsuda, B., Singer, K., & Thomas, J. (1997). *Standards of care for youth in sex offense specific residential treatment.* Holyoke, MA: NEARI Press.

DeBlois, D., & Sanders, C. (Directors). (2002). *Lilo and Stitch* [Motion picture]. United States: Walt Disney Feature Animation.

Delson, N. (2003). *Using conscience as a guide: Enhancing sex offender treatment in the moral domain.* Holyoke, MA: NEARI Press.

Donner, R. (Director). (1992). *Radio flyer* [Motion picture]. United States: Columbia Pictures Corporation.

Erooga, M., & Masson, H. (1999). *Children and young people who sexually abuse others: Challenges and responses.* London: Routledge.

Frank, A. (1958). *Anne Frank: The diary of a young girl.* New York: Pocket Books.

Gilliam, T., & Jones, T. (Directors). (1975). *Monty Python and the holy grail* [Motion picture]. UK: Michael White Productions.

Hanks, T. (Director). (2001). *Band of brothers* [Mini-Series]. United States: DreamWorks SKG.

Isaac, C., & Lane, S. (1990). *The sexual abuse cycle in the treatment of adolescent sexual abusers.* Orwell, VT: The Safer Society Press.

Kahn, T. J. (2001). *Pathways: A guided workbook for youth beginning treatment.* Orwell, VT: The Safer Society Press.

Kendall, P. C. (1991). *Child and adolescent therapy: Cognitive behavioral procedures.* NY: Guilford Press.

Klorer, P. G. (2000). *Expressive therapy with troubled children.* Lanham, MD: Rowan & Littlefield.

LaGravenese, R. (Director). (2007). *Freedom writers* [Motion picture]. United States: Paramount Pictures.

Lane, S. (1997). The sexual abuse cycle. In G. D. Ryan & S. Lane (Eds.), *Juvenile sexual offending: Causes, consequences and correction* (pp. 77–121). New York: Jossey Bass.

Lee, J. (Producer). (2002). *Jibuero* (The Way Home). [Motion picture]. Korea: CJ Entertainment.

Liebman, M. (1986). *Art therapy for groups.* Cambridge, MA: Brookline Books.

Longo, R., & Bays, L. (1999) *Enhancing empathy.* Holyoke, MA: NEARI Press.

Longo, R. E., & Longo, D. P. (2003). *New hope for youth: Experiential exercises for children and adolescents.* Holyoke, MA: NEARI Press.

Longo, R. E., & Prescott, D. S. (2006). *Current perspectives: Working with sexually aggressive youth and youth with sexual behavior problems.* Holyoke, MA: NEARI Press.

Mitchell, M. (Director). (2005). *Sky high* [Motion picture]. United States: Max Stronghold Productions.

Nathan, A., & Mirviss, S. (1998). *Therapy techniques: Using the creative arts.* Ravensdale, WA: Idyll Arbor.

O'Connor, G. (Director). (2004). *Miracle* [Motion picture]. United States: Pop Pop Productions.

Ramis, H. (Director). (1993). *Groundhog day* [Motion picture]. United States: Columbia Pictures.

Robertie, K., Weidenbenner, R., Barrett, L., & Poole, R. (2007). A super milieu: Using superheroes in the residential treatment of adolescents with sexual behavior problems. In L. Rubin (Ed.), *Using superheroes in counseling and play therapy* (pp. 143–168). New York, NY: Springer Publishing.

Sonnenfeld, B. (Director). (1991). *The Addams family* [Motion picture]. United States: Orion pictures Corporation.

Stickrod, A., Hamer, J., & Janes, B. (1984). *Informational guide on the juvenile sexual offender.* Eugene, OR: Adolescent Sex Offender Treatment Network.

Story, T. (Director). (2005). *Fantastic four* [Motion picture]. United States: Twentieth Century-Fox Film Corporation.

Stuart, M. (1971). *Willy Wonka and the chocolate factory* [Motion picture]. United States: David L. Wolper (Director). Wolper Productions.

Van Sant, G. (Director). (1998). *Good will hunting* [Motion picture]. United States: Be Gentlemen Limited Partnership.

Washington, D. (Director). (2002). *Antwone Fisher* [Motion picture]. United States: Mundy Lane Entertainment.

Wedge, C., & Saldanha, C. (Directors). (2002). *Ice age* [Motion picture]. United States: Twentieth Century Fox Animation.

Winick, G. (Director). (2004). *13 going on 30* [Motion picture]. United States: Revolution Studio.

Zemeckis, R. (Director). (1985). *Back to the future* [Motion picture]. United States: Amblin Entertainment.

Zwick, J. (Director). (2002). *My big fat Greek wedding* [Motion picture]. United States: Big Wedding.

CHAPTER 7

Little Miss Sunshine and Positive Psychology as a Vehicle for Change in Adolescent Depression

Dora Finamore

Adolescent depression is at epidemic levels and ignoring symptoms can increase the risk for suicide. In fact, studies report, "Depressive disorders, including Major Depressive Disorder (MDD), Depressive Disorder Not Otherwise Specified (NOS), and Dysthymia, affect up to 2.5% of children and 8.3% of adolescents" (Singh, Pfeifer, Barzman, Kowatch, & DelBello, 2007, p. 1). Additionally, "epidemiological studies suggest that by age 14, as many as 9% of youth have experienced at least one episode of severe depression" (Lewinsohn, Rohde, Seeley, & Fischer, 1993). In a recent meta-analysis, Horowitz and Garber (2006) determined that 1%–8% of children and adolescents at any given time are suffering from depression, increasing the risk for later adult mood disorders by up to 72%.

The symptoms of depression may not be easily distinguishable from what might otherwise be considered normal adolescent angst. Researchers are discovering that contrary to popular opinion, negative thinking may not be a normative adolescent experience and that teaching young people how to protect themselves from depression requires active intervention such as helping them to develop a resilient cognitive schema. As Rutter asserts,

> Protection does not reside in the psychological chemistry of the moment but in the ways in which people deal with life changes and in

what they do about their stressful or disadvantageous circumstances. Particular attention needs to be paid to the mechanisms operating at key turning points in people's lives when a risk trajectory may be redirected onto a more adaptive path. (1987, p. 329)

Through positive psychology as recently propounded by Martin Seligman, youth's greatest assets can be identified and channeled toward healthy decision making, well-being, and those qualities that foster resilience (Snyder & Lopez, 2002). Positive character traits are what Seligman considers to be virtues and strengths and include *wisdom, courage, love, justice, temperance,* and *spirituality.* Embodied within these core virtues are 24 additional strengths including hope, optimism, future-mindedness, social intelligence, and emotional intelligence that can be utilized as resources for self-awareness, growth, and change. Another focus in positive psychology is on *flourishing,* defined as "a state in which an individual feels positive emotion toward life and is functioning well psychologically and socially" (Keyes & Haidt, 2003, p. 294).

So, what do positive psychology, adolescent depression, and the movie *Little Miss Sunshine* (Dayton & Faris, 2006) have in common? In this not-so-typical cross-country family road trip, one of the main characters, Dwayne (Paul Dano), seems to typify the plight of the contemporary angst-ridden adolescent. The anger-fueled, Nietzsche-reading adolescent maintains his adamant vow of silence and scribbles his thoughts on a small notepad he carries. He will not speak until he is accepted into the Air Force Academy. When Olive, the protagonist, is invited to her dream beauty contest after the winner is fired for taking diet pills, the family pulls together to make the trip from New Mexico to California. Olive is still in the restroom at a gas station when her grandfather realizes she is not in the VW van. Proclaiming that no one gets left behind, once he realizes that Olive is left behind in a rest stop, the father (Greg Kinnear) swiftly turns the yellow bus around to retrieve her. Instead of being portrayed as a frightened, unglued, and crying child, Olive is depicted as a centered, resilient, confident, and unruffled 7-year old, just waiting, confident in the knowledge that her family will return for her.

After viewing the movie for the first time, I felt certain it could be of use with one particular adolescent client who was suffering with depression and anxiety rooted in abandonment issues. The client reminded me of Dwayne and I hoped to facilitate her healing by helping her identify with Olive, the character displaying the qualities of positive psychology. Little did I realize Bailey, a brave young client who you will meet later in this chapter, had bigger plans.

ADOLESCENT DEPRESSION

Numerous individual, social, and cultural factors contribute to the increasing prevalence of depression and other mood disorders in young people (Reyna & Farley, 2006). It is also well documented that brain maturation does not reach completion until well beyond adolescence, which may further contribute to the increasing prevalence and longevity of mood disorders in young people (Sowell et al., 1999).

North America's college counseling centers report an increase in troubled students, according to psychologist Robert Gallagher of the University of Pittsburgh. His 2001 survey of counseling centers shows that 85% of colleges report an increase during the past 5 years in students with severe psychological problems (as cited in Peterson, 2002). Peter Lewinsohn (as cited in Marano, 2003) at the University of Oregon notes,

> Not only do adolescents experience major depression at the same rates that adults do, three quarters of depressed adolescents experience further psychiatric disorders. The focus on treating adolescent depression includes identifying thinking errors and negative thoughts and coming up with more positive and realistic thoughts; and increasing problem-solving skills. (p. 1)

Given that depression may thus be so easily triggered by both neurological and psychosocial factors, one would think treatment challenges in this domain to be insurmountable. However, depression can be treated before the brain fully develops. We have the ability to reach young people and help them achieve emotional stability, build coping skills, and increase well-being. However, there are many risk factors for depression that must be identified before effective treatment can commence. One such factor is a pessimistic outlook on life. Brent and Birmaher (2002) describe

> a 16-year-old boy [who] is brought by his parents to his primary care physician because of a decline in school performance, which began at least three years earlier and has become more severe in the past year. He reports boredom, a lack of enjoyment and motivation, poor self-esteem, a feeling of hopelessness, difficulty sleeping, poor concentration, and passive thoughts of suicide without a plan. (p. 1)

Treatment for adolescent depression has come a long way; yet, it still challenges many clinicians to develop effective strategies that move beyond the traditional pathology-oriented perspective that focuses upon the negative elements typically associated with depression, including pessimism, hopelessness, and anger. A burgeoning literature supports the use of positive-based strategies in working with depressed teens (Aspinwall & Staudinger, 2002).

POSITIVE PSYCHOLOGY

In 1998, a small group of researchers led by former APA president and earlier proponent of the concept of learned helplessness, Martin Seligman, met in Akumal, Mexico, in order to brainstorm ideas related to the burgeoning field of positive psychology. Along with other researchers including Mihaly Csikszentmihalyi, Ed Diener, and Ray Fowler, they solidified a new movement in psychology that would soon generate worldwide research interest and efforts in order to answer the seemingly simple question, "What makes people happy, flourish and thrive?" Seligman (1998, 2002), had long asserted that traditional mental health researchers focused on the most negative aspects of humanity. The group proposed that positive psychology should be "the scientific study of the conditions and processes that contribute to the flourishing or optimal functioning of people, groups, and institutions" (as cited in Gable & Haidt, 2005, p. 103). Their theory centers around six core virtues and 24 signature strengths including creativity, curiosity, love of learning, bravery, persistence, integrity, vitality, love, kindness, social intelligence, leadership, forgiveness, and mercy; humility, modesty, prudence, self-regulation, appreciation of beauty, gratitude, hope, humor, playfulness, and spirituality (Snyder & Lopez, 2007).

The Templeton Foundation, noted for its support of empirical research in science, religion, and philosophy, took notice of Seligman during his keynote address at their 1997 conference and was particularly impressed by the passionate reception he received by the audience (McGuire, 1999). Sir John Templeton, a noted philanthropist knighted by Queen Elizabeth, rose from the audience and asked Seligman how his foundation could help promote positive psychology. Soon after the conference, Seligman and his colleagues were offered an unparalleled $200,000 grant to facilitate research in positive psychology. Not only was the foundation interested in research into happiness, but also how people flourish in all areas of life. Their groundbreaking research would subsequently reveal that building upon and utilizing one's signature strengths can help prevent depression (Peterson & Seligman, 2004) and that there is a remarkable cross-cultural consistency in the 24 character strengths (Seligman, Steen, Park, & Peterson, 2005).

The main focus of positive psychology is on prevention, not cure as in traditional psychology approaches. According to Dieser (2005),

The primary idea is that positive psychology can be used in a preventative manner, instead of following the medical model approach of focusing on a person's illness. Positive emotions have many healthy consequences, such as friendship, love, creative thinking, and physical health. People who are happier spend more time with people in free time and leisure pursuits. Acquiring a rich social life can help raise the amount of happiness a person experiences. (p. 242)

It was Seligman's own personality traits that facilitated his continued work in experimenting to find more effective treatment for depression. Ironically, it was Seligman's young daughter Nikki who inspired him to take stock of his own pessimistic thinking. This epiphany led to the 1999 Mexico summit, as a result of which it was asserted that

this new positive psychology was a far cry from run-of-the-mill psychology which had little knowledge of what "makes life worth living" and was more interested in diagnosing and fixing damage and disease. Six years on, many more psychologists are rallying behind this banner. So too are those in other disciplines such as economics, population health, business, education and other areas where human development and flourishing matter. (Seligman & Csikszentmihalyi, 2000)

Psychological wisdom suggests that while much of personality is inherited, environment also accounts for a significant portion of variation in human behavior. According to Sheldon and Lyubomirsky (2006), a significant percentage of our happiness can be affected by intentional activities, setting goals, making choices, and developing self-regulation. Lyubomirsky's (2001) earlier research is consistent with Seligman's work in the area of positive psychology in that,

My empirical findings over the years have revealed that chronically happy and unhappy individuals differ systematically and in a manner supportive of their differing cognitive and motivational strategies they use. Truly happy individuals construe life events and daily situations in ways that seem to maintain their happiness, while unhappy individuals construe experiences in ways that seem to reinforce unhappiness. (p. 241)

Flourishing and flow are two concepts that form the foundation of positive psychology, or living a life of meaning. As Csikszentmihalyi (1997) states, "The metaphor of flow is one that many people have used to describe the sense of effortless action they feel in moments that stand out as the best in their lives. Athletes refer to it as 'being in the zone'" (p. 29). In January 2003, *Time Magazine* devoted an entire issue to happiness.

Then in January 2005, *Time* once again focused on happiness, this time including the connection among causal attributions, pessimistic thinking, and depression.

Positive Psychology in Education

In 2004, historically traditional Harvard University offered its first course in positive psychology. It has since become the most popular course in Harvard's history. According to Tal Ben-Shahar (as cited in Lambert, 2007), over 850 students registered for the class, surpassing even introductory economics. What would motivate college-age adolescents to take such a course in happiness? The excitement and enthusiasm for positive psychology was evident from the beginning of the positive psychology movement. In 1992, Seligman and colleagues received the needed monies to expand their research. Seligman's group was awarded a $2.8 million grant from the Department of Education to augment a ninth-grade language arts curriculum with an emphasis on human strengths and positive emotions contained within the course literature. The grant was designed to fund a long-term study to trace the lives of students who took the course, and compare outcomes to those of students who took the same course but without the positive psychology enrichment.

Teaching positive psychology to youth has tremendous preventative potential for bolstering resilience. The same may be said for warding off depression by teaching students the principles of positive psychology and bolstering coping skills through teaching positive-oriented problem-solving strategies. Seligman discussed how teaching positive emotions in early childhood is highly effective and facilitates the upward spiral of positive well-being. Part of helping adolescents is offering hope where none is often perceived. In this context, Fisher (2007) noted,

> Hope is a thinking process in which the person clearly conceptualizes goals, but also perceives that s/he can produce the pathways to these goals (called pathways thinking) and can initiate and sustain movement along those selected pathways (called agency thinking). While hope theory has an emphasis on conceptualizing, the initial change for the clients happened without their conscious goal-setting or planning.

One of the important elements of positive psychology is an emphasis on learning how to think optimistically in order to better manage so-called negative emotions, such as anger and depression. Popular culture is a powerful carrier of the expressions of both negative and positive emotions through music, literature, art, the Internet, and film. Movies and the Internet seem to be ready-made vehicles for helping adolescents learn about and cope with negative emotions, given their reliance on it in day-to-day life. With the advent of technological devices such as high memory iPods, and MP3 devices, adolescents now have instant and ongoing access not only to music, but to movies. Given the ubiquity of emotional messages and content in movies and adolescents' ready access to them, it makes sense to incorporate movie watching into the therapeutic encounter. Exercise 7.1 provides an exercise that can be done at home based on positive psychology and the movies.

LITTLE MISS SUNSHINE AND POSITIVE PSYCHOLOGY

Happiness serves hardly any other purpose than to make unhappiness possible.

—Marcel Proust

Clearly, research supports the utility of positive psychology in helping young people learn to identify their character strengths, develop and cultivate traits for resiliency, and overcome depression by modifying their cognitions and emotional responses. In *Little Miss Sunshine*, the Hoover family, while clearly a deeply dysfunctional one, also displays many of the strengths consistent with Seligman's positive psychology. Each one of the clan portrays *authenticity*, albeit eccentric. Olive displays wisdom, courage, love, justice, temperance, and perhaps even spirituality. Even the Hoovers' vehicle (which serves as the backdrop for most of the movie) can be viewed as a metaphor for triumph in the face of adversity and dysfunction. It displays perseverance and tenacity in its struggle to keep its engine running, relying as much on industry and fortitude as gasoline.

The family decides to travel 800 miles to support their young daughter Olive in her quest to enter a child beauty contest. Adolescent son Dwayne, selectively mute and clearly discouraged, shows determination and motivation by lifting weights and keeping physically fit behind closed doors in hopes of one day becoming an airline pilot. However, Dwayne refuses to speak as a passive-aggressive protest against the family he reportedly hates; not unlike words heard by many of today's adolescents and what we as clinicians sometimes hear in the privacy of our therapy rooms.

Greg Kinnear, the father (Richard) in the movie, demonstrates enthusiasm and optimism in spite of an unsuccessful career touting a nine-step "winners" program and receiving yet another rejection from his publisher. After rushing the patriarch of the family (Alan Arkin) to the hospital on the way to the pageant, death becomes part of their reality as Grandpa passes on! This loss is felt and displayed compassionately by everyone, especially Olive, who was taught the "moves" for dancing in the pageant by Grandpa. Again, the mantra, "No one gets left behind," is poignantly and humorously demonstrated. Richard finally reveals the strength of courage, leadership, love, and perseverance (what he has been peddling for so long) and steals the body from the hospital with the help of the family to assure that Olive makes the deadline for the beauty pageant. Only after doing so does he give his father a respectful burial. Clearly, valor, creativity, open-mindedness, teamwork, love, optimism, future-mindedness, faith, hope, humor, and playfulness are evidenced by all family members, especially when they are stopped by a police officer for a traffic violation (a nonstop honking horn) with Grandpa in the back of the van, rigor mortis quickly setting in.

The family pulls together in facing life's challenges head on and in the moment. The mother, Sheryl, epitomizes positive psychology's principles, never wavering from her optimism and in-the-moment experience. Although the movie and ending are bittersweet, the love, hope, and motivation of the family wins out and Olive perseveres. She makes the deadline for the competition and with innocence, grace, and zest, dances a bawdy, hysterical striptease-like dance, to the horror of the judges. As the judges try to get Olive to stop her performance, one by one, the family jumps onstage to support and encourage her to finish what she so brave-heartedly started. The family pulls together in the final show of support; one Grandpa would have loved!

This last scene serves as a metaphor for the entire movie and the family's strengths. The family in their attempt to protect and shield Olive from harsh criticism, hurt, and humiliation, jump onstage in mutual support and a bit of anarchy while dancing to the song that Rick James immortalized, *Superfreak* (Miller & Miller, 1981). The movie demonstrates that try as we may, we parents cannot always protect our children, but we can display valor and courage trying. The point is even though families are far from perfect, hope lies in the willingness, grace, courage, optimism, and selflessness to learn from adversity, grow together, and be authentic! These qualities can serve as a vehicle for working with adolescents in therapy and teaching those skills to build optimism and resilience (Finamore, 2008). Psychotherapists can model and teach families that "No one gets left behind." Despite Olive's losing the contest, optimism, hope, and love shine through as the family literally pushes the van for a jump start while running alongside in order to get back home.

CASE STUDY

Bailey, a thin child with big brown eyes, was brought to therapy by her maternal grandmother. The grandmother had raised Bailey since age 7, when her parents were jailed for drug dealing and armed robbery and were subsequently sentenced to 20 years in prison. She was an only child and her grandmother was young enough (44) to have the energy needed to take responsibility for Bailey. The presenting problems were generalized anxiety, somatic complaints, school refusal, and difficulty sleeping. However, I also wanted to rule out depression based on her unstable family history, so Bailey completed a Beck Depression Inventory-Youth Version on which she scored in the moderate range. She often voiced somatic complaints in an effort to persuade her grandmother to let her stay home from school.

In school, Bailey was a good student, often demonstrating her leadership and resilience by being chosen for AP classes and extracurricular clubs (school newspaper editor). She had friends and did not seem to have any behavioral problems at school. In therapy, Bailey bit her nails and admitted this was a lifelong habit. She seemed unable to sit still in my office during the first two sessions, but soon thereafter, we seemed to develop a strong therapeutic alliance, evidenced by her eagerness to return. Her grandmother took excellent care of her and made sure Bailey had a thorough physical by her pediatrician before seeking counseling. The pediatrician concluded that her school refusal and sleep problems were probably related to her anxiety and depression, brought on by the trauma she had experienced living with her biological parents.

Up to age 7, Bailey had moved with her parents many times and was often left in the care of friends and relatives. Her parents would sometimes disappear for days with little regard for the developmental and emotional impact the chaos might have on a child. Bailey's parents were very young; in fact, they were 17 when she was born and had dropped out of high school in their last year. They never tried to contact Bailey while they were in prison, and although she expressed sadness, she seemed to take their lack of contact in stride. Her grandmother displayed a strong character, with a solid sense of the future; one of optimism for herself and Bailey. She had been married for 18 years, and was left financially secure, although not wealthy, when her husband died 7 years before. She worked full-time in the local library, and appeared to enjoy the work. She had a deep and abiding love and concern for Bailey that was observed during the first session of therapy, through subsequent phone conversations, and from what the client shared in session. The feelings of warmth and love were mutual between Bailey and her grandmother. Despite these relationship qualities, Bailey demonstrated some significant disturbances in functioning.

In my work with Bailey, one of the most important features of therapy revolved around a strong therapeutic relationship, one we had developed over 3 months. She was guarded at first (naturally) and a bit discouraged from the many hurts and disappointments she had experienced at the hands of adults. Positive psychology seemed a likely way of gently helping her open up to the hope and possibilities of a good future while offering and encouraging some symptomatic relief almost from the first session of therapy. She demonstrated Seligman's strengths and virtues in school life while her inner life reflected anything but the American dream, much like the film. Bailey seemed open to the idea of using a counseling strategy that focused on the strengths or positive aspects of personality rather than her past. She seemed curious about watching a movie in therapy since her past experience in counseling at age 8 was short-lived and, according to Bailey, "did not work." I felt the movie could be a catalyst to help Bailey reach the deepest parts of her emotional suffering while focusing on solutions.

Bailey had a pretty good idea of Seligman's 24 strengths and virtues because we had worked together first reading parts of the book on positive psychology, learning the model and exploring the strengths in relation to her life problems. Over the course of 3 months, she also read Seligman's *Authentic Happiness* (2002) and completed the VIA (Virtues in Action) survey on the Web.[1] Together, we completed the survey, which identifies strengths such as valor, openness to experience, creativity, resilience, optimism, and so forth.

The six characters in *Little Miss Sunshine* seemed to reflect many of this adolescent's relationships and struggles. When we initially and briefly watched the opening scene where Olive is mesmerized watching a beauty pageant, my client remarked, "Look at the little girls' eyes. She looks so happy." I knew we were on to something that could be a catalyst for communication and change. In working with this young person, who had experienced too much trauma for any human being, thoughts of humility and Seligman's strengths of love, kindness, and social intelligence were clearly reflected as she shared her stories and life events that paralleled the struggles and neuroses and creativity of the characters in the movie. Bailey also displayed social intelligence, love, tenderness, and deep understanding of what it means to be human; ironic since she had suffered many emotional traumas including abandonment by both parents. There was an authentic, albeit angry quality to her description of life in general, displaying a pseudomaturity for a young girl. And yet this young adolescent managed to rise above the hurts in a way that had her focused on the future and mindful for those that cared and nurtured her after she was abandoned. Most striking was her humanity for the parents who left her. She was able to share her feelings and her sadness, but at the same time, live a life of gratitude and satisfaction, staying in the moment of each experience and not dwelling on the past. However, her mood was labile at times and her symptoms reflected deeper feelings that required expression and release so she could continue to thrive.

She gleefully shared her enthusiasm for movies, in particular horror movies. This enthusiasm for horror movies may have been a medium for Bailey's anger, sadness, and fears resulting from her traumatic past or identification with the characters. As the weeks passed, Bailey seemed to ease into some level of comfort and looked forward to our sessions. As the therapeutic alliance grew stronger, I decided it was time we watched a movie together, and she agreed.

At first, Bailey minimized her problems, professing, "Everything's okay." She acknowledged receiving good grades and feeling happy with her life. When the topic of her parents came up she became agitated, and on edge. It was a difficult subject for her, one she avoided. This shy, quiet young girl suddenly became stiff, angry, and emotionally withdrawn. Like many adolescents, Bailey came to therapy against her will. She was quiet and reserved at first, much like many 13-year-olds with whom I have worked, but she endured. She smiled sometimes, gritting her teeth but asking to return. As our work proceeded, I moved away from the topic of parents and on to movies that she loved. I noticed the energy in her changed; she no longer was withdrawn and angry, but excited and more comfortable. I took it as a clinical cue to move forward. Having worked with adolescents for many years, it was not unusual to work unconventionally. I naturally assessed the situation and looked for a way to connect, and to help this young woman start to heal and grow from the pain she had been holding.

Since Bailey reported being an avid fan of movies, it seemed a natural communication vehicle for both of us. I explained to Bailey that the first time we watched the film we would not comment, just watch and listen. Her grandmother agreed for her to have two back-to-back sessions so we could watch *Little Miss Sunshine* in its entirety. The only requirement was for Bailey to go home that night and write one page, commenting on each character. The next week, we began to process the experience and her reflection, highlighting the struggles and strengths of each character in the movie and working with Bailey to identify her growth. Bailey appeared to enjoy the opportunity to critique everyone else's behavior for a change and slowly warmed to any connections I might make. In fact, she particularly enjoyed acting out the characters. She seemed to have a keen awareness of each character and identified most with Dwayne, the withdrawn, selectively mute, and depressed adolescent; what a surprise! My therapeutic strategy was to continue delving into the characters, highlighting each character trait that reflected the strengths identified in positive psychology. The film seemed to capture them all quite nicely. And Bailey was able to share her positive traits of creativity and fun.

During the fourth session, Bailey began to identify her strengths and as we watched the film we were able to relate many of the different character's problems to the client's and her parents. She never denied any of the problems in her life, and neither did any of the characters in the film. But she did have trouble talking and sharing her feelings beyond the surface. Much like the characters in the film (that would by most standards be labeled dysfunctional), my client and the main character, Olive, demonstrated resilience and positive character strengths in the face of uncertainty, instability, and daily struggles to survive. However, amidst the positive personality characteristics, Bailey also exhibited several problematic symptoms that blocked her growth.

At the beginning of each session, Bailey seemed a bit guarded, so we would take 10 minutes reestablishing trust and bringing in some levity and sarcasm, to which she seemed to relate. I acknowledged her reluctance and agreed how weird being in therapy could feel; after all, her parents were the ones with the problem—not her! I agreed that she probably knew what was best and that no one really knew what her life was like. In fact, I confirmed to Bailey that it was silly how anyone, even a trained therapist, could think otherwise. I was merely there to help her explore where she wanted to go in life and to help her see all the possibilities and options ahead. Besides, Bailey had agreed to attend therapy for 16 sessions, so we were going to make the best of it. Why not have fun in the process?

By the sixth session, her fears, despair, and anguish began to emerge. As we discussed the character of the grandfather and his addiction to heroin, Bailey became tearful and shared how hurt and frightened she had been over her parent's drug use. In particular she expressed anger when her parents went on a drug binge when she was 5 years old. They had friends over and were drinking and loud. She awoke from a deep sleep to find several people stoned and dazed. She tried to go back to sleep but her anxiety kept her awake. She crawled under the bed, sucking her thumb, feeling scared and confused, rocking herself to sleep. When morning came, she walked out and found everyone gone, including her parents. She waited until that afternoon to call her grandmother. Her grandmother came and picked Bailey up, gathered some clothes and called the police. Child Protective Services interviewed Bailey. Her grandmother tried to assuage her fears but Bailey feared her parents would never come home, or worse, would die. This is the time she remembers feeling the first symptoms of panic.

She never told her grandmother, but she felt like she had a 500-pound weight on her chest, felt shaky and "sweaty," had a sense of "not being in her body," or depersonalization; with a profound sense of dread. These symptoms are characteristic of severe anxiety and/or panic. Bailey was curious enough and bright to understand this was her body's way of escaping from perceived intense fear when I explained the physiological reason she had experienced these symptoms. Reframing this experience into a normal response seemed to ease her discomfort and provide confirmation that she was not crazy! This abandonment by Bailey's parents would happen many times. Her grandmother would always be there for the rescue. She recognized how Olive's father in the movie reflected her grandmother's spirit of "No child gets left behind," although the pain on her face showed the loss felt.

There is no doubt that the adolescent years bring a sense of loss. Our work together helped Bailey see that everyone experiences some sense of loss and that with time, she could heal. When the grandfather in the film dies, it is not clear if he dies from a drug overdose or of natural causes. Bailey was convinced he died of a drug overdose. Although the character Olive is unaware of her devoted grandfather's addiction to heroin, Bailey noticed the love Olive felt and the care she received despite the hardship witnessed by her grandfather. At first she could not understand how someone addicted to heroin could make time to show love and care for someone else; and yet, it happened. Olive's grandfather was devoted to her. He taught her all of the "moves" and prepared her in earnest for the beauty contest. This opened up a discussion about Bailey's parents' behavior. Her masked anger for them slowly began to change. She admitted feeling resigned that they would likely stay in jail for a long time, at least until she was in her 20s, but she also acknowledged their willingness to allow her grandmother permanent custody. This agreement provided stability for Bailey, a life unfamiliar before coming to live with her grandmother. This seemed to start a change in Bailey's attitude. She seemed to even identify a few strengths in her parents (openness, courage, love). But she still refused to speak to them by phone and was guarded about her future in their care. Bailey could be very pessimistic at times about her life. There were times when Bailey even romanticized about the idea of death and wrote a few poems on the topic. We explored the topic to rule out any ideation or plan.

It is natural for adolescents to think about death; some even obsess about the idea. After all, they are in the throes of experiencing the death of their childhood. In the case of Bailey, she had never really experienced much of a childhood until she came to live permanently with her grandmother at age 7. In some ways she was too mature, a kind of pseudomaturity that comes from early childhood trauma. The character Dwayne displayed characteristics that appealed to Bailey. She even took notice of the special relationship between Uncle Frank and Dwayne. Uncle Frank was a mess. He was living with the family after trying to commit suicide. Although depressed, he demonstrated strength throughout the movie. His repeated exclamation of, "I am the number one Proust scholar in the world," became comical and seemed to be a catalyst for healing and open communication between Frank and young Dwayne. I think that Dwayne related to Frank because they both shared similar internal experiences. Frank saw himself in young Dwayne and vice versa.

Dwayne, selectively mute by choice and clearly discouraged, displayed a sense of future-mindedness in his determination and motivation in caring for his body (lifting weights and keeping physically fit behind closed doors). It was as if he was hanging on to the hope that his future would fulfill his dreams (becoming an airline pilot). However, his family was unaware of his deepest feelings. Dwayne refused to speak as a passive-aggressive protest against the family; it seems he may have been trying to get their attention! Frank, Dwayne's uncle recently released from a mental health facility after a suicide attempt, starts to connect with Dwayne on a deep level. It appears there is understanding between them almost without words. Together they are able to provide a catalyst for the motivation to live. With Bailey, the somatic complaints, insomnia, anxiety, and depression were symptoms of a similar inner life.

During the middle of therapy (sessions 8–12), Bailey realized the relationship she shared with her beloved grandmother was similar to the relationship between Frank and Dwayne. Her grandmother had suffered from anxiety and depression during her early 20s and 30s but had joined a group therapy program subsequent to being hospitalized after the first major episode. She made friends, started working as a facilitator in a client-centered facility, and was able to learn how to cope with life's adversities, and that she was not alone. This served as a catalyst for her motivation to finish college and earn her degree in library science. Her grandmother had been abandoned by her husband (Bailey's grandfather) at age 20. Bailey never imagined her grandmother would have experienced such difficulty; she always perceived her as being strong, and confident, a take-charge person. Bailey shared how seeing her grandmother struggle, and yet take control of her life, provided the chance to be happy.

During session 12, Bailey seemed calmer and more settled. She was sleeping fairly well. She stopped complaining of stomach pains, and her grandmother reported more cooperation for attending school. It seems Bailey may have turned the corner after learning about her grandmother's struggles and her commitment to have a better life. With motivation, care, and support, people can change their thinking and take action to be happy despite setbacks. Our work was coming to an end. Bailey remained active in school activities and had friends. By session 15, she remarked, "I think we are finished; I am happy right now and sleeping well." We agreed to meet one more time. I assured her if the need arose in the future she could always return. I affirmed Bailey's feelings about the good work she had done and that her commitment to growth and identifying her strengths (much like her beloved grandmother and Olive) were the skills that would carry her into the future.

NOTE

1. For the Virtues in Action survey, see http://www.authentichappiness.sas.upenn.edu/Default.aspx.

Exercise 7.1: Film Exercise

Choose a film to watch with your parents or caregivers, and make it a fun night at the movies. Serve popcorn, and refreshments. Make a special invitation on the computer, using whatever film best depicts the issue or problem and reflects a current situation in your family. You can find many film reviews at Netflix, for example. Ask your parents (or caregivers) to make a list of all the character's strengths and struggles in the film when the movie is over. Then ask them to meet the next evening to role play the character in the film that they identify with. This should help open up a discussion of any current struggles and also the strengths of each person. It should provide some laughs too. The point is, use it as a tool to spend time together having fun and fostering communication. Try and pick one with a positive ending, not one that focuses on the negative, in keeping with Seligman's positive psychology principles.

REFERENCES

Aspinwall, L. G., & Staudinger, U. M. (Eds.). (2002). *A psychology of human strengths: Fundamental questions and future directions for a positive psychology*. Washington, DC: American Psychological Association.

Brent, D. A., & Birmaher, B. (2002). Adolescent depression. *New England Journal of Medicine, 9*(347), 667–671.

Csikszentmihalyi, M. (1997). *Finding flow: The psychology of engagement with everyday life*. New York: Basic Books.

Dayton, J., & Faris, V. (Directors). (2006). *Little Miss Sunshine* [Motion picture]. United States: Big Beach Films.

Dieser, R. B. (2005). Authentic Happiness: Using the new positive psychology to realize your potential to realize your lasting fulfillment. *Therapeutic Recreation Journal, 39,* 241–248.

Finamore, D. (2008). Resilience. In *The encyclopedia of counseling*. California: Sage Press.

Fisher, S. (2007). *Tell me something good: Applying validated positive psychology interventions*. Retrieved March 25, 2008 from http://pos-psych.com/news/sherri-fisher/20070305128

Gable, S. H., & Haidt, J. (2005). What and why is positive psychology? *Review of General Psychology, 9*(2), 103–110.

Horowitz, J. L., & Garber, J. (2006). The prevention of depressive symptoms in children and adolescents: A meta-analytic review. *Journal of Clinical and Consulting Psychology, 74,* 401–415.

Keyes, C. & Haidt, J. (Eds.) (2003). Flourishing: Positive psychology and the life well-lived. Washington, DC: American Psychological Association Press.

Lambert, C. (2007, September-October). Psychology explores humans at their best. *The Science of Happiness*. Retrieved July 1, 2007, from http://www. harvardmagazine.com/2007/01/the-science-of-happiness.html

Lewinsohn, P., Rohde, P., Seeley, J., & Fischer, S. (1993). Age-cohort changes in the lifetime occurrence of depression and other mental disorders. *Journal of Abnormal Psychology, 102*, 110–120.

Lyubomirsky, S. (2001). Why are some people happier than others? The role of cognitive and motivational processes in well-being. *American Psychologist, 56*, 239–249.

Marano, H. E. (2003). A long arm: Teen depression. Retrieved July 11, 2007, from http://psychologytoday.com/articles/pto-20030807–000007.html

McGuire, P. A. (1999). Templeton positive about largest psychology award. *APA Monitor Online*. Retrieved June 2, 2007, from http://www.apa.org/monitor/may99/research.html

Miller, A., & Miller, J. (1981). Superfreak. On *Streetsongs* [CD]. Detroit: Motown Records.

Peterson, K. S. (2002). *U.S.A. Today*. Retrieved July 1, 2007, from http://www. usatoday.com/news/health/mental/2002–05–22-college-depression.htm

Peterson, C., & Seligman, M. E. P. (2004). *Character strengths and virtues: A handbook and classification*. New York: Oxford University Press

Reyna, V. F., & Farley, F. (2006). Risk and rationality in adolescent decision making: Implications for theory, practice, and public policy. *Psychological Science in the Public Interest, 7*, 1–44.

Rutter, M. (1987). Psychosocial resilience and protective mechanisms. *American Journal of Orthopsychiatry, 57*, 316–329.

Seligman, M. E. P. (2002). *Authentic happiness: Using the new positive psychology to realize your potential for lasting fulfillment*. New York: Free Press.

Seligman, M. E. P. (1998). *Learned optimism: How to change your mind and your life*. New York: Pocketbooks (Simon & Schuster).

Seligman, M. E. P. (2002). Positive psychology for ninth graders. *Authentic Happiness Newsletter*. Retrieved June 9, 2007, from http://www.authentichappiness. sas.upenn.edu/newsletter.aspx?id = 53

Seligman, M. E. P., Steen, T. A., Park, N., & Peterson, C. (2005). Positive psychology progress: Empirical validation of interventions. *American Psychologist, 60*(5), 410–421.

Seligman, M. E. P., & Csikszentmihalyi, M. (2000). *Center for confidence*. Retrieved June 10, 2007, from http://www.centreforconfidence.co.uk/pp/overview.php?p = c2lkPTEmdGlkPTAmaWQ9MjMy

Sheldon, K. M., & Lyubomirsky, S. (2006). Achieving sustainable gains in happiness: Change your actions not your circumstances. *Journal of Positive Psychology, 7*, 55–86.

Singh, M. K., Pfeifer, J., Barzman, D., Kowatch, R. A., & DelBello, M. P. (2007). Pharmacotherapy for child and adolescent mood disorders. *Psychiatric Annals, 37*, 465.

Snyder, M. B. (2004, March). *Senior student affairs officer round table: Hottest topics in student affairs*. Session held at the annual meeting of the National Association of Student Personnel Administrators, Denver, Colorado.

Snyder, C. R., & Lopez, S. J. (2002). *Handbook of positive psychology*. New York: Oxford University Press.

Snyder, C. R., & Lopez. S. J. (2007). *Positive psychology: The scientific and practical explorations of human strengths*. California: Sage.

Sowell, E. R., Thompson, P. M., Holmes, C. J., Jeringan, T. L., & Toga, A. W. (1999). In vivo evidence for post-adolescent brain maturation in frontal and striatal regions. *Nature Neuroscience, 2(10)*, 859–861.

Wallis, C. (2005). The new science of happiness. *Time Online*. Retrieved July 15, 2007, from http://www.time.com/time/magazine/article/0,9171,1015832,00.html

CHAPTER 8

Movie Metaphors in Miniature

Children's Use of Popular Hero and Shadow Figures in Sandplay

Linda B. Hunter

Sandplay therapy is the playful and creative expression of a person's inner life, a form of Jungian "active imagination" that can be used productively by anyone, regardless of verbal or cognitive capacity. Primary among its healing mechanisms is the access offered to what Jung understood as the collective unconscious, the reservoir of archetypes that connect humans to the spiritual and conceptual resources of the world.

The miniature figures used to build sandplay scenes express archetypal abstractions as concrete, tangible symbols from different cultures and times that become metaphors woven into stories told in the sand. In our world of Disney movies and television cartoons, characters from mythology and fairy tales have become alive and familiar to most children. In a sandplay therapy setting, these characters are often chosen from among the multitude of figures made available to express profoundly significant and personal meanings.

In this context where popular culture meets play therapy meets deep strata of universal meaning, the natural language of the child, which is play, finds a greatly expanded vocabulary of what we may call *toy words* with which to do healing work.

Through the contact with sand and miniatures that sandplay makes available, children find access to the depths of the psyche, the collective unconscious where meaning and healing are generated. What their spirit can believe in, and their mind can imagine, their body can express through creative play. What they express becomes their story which, if carefully observed through eyes, ears, and intuition, can help adults to truly understand the inner life of children.

SANDPLAY

Explored initially by children in the playrooms of Margaret Lowenfeld (1979) in 1920s London and developed into a therapeutic modality by Dora Kalff in Switzerland, this use of miniature toys and sand contained in trays taps into the most natural and spontaneous play of children. In almost any setting (home, school, park, child care, and camp), children will amuse themselves by playing with any available small toys. Miniature toys, displayed in a way that is clearly and easily accessible, make a new space familiar and comfortable, invite fantasy play in children of all ages, and build rapport and a bridge to the therapeutic situation.

In sandplay, the child easily leads the way, choosing not only the content but the pace, the process, and the outcome of the play. Individualized styles are accepted and encouraged: the child can be silent or narrate every move; independently play or initiate extensive interaction with the therapist; spontaneously play by leaving toys in a jumble where they happen to fall, or carefully and artistically create an expressive image.

Sandplay is purposeful imaging guided by the unconscious—hands placing miniature objects—which will come to consciousness when the time is ripe and in the meantime will do its work in the unconscious (Bradway, 1986). The process of healing takes place while playing with sand and figures, without the need for interpretation, verbalization, or conscious awareness. Whatever the child's style or abilities, success is guaranteed. No talent or technique is needed. Anything created is easily changed.

The sandplay process involves the whole child: the senses of touch, vision, and hearing; emotions; thoughts; behavior. Using both hands simultaneously connects two lobes of the brain, thinking and imagination. Because the body, heart, and mind are all engaged, this is actual experience that creates neural pathways, develops new memories, and builds internal resources that can be called upon in later real-world situations. Many children, even the most anxious or angry, hyperactive or distractible, seem to be able to concentrate their attention, to work with a kind of meditative focus that gives them access to a deep level of their psychic functioning.

Sandplay makes the abstract (ideas, emotions, beliefs) concrete. As opposed to virtual forms of play, figures are tangible; symbols can be handled as well as seen. Images can be combined into clusters that communicate visually and simultaneously many meanings, as opposed to the linear-sequential restrictions of verbal therapy.

Sandplay therapy provides a space that is both free and protected, contained by the presence of the therapist, by the dimensions of the sand tray and by the extensive but limited range of figures available. By being given structure and form, experiences become meaningful and hidden aspects of the child's self can be expressed and acknowledged. The terrific pressure of fantasies and emotions decreases as they are creatively expressed.

The process of making scenes and stories with miniatures allows the child to be in complete control of what he or she does, while limiting responsibility to a tiny, manageable world. Imagination can be given free rein, behavior rehearsed, and obstacles defined and overcome. Resources can be discovered and utilized and fears can be faced. Conflicts can be resolved, solutions generated, and relationships explored. All this can be accomplished on a symbolic, unconscious, nonverbal level, allowing the revelation in silence of unspeakable events and horrifying secrets while concealing from the child's conscious mind what he or she is not ready to handle. Thus deeply troubling situations can be worked on without retraumatizing or disturbing functional defenses. Potentially damaging posttraumatic secret rituals are released into the sand tray (Gil, 1991). Worst fear scenarios can be played out with different endings, with humor, and with hope. Chaos can be lived with and directed to creative purposes (Capitolo, 2002).

The tray absorbs the fear, anger, and hurt as these feelings are revealed in the scenes. Shadow elements can be brought out into the light, be handled, seen, acknowledged, and integrated. Superheroes and other allies can be introduced to balance the shadow power, and used to help fight internal battles (Kalff, 1980). Aggression and anger played out in miniature stays within the comfort and acceptance levels of most therapists and the controllable anxiety levels of most children. Thus limit-setting is rarely necessary in sandplay, making the modality extremely useful with the angry or aggressive child.

Creativity, imagination, and visual, right-brain learning are fostered by the materials and the freedom to use them in almost any way children choose. The process naturally leads to a positive sense of control over their small world and a sense of responsibility for their actions/creations. The tray and its contents provide a reflective mirror which the child self-creates and thus becomes able to own. An intimate therapeutic relationship can develop with less dependence, because it is buffered by the tray.

Sandplay encourages a number of developmental growth factors. Choice making is an integral part of the sandplay process: deciding which figures to use, how to use them, what to save, change, destroy, remake. Choices become more conscious and mindful as the work proceeds. Problem-solving skills are honed through developing new and creative solutions, from how to keep the sand tunnel from collapsing to how to express anger in powerful but nonaggressive ways. Mastery is practiced through the opportunity to act out negative situations in the miniature metaphor. A sense of constructive power replaces victimized vulnerability. The positive power of magical thinking—the sense that what we believe affects our world and our own efforts make transformation possible—can, in the sand tray, become tangibly real.

Self-discovery leads to age-appropriate identity formation through exploration that is stimulated and encouraged by the diversity of figures. The opportunity to safely express and explore all aspects of who they are and hope to become allows children to observe, respect, and value themselves, to develop a meaningful sense of autonomy and self-esteem. Thus the tiger and the rabbit find ways to coexist, compete, and play. The Buddha, the Beast, and the divine Baby are recognized as valid players in a child's psyche.

Ego development can be observed. A healthy ego is symbolically able to give assistance and guidance as a police officer or Indian chief. Soldiers, bodyguards, athletes, and power figures often represent the positive ego. As ego strength grows, the masculine shadow symbols take on less menacing form, and the feminine elements appear as women instead of as dragons (Henderson, 1964). As children show their strengths to the observer, they begin to integrate them into a more positive self-concept. Once children have imagined positive, resourceful solutions, they are much more likely to achieve them.

Children work with the sand and the figures on normal developmental tasks, an opportunity often missed in troubled childhoods. The search for object constancy becomes miniaturized hide-and-seek, burying and retrieving in the sand. Categorizing, learning about similarities and differences, forming connections (family groups of like animals) and separations (opposing sides of battles), is facilitated by the multitude of miniature figures.

The tray contains the scene and provides boundaries for the work being done. The tray creates a tangible special play space in which the child's world is displayed. The empty space within its borders activates the child's imagination, inviting the placement of figures. The visible containment helps children to accept, create, and expand limits in their lives. Overly rigid self-boundaries become more flexible as gates appear and vehicles are able to move. Overly fluid boundaries become protective and clear as fences, signs, and roadways direct traffic.

The miniature collection combines both realistic and fantasy images of all kinds, offering an abundant, rich vocabulary for the child's language of play: bridges, birds, and babies; treasure, toilets, and turtles; fire, fences, and flowers; scary shadow figures (monsters, sharks, dragons) and nurturing, protective power figures (strong men and women, lions, dolphins); keys, weapons, shells, and coins. Miniature weapons can be used to represent violence and protection without play becoming overtly aggressive (Hunter, 1998).

With all these elements displayed, children feel permission and encouragement to explore and reveal both the ugly and the beautiful, the scary and the safe, the painfully broken and the magnificently whole aspects of their lives.

Collections can be tailored to special populations (cultural items, ethnic figures); different ages (sturdy, colorful, and large for preschool; intricate, ambiguous, and natural figures for adolescents); and made portable to carry to schools, homes, hospitals, or camps. Thus with some thought, energy, and creative flexibility, sandplay can be widely and effectively provided to diverse populations and settings and engage even those who intend to be resistant.

Sandplay facilitates storytelling, making it possible for even very young children to identify characters, conflict, possible allies, and paths to resolution in their life stories. By observing and listening with respectful nonjudgmental attention and mindful awareness of the whole child, the play therapist is able to accept the expression of the child's feelings and fantasies without minimizing or overreacting, and appreciate how imagination and creativity lead to growth and mastery. By responding within the child's choice of metaphor, the therapist is able to build a cotransference relationship based on mutual respect, learning, and caring (Bradway & McCoard, 1997). Entering the world of and developing empathy for the troubled child is considerably less problematic when buffered by sand, tray, and miniatures. Having a meaningful product (photographs used as a visual record of the child's creations) clearly shows changes taking place over time and deepens the therapist's understanding.

JUNGIAN THEORY

Carl Jung (1971) added to Freud's formulation of the personal unconscious active in the psyche with the concept of the collective unconscious populated by archetypes. These inherited a priori patterns of thinking and instinctual behavior become the structural forming elements in the unconscious out of which patterns emerge. They arise from universal experiences, are expressed in metaphors, contain both positive and negative aspects, give shape to the fantasy lives of individuals, and actively and continually influence our thoughts, feelings, actions, imagination, and perceptions. A problem is transformed by reaching to its archetypal core.

Archetypal motifs found in legends and mythologies repeat in similar and even identical form the world over. Jung (1964) considered them of immense value to the psyche of all peoples; a force for bringing the world together and deepening empathy.

Archetypes find expression through symbols. Symbols emerge from the interaction between an archetype and a particular culture. Many different symbols at different times describe the same archetype, in terms that are simultaneously unique and universal. Through consideration of a symbol, problems can be solved, what is stuck can find a new path, opposites can move together. Through personal symbol journeys, we find connection with the collective.

The inclusion in a sandplay miniature collection of mythological and fantasy figures representing diverse cultures and historical eras connects children to the collective unconscious of archetypal symbols and the accumulated wisdom of humankind (Kiepenheuer, 1990). Archetypes are clearly involved when the images used have little or no connection to ordinary life, or represent cultures or religions to which the child has had no direct access (Jung, 1964).

Disney movies with their Burger King plastic images of mythological and fairy tale figures have brought archetypal personalities and symbols into everyday childhood play. Both the terribly evil and the wonderfully good mother and father characters are available for expressive play. Hero, shadow, trickster, and wisdom images abound. While children may initially choose these figures with the movie scenario in mind, the story is quickly shaped into something personal and relevant to the individual child's needs and life.

A basic element of Jungian theory that is visibly and powerfully worked on in sandplay is what he termed the shadow. The shadow in Jungian thought comprises personal qualities that are unacknowledged and unaccepted by the individual. These are often represented by images of the enemy, the ugly, violent destructive power, and the negative side of the archetypes: terrible mother; demon child; destructive father; the villain (Darth Vader, Lex Luthor, Joker). The shadow is a complex concept that includes elements unique to the individual and common to the collective. The shadow is often projected on others and takes form as the monster in animal, human, or fantasy shape, active negative energy that calls forth a response in the child to escape, combat, tame, or transform.

A goal of Jungian therapy is to safely examine the contents of the shadow, and then embrace and integrate the opposites it contains. In sandplay, work with opposites is often expressed as conflict. The play of young boys with fighting figures safely allows the energy of the "bad"—of anger, aggression, and defiance—to be separated from its quality of badness and used to fight for the good. As the work progresses and moves toward integration, the battle often becomes a metaphor, a sports contest instead of war. Aggression becomes competition; players can be friends as well as opponents. The purpose of the conflict becomes winning rather than killing.

CASE APPLICATIONS

Popular figures and themes from movies, TV, and comics often find their way into children's sandplay scenes. In this way children connect to the resources of the collective unconscious, knowing on some level that through this work the journey that compels them can take place and that, as Joseph Campbell writes: "We have not even to risk the adventure alone, for the heroes of all time have gone before us. . . . Where we had thought to travel outward, we will come to the center of our own existence. And where we had thought to be alone, we will be with all the world" (Campbell & Moyers, 1988).

Cowboys and Indians

The classic American movie Western theme shown around the globe provides a metaphor for conflict, the significance of which has evolved as diversity becomes more integral to our everyday lives. As peoples all over the world have struggled to maintain their land, independence, and indigenous values, the American Indian has come to represent the defense of a more peaceful and natural human existence in contrast to the intrusive forces of expansion, development, and technology. This was clearly represented in the Balkans in the years following the wars of ethnic cleansing in that area, as children in peace-building camps created sandplay battles on the theme of defense of land and way of life, often using the American Indians and alien invaders as metaphors for the struggle in their countries: The bad guys want to take away the Indians' totem and life. The animals and Indians fight them off. Modern people and their robots have come to take the Indians' land and holy objects.

Smurfs, Fraggles, and Other Wee Folks

The smaller, gentler characters from cartoons are often used by younger children to concretize ideas and feelings with which they are struggling.

A small 7-year old African American boy in residential treatment was demonstrating extremely disturbed behaviors. His first sandplay session, just after arriving in placement, illustrated the tension he was feeling and his ability to project a conscious image.

The story begins with what he called a "nice town" of small, gentle cartoon characters: Smurfs, Cabbage Patch kids, Fraggles. Anything that could represent violence is explained another way such as missiles that are "made into fireworks" presided over by Mickey the Magician. A "new guy in town" (Cat in tuxedo) is having trouble fitting in and is playing jokes on others. The only angry figure is Donald Duck "getting mad at" a little Fraggle girl. A Sesame Street policeman "makes sure that no one gets too close to the fireworks." ET quietly calls home from behind a tree.

Soon this safely gentle world begins to break up and he decides to "play all the cartoons together." He enjoys picking out the characters he recognizes and dividing them into "bad guys and good guys." He creates a home for them all to coexist, taking turns and relating across differences. A large figure of Aladdin's genie, smiling with hand upraised, holds center stage.

After weeks of significant work with animals and battles, monsters and large powerful symbols, he returns to the cartoon characters and theme of a diverse family trying to get along. He gives different family members the autonomy to "do what they like best": "He wants to be president (Pink Panther with briefcase) . . . This one is named Mario and he is good at his work, climbing trees . . . This one likes ducks so he looks like one (Donald). . . . She likes mice and wants to be a cheerleader (Minnie). . . . This one likes painting (Smurf). . . . He likes to think (Goofy). This one is the grandfather (Smurf) of everybody and this is the mother (Smurf with pie). It's a whole big family even though they all look different."

After more profound work exploring spiritual and emotional issues, in his last session he returns to the small gentle cartoon figures combined into an extended "Halloween family." Nuclear families are more defined although the system remains open and flexible: "The Mickey Mouse family lives with the Smurf family. . . . The Cabbage Scratches (sic) don't live there, they just go and take showers." Individuals are accepted for diverse identities. "One has a job being a ballerina, one has a job fishing (Smurfs), one is always mad at himself (Donald). Snow White is here, she's Popeye's girlfriend, and her enemy (the evil queen) is over here. The new man (cat in tuxedo) is moving to the village and the others like him now." The range of familiar figures gave him the tools to explore powerful issues of social relationships, boundaries, rejection, and acceptance.

MEETING THE SUPERHEROES

As they intensely struggle to find a masculine identification that allows them to integrate power, competence, and assertiveness into a positive view of their young manhood, identification with power figures can help boys to overcome in imagination the limits of age and ability, find inner strength along with an imaginary friend, and increase self-confidence (Mills & Crowley, 1986). In sandplay, children use strong power figures representing a wide range of emotional, social, and behavioral possibilities to represent many aspects of the internal and external conflicts and struggles they are experiencing.

Good Guys Versus Bad Guys

Many boys are working on building an archetypal father. Just as in fairy tales, real fathers are frequently ineffectual or missing, offering neither protection nor support as the child ventures to explore a wider world. Power, often aggressive and intrusive, is an intimate part of male identification. In comics and movies, as well as in life, connection to violence is frequently at the inner core of masculine identity (Shaia, 1994).

A 9-year-old African American child uses an array of movie images to represent humans fighting nonhumans in a war of opposites: conscious versus unconscious, ego versus instinct, good versus bad. Whenever a different kind of creature, an unconscious image, or an instinctual drive shows itself, it must be attacked and destroyed before its scary "otherness" gets loose in the world.

Another boy expresses the helplessness and hopelessness he experiences by plunging both the heroes and their enemies up to their necks in quicksand, an apt metaphor for the world in which many young black males from the inner city find themselves, where unseen danger lurks to pull them down, and the more they struggle, the more impossible it is for them to extricate themselves. Outside help is needed.

In a third scene, good guy–bad guy twosomes confront each other in battle stance. Fighting between the dueling pairs is intense, bloody, very graphic, and generally deadly although not permanently so. Each combatant uses his own special weapon: "breathing fire, hurling stones, squirting blood." In the course of the unfolding drama, the best weapon of all is discovered. "The little one can beat the big one 'cuz he grows when he gets mad." A very small 7-year-old African American child who throws very large, dangerous tantrums, has thus explained to himself and to me that getting mad allows him to feel big and strong enough so that eventually the "good guys will win."

An 8-year old African American boy who had accidentally shot and killed a cousin and been ostracized by his extended family has moved to the point in his sandplay process where he can fight for a positive future. His tray is filled with dueling pairs who are carefully matched in size and strength (Ninja Turtle and Superman; Wonder Woman and GI Jane; Swamp Thing and Hulk Hogan wrestler). They are fighting individual contests of skill and strength. There are no weapons and no killing. The winning team, the good guys, will get the prize, which is a baby coming down from the "space ship" with a "secret crystal."

Another boy's process shows how the good-versus-bad conflict can evolve toward healing. In the first version of this tray, after a hard-fought battle, the good and bad forces were left separated by a high "alarm fence" made of fencing and a thick sand wall with a slinky on top to make it razor sharp. The fence was there to protect the good guys (Superman, Wonder Woman, etc.) from surprise attack by the bad (Footsoldier, Star Wars soldiers, wrestlers, etc.). After finishing this picture, this 8-year-old African American boy went back to the shelves, chose another figure and then accidentally dropped and broke it. He was most upset, sitting on the floor, berating himself for his stupidity. When he was quiet for a moment, I commented that he sure gets angry with himself when he makes a mistake. He was silent for a while, then got up and slowly went to the tray saying, "Don't need this no more." He took out the fence separating the two sides and replaced it with a river crossed by a bridge. In this final version of the tray the conflict is bridged. When the prone figures revive to fight the next round in the ongoing battle that is these boys' lives, the two sides will be connected to each other rather than walled off. This boy is no longer so sure that the impulsive, angry "bad" will overwhelm the emerging "good."

Batman and Company

Among the powerful masculine cartoon heroes known to use violence to help the good and destroy the bad, Batman is frequently the first figure a boy will select from the shelves. Two different figures in my sandplay collection illustrate the two sides of what Batman represents for the children who include him in their sand worlds: the standing tall and straight protector of victims and defender of good; and the black-cloaked Batman in action, the dark and mysterious knight from *Batman Returns,* the orphan seeking revenge for his parent's death, personifying the possibility of violence as a solution to the pain children feel.

Bats are mammals that live in the air and direct their movements by internal radar. They are night creatures that prefer dark places and hang upside down. Ambivalence and inversion are suggested. Batman has the powers and contradictions of bats combined with human feelings. Ambivalence is further emphasized by Two-Face, a half white, half black figure of a man with a regular face on the white side and an angry distorted blue face on the other. He is pointedly used to represent the ambiguous role that some boys' fathers play in their lives. Robin is the hero's apprentice, a shaman-in-training with his cape, not quite ready to fly. He is a great symbol for the preadolescent boy who is struggling with defining his masculine powers, showing both the helplessness and the hope that many boys feel in their young male role.

Superman

The preeminent masculine hero figure, Superman, fights, sits, stands, lies tied down, flies in the center of many sand trays. As the first true superhero, the archetypal warrior, Superman combines diverse powers in one individual. While Hitler used the term *superman* to genetically select for power and racial purity, the American version is a compassionate and intuitive champion of the vulnerable, combining pride and goodness as he learns to use his special powers to protect and rescue (Sugatt, 1999). His background is relevant to the life of many boys. He is sent away from his home and family and into a strange world that he has trouble understanding. He has times of depression and resentment, fearful and wary of his powers, which set him apart from those who would be his friends. On his journey he transforms from the warrior to the teacher. Superman reflects both a narcissistic tendency to inflation and the compassionate strength that begins to surface as boys discard their masks of the nasty trickster.

Teenage Mutant Ninja Turtles

Many children use these curious composite cartoon figures to represent complex concepts and feelings. This modern myth is about resiliency and the weak becoming powerful, about diversity and integration of opposites. As children, these turtles, found helpless in a sewer, are adopted and mentored by another unlikely hero who frequents such lowly places, a wise and skillful rat. He trains them in the techniques of violence and qualities of compassion and loyalty. Amid many mischievous antics, they become the Teenage Mutant Ninja Turtles who use their powers to help the good and punish the bad, and to protect themselves, each other, and their mentor/father. They are in many ways superheroes for our era and for children whose lives begin in the sewers of our affluent world and who must learn early to rely on themselves (Hunter, 1998).

The Ninja Turtles' strange appearance and green skin color, their names inherited from great Renaissance artists, and their playful teenage personalities make them great images for minority "tween" boys as they practice their kicks and ride motorcycles. They show up on both the bad and good sides of conflicts, representing fighting skill, sometimes violent and deadly, sometimes quiet, with equally skillful opponents from other stories.

The Green Hulk

This large half-clothed figure, whose power and green color are triggered by anger, frequently represents the angry, confused parts of boys' personalities and relationships.

In one tray a tiny ninja in white clothes, surrounded by equally small knights with swords, confronts a giant figure of the Green Hulk. It is clearly a fight of David and Goliath proportions. When the small warriors have won and killed the giant they will "take off his skin and eat him," removing his difference and his badness, and ingesting his strength. This 11-year-old African American deals with complex issues of skin (color)/deep badness and inner goodness as he metaphorically expresses the concept: "The demon that you can swallow gives you its power" (Campbell & Moyers, 1988).

This same image figures prominently in the initial trays of a 9-year-old Hispanic boy. In his first tray every one of the many figures used has a weapon and must be constantly on guard because there is no way to know who is a bad guy. Opposites are jumbled up together everywhere, including Swamp Thing, Ninja Turtles and their enemies, and diverse Star Wars characters. The creator of this scene has carefully buried a treasure chest behind the large Green Hulk figure. He says that the "good" figures know a treasure is hidden but don't know what or where it is. This is a carefully chosen and created image of the internal chaos of *knowing* you're bad because everyone has always told you that, yet suspecting that there is a "treasure" of goodness somewhere and some good parts to find it with.

In his second tray the good guys on the left confront the bad guys on the right. The two sides are now clearly defined and separated by a fence, a sand wall, and a river with sharks and alligators in it. Perhaps they could stay safely separate except that the bad guys have placed the treasure chest between the "fire devil" and the Green Hulk. The good must attack since the battle is to decide whether the bad or the good will possess the treasure, the totality of the person.

The Green Hulk takes a stand on the good side of another confrontation created by a 12-year-old African American boy who built weekly sand trays in his class for emotionally handicapped (behavior problem) students. American flags, airplane, fire truck, and male power figures stand braced around the Twin Towers, confronting the attacking world-globe.

Swamp Thing

Swamp Thing, an introverted good guy cartoon figure, green and brown like a tree, whose power comes from nature and is only used to protect himself or others, is placed by one boy in the center of a garden home, surrounded by wonderful and playful things. White fences protect him but with a wide open inviting entrance and a one-way sign pointing in. Within that central enclosure this green and brown tree-man stands wearing a whimsically placed black hat, emphasizing perhaps the thinking function in this otherwise instinctual image, acknowledging the "tension between opposites of primitive and civilized" (Jung, 1959, p. 266). As the "wild-man," or "green-man" (Johnson, 1999) this figure represents connectedness to the natural world. This child who, like Adam, was expelled from his home in punishment for his sin, an act of unintentional violence, has perhaps returned to the primeval garden.

ENTER THE BEAST

The Beast symbol points to spirit confined, the kind, intelligent, princely essence underneath the lion-like angry monster persona. A large figure with arms outstretched makes a strong statement about the painful curse that angry and impulsive action brings into the lives of many boys in therapeutic treatment. Another, much smaller Beast figure is studying himself in a mirror after he has met Beauty, perhaps to see himself as others see him now that hope has come into his life. Use of either image implies that boys also are seeking someone (a therapist perhaps) who can look with caring beneath their troubled and troubling behavior and free them from the punishing curse that limits and confines their life.

THE TRICKSTER

The counterpart to heroic masculine figures in movies, Jungian worldview, and many sand trays is often what Jung calls the Trickster archetype. The Trickster is "not really evil but does atrocious things from unconsciousness and unrelatedness" (Jung, 1959, p. 264). The Trickster represents the "shadowy destructive aspects in the human psyche as well as seeds of healing and light" (Porat & Meltzer, 1998, p. 54). It is that aspect of our own nature that is "ready to bring us down when inflated and humanize us when pompous" (Singer, 1973, p. 289). Tricksters bring in the spirit of disorder, the disregard of boundaries (Weller, 1999).

A 9-year-old African American boy who caused the accidental death of his best friend struggles in sandplay to extricate himself from enmeshed identification with the negative Trickster. An early tray shows a prone figure of Batman's perennial shadow/enemy, Joker, banished to a far corner by animals who "growl at him and he runs away from them."

The evil Joker is the Trickster who laughs as he destroys and attacks. He represents the bad side that always loses yet constantly reappears to fight again, mirroring the young boy's ongoing struggle to contain destructive impulses. The Trickster aspect of this boy's personality—getting others into trouble, trying to escape from rules and get special privileges—gets him rejected like Joker. His task is to change Trickster energy into positive, playful interactions.

In a later tray, he places Bart Simpson on the negative side of a bifurcated good-bad scene, bringing in a clownish Trickster mentality that he is beginning to recognize as part of his shadow. The clown "messes up what is supposed to go smoothly, incarnates mistakes that performers can't make" (Larsen, 1990, p. 263). With pranks and sarcasm, he changes terrible emotions into something to be laughed at, creates a bridge between sadness and laughter (Navone, 1998). In Afro-American folktales, the Trickster uses "outrageous actions and unbridled egotism in response to deprivation and death, exaggeration, selfishness, and reprehensible cutting up" to bring meaning to insignificant or painful events (Abrahams, 1985, p. 8).

Other Trickster symbols also appear. TV wrestlers, who use performance skills to seem more violent than they really are, demonstrate physical agility and strength but add an element of Trickster farce since viewers know that many of their aggressive moves are fake. This same boy's work with these wrestlers seems to be a way of mastering the tragedy of having his fake aggressive play with his friend turn out to be so real and lethal.

Casper, the Friendly Ghost

Another Trickster element that appears significant in this boy's sandplay is Casper, the friendly ghost "monster," flying over the scene terrorizing those below: "The monster ate the horse up. He comes to the ground and eats people. Then the sharks come and he eats them up too." Used by this black boy, this is the white shadow figure, the ghost, perhaps of his friend. In Apache lore, people who have died before their time, or violently, hover in darkness, waiting for vengeance by driving the living crazy, or to suicide (Boyer, 1979), just as this boy heard his friend's voice calling him to die. As a Trickster, Casper looks friendly but will gobble you up. Life is not what it appears, so all must protect themselves.

Freddy Kreuger

This evil-looking movie character, Freddy Kreuger holding a skull, is used in diverse ways. The boy who killed his friend picks the figure from the shelf but decides not to use it because he "is mean, can't be in it, he's too scary. I don't like scary people." His avoidance and denial of death issues indicate necessary defenses in his first session, perhaps even positive ego strength to not be compelled by threatening unconscious material.

Another boy chose to place this large image in a beach scene bending over the figures of a young boy and girl sleeping on a bed. His comment concerning this character was: "I like him. He gives me nightmares. I think that's why they have him, to give people nightmares."

A third boy, 11 years old and in family therapy, looks with compassion at the ugly wounds on this figure's face and decides that "he got hurt in the war," as his family members have been hurt by the wars raging in his family.

A 7-year-old black girl in a crisis stabilization unit includes this figure in her struggle with identity, focusing her rage on herself. Three figures are placed in a triangle with Freddy Kreuger looking at the figure of a black girl wearing only a diaper with a finger puppet monster covering her face. A white girl figure with blond hair wears a fancy dress in the third corner. A candelabra in the middle casts the light that projects the shadow quality of this scene. A large rubber knife and a realistic looking toy gun lie to either side of the trio, emphasizing the danger.

STAR WARS

The metaphor of *Star Wars* portrays clearly that the boy (Luke) cannot become a hero until he searches for and fights his own shadow, which is his dark father (Darth Vader), the essence of his male inheritance (Rise, 1994). It is a modern oedipal situation that reflects the actual reality for many boys: an abusive, dangerous father, who has abandoned his son for the power brought by connection to the forces of evil (drugs, crime), who must be acknowledged, then overcome (killed), so that the child can be free to grow (Hunter, 1998).

This multifaceted myth provides significant images that children use to express a range of symbolic meanings.

The friendly, knowledgeable helper robot figures, C3PO and R2D2, are placed in the sand scenes of many children. Robots are considered a symbol of children in placement (A. Bailey, personal communication, October 5, 1994), having to repress their individuality and vitality in order to conform to the requirements of a facility. Traumatized children often feel like robots as protective numbing desensitizes them to their human vulnerability.

Princess Leia is frequently used as an anima/sister figure, young, positive, strong feminine energy sometimes confronting the devouring feminine in the shape of a dragon, dinosaur, or alligator. The Leia, Han Solo, and Luke characters are brought into sand scenes to illustrate the positive loyal support and sometimes negative demands of sibling and peer relationships.

The diverse beings found on the good side of the galactic battles help children explore issues of diversity and difference in their own lives. Chewbacca's struggles with speech, the Ewoks' small stature, and Yoda's strange appearance can be used to symbolize the friendship and respect that exist despite these social challenges. Perhaps the most powerful message of this myth for struggling children is knowledge that what ultimately prevails over the evil elements is the "Force" of courageous inner resources and determination (Crowley & Mills, 1989).

THE ARCHETYPAL FEMININE: WICKED STEPMOTHER—FAIRY GODMOTHER

Much therapeutic work in sandplay mirrors fairy-tale themes in which the real help as well as real trouble comes from women figures, thus representing the importance of the mother in a young child's life (Lurie, 1990). Many children who have not had adequate mothering tend to relate more to the archetypal feminine than to the real. The terrible mother is often portrayed as the witch, the evil queen, or ugly creatures. The loving mother shows up as an angel or nurturing animal. The fairy godmother is the positive feminine power to transform, as in making Pinocchio into a real boy, or changing the Beast back into a prince.

The boy who accidentally killed his friend works intensely on mother issues.

In an early tray, the queen who we know to be evil in another story, arms and cape outstretched, stands in the center as the "protector of everybody." The great mother, both terrible and nurturing, raises her arms in a shamanic gesture of magic or blessing. Here is a powerful illustration of contrasting levels of meaning. The image of protection that is personal and conscious to the builder stands in opposition to the fairy-tale, universal unconscious meaning of this figure as actively intending to kill the child. When this wicked stepmother gives Snow White poisoned food, offering death instead of life, the maternal relationship produces chaos and confusion in the child's psyche rather than order and meaning. However, when the terrible mother condemns Snow White to death, she also moves her toward growing up, finding her own strength (Dougherty, 1995), and individuation.

In a later tray, this same figure is reinforced on the left by another wicked queen with horns on her helmet and a dagger in her hand. Her alter image, under the right wing of the protector, is the fairy godmother, westernized compassionate Kuan Yin energy, with butterfly wings and a golden wand. Thus, "good" nurturing feminine figures on the right, the conscious, side of the tray, are shadowed by the "bad" threatening figures on the other. The evil side of the protector, mother figure is revealed.

Snow White's dwarves also have a role to play in this boy's story. Two of them cooperate to move themselves by their own power. Their energy brings treasure up from deep within the matriarchal earth, unconscious content struggling toward the light, the gold hidden in the shadow realms (Jung in Weinrib, 1983). They provide refuge to Snow White as she flees from death at the hands of the terrible mother, preserving her beauty and goodness until it can be safely reawakened. Their presence tells us that the child's process will require digging deep and working hard and will probably result in finding something valuable.

The time Snow White spent living with the dwarves could equate to the child's time in treatment, where if he works hard, takes responsibility, and finds solutions to conflicts, his ego will mature and he moves into adolescence. His task of acknowledging both positive and negative aspects of the mother and discovering his own path to meaning and order in life is further complicated by the trauma of having given death to a friend when he thought he was offering play. Finding compassion for the good part of the evil queen is perhaps part of finding compassion and forgiveness for himself.

Another female movie figure clearly symbolizes the Terrible Mother. A boy torn by family conflict created a series of sand tray scenes portraying attack by threatening figures surrounding the intended victim. Eventually, the central figure became Cruella, the evil mistress of *101 Dalmatians*, whose only interest in the puppies is to make a coat from their skins. The figure has half-white, half-black hair, a malevolent smile and hands covered with red blood, an apt image for this boy's rejecting stepmother. Instead of having her killed, however, his story brings in the police to take her off to jail and free the dogs.

OTHER ASPECTS OF THE FEMININE ARCHETYPE

Wonder Woman brings in the feminine counterpart to Superman, the Amazon whose strength is used positively to assist those in need. She represents feminine strength used in masculine ways—wrestling, riding horses, keeping animals (instincts) under control.

The Pocahontas character takes on diverse roles in the children's stories. For a boy in the Balkans, she became a peaceful warrior. His early scenes portrayed his town at war with civilians lying dead and dismembered under attack from soldiers. A later scene placed Pocahontas leading numerous animals (spirits of the people who had been killed) to a meeting with the chiefs of several Indian tribes. They are at first afraid and plan to attack her but then they listen to her message of peace and ultimately "peace happens."

Another boy, who was a baby when war devastated his country, spent his childhood in an orphanage. He worked hard over 6 years of sandplay in camp to resolve abandonment issues and imagine the concept of family, using multiple evil movie witch figures to express his view of Mother. As a young adolescent, he progressed to creating family scenes in which Pocahontas is the loving mother surrounded by many children with Aladdin as the father.

An 8-year-old girl in a school sand tray group used two identical figures of Pocahontas to express a terrifying experience that had led to psychiatric hospitalization the night before her group session. The female figure lies vulnerably on her back in the center of a circle of threatening reptilian creatures, creating what Grubbs (1994) has termed a mandala-shaped "wound tray," releasing the hurtful material. The second Pocahontas figure lies outside the circle on her side facing, but removed from, the dangerous center, a vibrant image of the psychic act of dissociation to cope with extreme stress.

A young teenage girl in a Crisis Stabilization Unit expresses fascination with the occult, demonic, and supernatural. Her sandplay scenes contrast "all that is good in the world," represented by Wizard of Oz's good witch Glinda and Pinocchio's fairy godmother, with the evil forces of Oz's bad witch and Aladdin's Jafar. Dragons, unicorns, and real animals of land and sea fight on each side of the battle for the crystal that is "the key to all power." As the work proceeds, the good women figures protect the small, capture the crystal and a large gold key that "unlocks the castle where the good fairies live," and move into the center of the tray.

Aladdin and Jasmine fly through the scenes on their magic carpet, watched by their genie, who smiles benevolently as he emerges from his lamp. The power of their young love gradually displaces Jafar from his dominant position in the tray.

The Little Mermaid, Ariel, becomes an identification figure for this girl, as she accepts the task of finding a way to live in both conscious and unconscious worlds. The movie figure of this young female moves from a side position surrounded and almost hidden by sea animals, to a stream-like path drawn in the sand, to a blue stream in which gold fish swim, and finally into the center of a large pool where she is truly in her element. Another figure of Ariel as human now takes her place on the land. The little mermaid has helped this troubled girl find her voice and imagine a way to survive in an alien environment.

CONCLUSION

Children's sand worlds are often complex and go deeply into power-ful realms. In following their hero's journey, we see them regress to the trauma that brought them into treatment, express it in action and images, in feelings and thoughts, and release the wounds that disabled them. We observe the meetings that occur as they travel: with the monsters and devouring animals of the shadow, with the helpful and wise characters of their resilience, with the masculine images of the father archetype and strengthening ego, and the feminine images of the mother archetype and the anima as they find the resources to transcend their disastrous personal histories. We follow them as they integrate the opposites they have encountered, and discover the treasure of the spirit within (Hunter, 1998).

On this journey, they receive help from characters familiar to them from popular cultural media. Among the movie and television renditions of fairy tales and modern myths, children gather powerful masculine and feminine forces to deal with the traumas they have experienced. They find allies to help them fight the inner demons that torment them, ways to integrate the opposites and conflicts in their lives, and arche-typal parents to compensate for absent or negative real ones. In symbolic sandplay terms, they find ways to balance the compassionate good mas-culine strength of Superman with the evil, jealous feminine power of the stepmother-queens; the nurturing magic of the fairy godmother with the evil tricks of the Joker.

Through these movie images children connect to the fairy tale stories that most relate to their life, the inner and outer pressures they expe-rience, and the solutions they need. They receive a powerful message: "a struggle against severe difficulties in life is unavoidable . . . but if one does not shy away but steadfastly meets unexpected and often unjust hardships, one masters all obstacles and at the end emerges victorious" (Bettelheim, 1976, p. 6).

REFERENCES

Abrahams, R. (1985). *Afro-American folktales: Stories from black traditions in the new world.* New York: Pantheon.

Bettelheim, B. (1976). *The uses of enchantment: The meaning and importance of fairy tales.* New York: Vintage Books.

Boyer, L. (1979). *Childhood and folklore: A psychoanalytic study of Apache personality.* New York: Library of Psychoanalytic Anthropology.

Bradway, K. (1986, September). *Sandplay: What makes it work?* Tenth International Congress for Analytical Psychology.

Bradway, K., & McCoard, B. (1997). *Sandplay—Silent workshop of the psyche.* New York: Routledge.

Campbell, J., & Moyers, B. (1988). *The power of myth.* New York: Doubleday.

Capitolo, M. (2002). Chaos theory and its application to the sandplay process. *Journal of Sandplay Therapy* 11(2), 37–53.

Crowley, R., & Mills, J. (1989). *Cartoon magic: How to help children discover their rainbows within.* New York: Magination Press.

Dougherty, N. (1995). Snow White. In M. Stein & L. Corbett (Eds.), *Psyche's stories: Modern Jungian interpretations of fairy tales.* Wilmette, IL: Chiron Publications.

Gil, E. (1991). *The healing power of play: Working with abused children.* New York: Guilford Press.

Grubbs, G. (1994). Into the wound: The psychic healing of abused children. *Journal of Sandplay Therapy* 4(1), 67–85.

Henderson, J. (1964). Ancient myths and modern man. In C. G. Jung (Ed.), *Man and his symbols.* New York: Laurel Books.

Hunter, L. B. (1998). *Images of resiliency: Troubled children create healing stories in the language of sandplay.* Palm Beach, FL: Behavioral Communications Institute.

Johnson, D. (1999). Fairy tale symbolism applied to sandplay. *Journal of Sandplay Therapy* 8(2), 65–86.

Jung, C. G. (1959). *Four archetypes: Mother, rebirth, spirit, trickster.* Princeton, NJ: Bollingen.

Jung, C. G. (1964). *Man and his symbols.* New York: Dell Publishing.

Jung, C. G. (1971). *The portable Jung.* J. Campbell (Ed.). New York: Viking.

Kalff, D. (1980). *Sandplay: A psychotherapeutic approach to the psyche.* Boston: Sigo Press.

Kiepenheuer, K. (1990). *Crossing the bridge: A Jungian approach to adolescence.* La Salle, IL: Open Court.

Larsen, S. (1990). *The mythic imagination: Your quest for meaning for personal mythology.* New York: Bantam Books.

Lowenfeld, M. (1979). *The world technique.* London: George Allen & Unwin.

Lurie, A. (1990). *Don't tell the grown-ups: Why kids love the books they do.* New York: Avon Books.

Mills, J., & Crowley, R. (1986). *Therapeutic metaphors for children and the child within.* New York: Brunner/Mazel.

Navone, A. (1998). The double birth. *Journal of Sandplay Therapy* 7(1), 27–60.

Porat, R., & Meltzer, B. (1998). Images of war and images of peace. *Journal of Sandplay Therapy* 7(2), 25–71.

Rise, C. (1994). Men's violence in sandplay. *Journal of Sandplay Therapy* 4(1), 19–35.

Shaia, A. (1994). A change in season: The renewed masculine. *Journal of Sandplay Therapy* 4(1), 13–17.

Singer, J. (1973). *Boundaries of the soul.* New York: Doubleday.

Sugatt, S. (1999). Superman: A modern myth. *Journal of Sandplay Therapy* 8(1), 77–88.

Weinrib, E. (1983). *Images of the self.* Boston: Sigo Press

Weller, B. (1999). Transformation of a teacher. *Journal of Sandplay Therapy* 8(2), 47–63.

PART IV

Video and Board Games

CHAPTER 9

Taking the Sand Tray High Tech

Using *The Sims* as a Therapeutic Tool in the Treatment of Adolescents

Deidre Skigen

Man is still the most extraordinary computer of all.

—John F. Kennedy

One's clinical techniques tend to change as a function
of the trends of the times, though one's goals remain the same.

—Gardner (1991)

It is a challenge to be in a public space and not hear a cell phone ring, observe a one-sided conversation, see children playing handheld video games or watch the lightning-fast fingers of a text messager. Portable technology is all around us and it is here to stay. In my practice, I see more and more children bringing their cell phones, GameBoys™, MP3 players, iPods, and laptops into session. I instituted a therapy room rule that all electronic devices needed to be shut off. To some of my clients this was a challenge. I had several adolescents devise creative ways to get around the rule and text message during session. I knew that video games had been used successfully in psychotherapy (Favelle, 1995). I retreated to the old adage: "If you can't beat them, join them" and so I did. Enter The Sims as the modern-day answer to the sand tray.

SAND, WATER, AND MINIATURES: A HISTORICAL AND THEORETICAL OVERVIEW

The history of sandplay follows a natural progression along with a series of integral historical events that allowed for its development. In addition to his landmark books *The Time Machine* (Wells, 1895) and *War of the Worlds* (1898), H.G. Wells penned two little-known books entitled *Little Wars* (1913) and *Floor Games* (1911). In them, and in particular the latter, he discussed in great detail the play time he spent with his sons creating inventive and complete miniature worlds. Wells instructed the reader on the ideal environment in which to play. He described the setup of a proper play area, from the location to the setting up of a proper floor, to lighting, and ventilation. He categorized the toys and building materials into two groups: structural objects that can be used over and over again and secondary objects that play a supportive role in the play. He and his sons transformed the linoleum floor into railway systems, twin cities, and exotic islands. Wells believed that this type of floor play and the infinite ways in which to create and play with elaborate and meticulous miniature worlds would fortify the imagination and serve the players well in adulthood.

Wells's book inspired Margaret Lowenfeld, a London physician, to create her "World Technique" or "Worldplay" (Boik & Goodwin, 2000). She was self-described as an unhappy and delicate child who was often ill and isolated (Mitchell & Friedman, 1994). Her parents divorced and she and her sister lived with their mother, who though sickly and herself dependent, encouraged both daughters to pursue careers in medicine. Margaret dedicated herself to extensive medical, military, and humanitarian service.

In attempts to expunge her own devils and answer plaguing questions, Lowenfeld opened the Clinic for Nervous and Difficult Children, one of the first clinics to address the psychological needs of children (Mitchell & Friedman, 1994). She said that

> All children are difficult sometimes, but some children are difficult all the time. Some children seem always to be catching something and never to be quite well. Some children are nervous and find life and school too difficult for them. Some children have distressing habits. This Clinic, which is in charge of a Physician, exists to help mothers in these kinds of trouble with their children, and also to help the children themselves. (Lowenfeld, cited in Mitchell & Friedman, 1994, p. 8)

Corresponding with the opening of the clinic, Lowenfeld remembered reading Wells' book. She modified the play described by Wells into a therapeutic model, which eventually evolved into the World Technique. She gathered miniatures, sticks, paper, toys, and various other objects. These objects were housed in what came to be known as the "Wonder Box" (Boik & Goodwin, 2000).

In the new clinic, the contents of the Wonder Box were placed in a cabinet, which became known as the world. The children would play with the toys on the floor. Eventually Lowenfeld added two zinc trays to the playroom. One contained sand and the other water. Now the children had a space to play in and create amazing sand stories (Boik & Goodwin, 2000).

> Here, in this child-created technique, Lowenfeld had found the instrument of her search. When children used miniatures in a shallow sand tray, their emotional and mental states of mind were communicated in a way that could be objectively recorded and analyzed. With the aid of this technique, she could now begin her work of exploring the child's mental processes. (Mitchell & Friedman, 1994, p. 9)

Lowenfeld felt that, "The process of such play seems to help children to express the inexpressible, to make visible that which is indefinable, elusive, a way of projecting the inner world of feeling" (Schaeffer & O'Connor, 1983; p. 157). Lowenfeld reflected that the sand pictures represented the child's unconscious life. The play provided a beautiful place where the child could convey what he needed to communicate to the therapist without having to use words (Mitchell & Friedman, 1994).

Dr. Lowenfeld provided thorough instructions on how to set up the play space. She began with a tray 29.5 × 20.5 × 2.8 inches that was filled halfway with coarse sand. She believed the specific size enabled the child to see the whole tray while keeping his head still. The interior of the tray is painted blue to simulate water. She believed the tray height should be waist high depending upon the height of the child. The extensive collection of miniatures and toys used in the sand tray should be within the child's reach in a cabinet (Mitchell & Friedman, 1994).

Lowenfeld categorized her technique in two parts. The first she called *the bridge*, which is to connect the adults and the children who live on opposite sides of the river. The second is *picture thinking* where the pictures serve as a way to communicate what is unable to be verbalized (Mitchell & Friedman, 1994).

In the 1930s, at the same time as Lowenfeld was developing the World Technique, Charlotte Buhler and her physician husband, Karl Buhler, developed novel observational approaches to measure and test children's developmental maturation. Some of their techniques of child observation are relevant today (Mitchell & Friedman, 1994).

Buhler's skill was as a researcher while Lowenfeld's was a clinician. Through their mutual respect for each other's work, they began creating norms for normal and psychologically impaired children and validation of the results from Lowenfeld's World Technique. Buhler is credited with creating the World Test (Mitchell & Friedman, 1994).

Dora Kalff was a Jungian analyst who worked with children. She heard Lowenfeld present her World Technique at a conference. She was intrigued and asked to study with Lowenfeld, who agreed. Kalff combined her Jungian training with her knowledge of the World Technique and developed sandplay (Boik & Goodwin, 2000) In sandplay, the individual makes a series of trays over a period of time. Kalff believed that what the patient made in the sand was directed by the unconscious. The therapist does not make interpretations at the time of the creation of the trays. If analysis is made, it is after the sandplay process is concluded and both the therapist and the sandplayer discuss the meaning of the trays. The healing power of the process is not placed on the outcome but on the nonverbal communication relayed through the picture created (Bradway, 2006). Kalff theorized "that Sandplay provided a natural therapeutic modality for the child, allowing the expression of both the archetypal and intra-personal worlds, as well as connecting the child to outer everyday reality" (Mitchell & Friedman, 1994, p. 50). The secure and contained play space formed and held by the therapist would allow the child to reconnect his "ego and Self" and thus "function in a more balanced and congruent manner" (Mitchell & Friedman, 1994). Sandplay enlists the child's imagination to create in a tangible medium. The trays are seen by the creator and the observer at the time of play (Bradway & McCoard, 1997). This process allows both the therapist and child to actually see the creation of the picture unfold in a mutually shared experience in a supportive environment.

Gisela Schubach De Dominico, PhD, a transformational healer and psychotherapist, studied with Dora Kalff. Margaret Lowenfeld's work was the subject of De Dominico's doctoral thesis. Building on their expertise, De Dominico conducted sandplay research with preschool children and developed the Sandtray-World Play model in the 1980s. She began training mental health professionals and educators in Sandtray-Worldplay and Dynamic Expressive Play Therapy. To this end she formed the Vision Quest into Symbolic Reality training program. She continues to share her knowledge and love for sandplay through workshops, lectures, seminars, and publications. For De Domenico, "trusting the psyche and its play products to faithfully indicate the clients' movement toward healing and growth" is the central idea embraced in her model (Boik & Goodman, 2000). She recognizes the importance of both the unconscious and the deep conscious in creating the sand picture. De Domenico advocates using different colored sands in trays of differing shapes. The focus is on the client's journey and the therapist acts as a co-explorer.

THE SIMS WORLD: A BRIEF OVERVIEW

In 1984, computer game designer Will Wright created *The Raid of Bungling Bay*, a game centered on a fortified island under attack by a renegade helicopter. Wright, who attended a Montessori school as a child, was an avid model builder. While making Bungling Bay, Wright realized that he enjoyed making the islands instead of annihilating them. It was then that he came up with the idea for SimCity (Electronic Arts Inc., 2007). Basically, SimCity is a one-person game. The objective is to create, build, and inhabit a city. The player designs the infrastructure, disasters, and rewards that are unique to his city and controls every aspect of the Sims' lives. A variety of scenarios and actual city maps are offered depending upon the edition.

In the world of video games, where action sells, it is not surprising that the first edition of SimCity for the Commodore 64 did not sell well. With competition from other wildly popular games at the time, SimCity looked tame. The game centered on construction of virtual worlds rather than their destruction. The player could neither win nor lose.

Wright met investor Jeff Braun at a pizza party in 1986. Braun was interested in entering the computer game industry and the two joined forces and founded the company Maxis in 1987. The company first published SimCity in 1989. The game was available for both the PC and Mac and was distributed by Broderbund. According to the Maxis Web site, "Sales are initially sluggish leaving Wright and Braun to handle all the tech support from Braun's apartment" (Electronic Arts, Inc., 2007). With strong word of mouth and a story in *Newsweek,* SimCity took off and Maxis could not keep the games on store shelves. With SimCity, Maxis had established a new genre for video gaming: System Simulation Games. Ironically they built such a good simulation game that it attracted the attention of the Central Intelligence Agency and the Defense Department.

Not long after, SimCity could be found in more than 10,000 classrooms as an educational aid. The public was clamoring for sequels. By 1994, SimCity 2000 was published. Loaded with new features, it was the top-selling video game in the world for 6 months. Now SimCity is on its fourth version.

In 1997, Maxis was bought out by Electronic Arts, Inc. The gaming creativity continued and EA released The Sims in 2000 to rave reviews and explosive sales. Expansion packs and add-on simulations with a variety of topics were soon published. In addition, the game is available for a variety of platforms including Xbox, Sony Play Station 2, Nintendo, and even mobile phones.

Will Wright, being the ever-imaginative gamer, developed Sims 2 with more realism and tech tricks. In this series, a player can delve deeper into the Sims' lives and feel a part of their world. "Like the toys of our youth, modern videogames rely on the player's active involvement. We're invited to create and interact with elaborately simulated worlds, characters, and story lines. Games aren't just fantasy worlds to explore; they actually amplify our powers of imagination" (Wright, 2006, p. 1). They provide the player with an opportunity to both create and tell a story of significance about themselves.

SIMSPLAY: THE GAME

Once you sit down at the computer screen, The Sims becomes your world, you create your Sims, and whether they thrive or perish is entirely up to you. This might seem like a daunting task at first, but with a little imagination and some video gaming know-how, you can create a wonderfully full life for your Sim. When you enter the game you are welcomed to the neighborhood and asked if you want to get acquainted with the system. If you are a first-time player you can take a tutorial to become familiar with the game basics.

Once familiar with the play, you begin a fully loaded game. First things first; you create your (Sim) character or in Simspeak, your avatar. You select the gender, age, skin tone, face, attire, personality, marital status, history, and job skills for all of the Sims. You can choose to enter an already existing family or create your own by adding family members (of your own design). You can also choose to go it alone for the time being.

There are a number of control features and game mechanics that necessitate learning so that the game can move along smoothly. The component of importance is the control panel. This is where all of the action is directed and monitored. It is located on the lower left side of the game screen. The panel is divided into sections. The lower left side is the action side. Here you control and monitor the game modes, floor plan, walls, game speed and time, views (zoom and rotation), household budget, and number of friends. The right side of the control panel contains the information on current Sims needs states.

Your Sim can function in five basic modes. Most of the time, your Sim will be in the live mode where the action happens. The other four modes are the Buy Mode, Build Mode, Camera Mode, and Options Mode. In the Live Mode you can speed up or pause the action. There are three speeds, normal, high, and ultra high. You can zoom in and rotate your view of your Sim's life. You assist your Sim in managing the household budgets, looking at job performance, adding or subtracting the number of family members, directing friends and romances they have and sustain. You can have your Sim take a tour around the neighborhood, make friends, go to work or school, have a dinner party, sleep, or basically accomplish anything you would in your own life. An essential part of the game, in this mode, is monitoring your Sim's current needs. Filling these needs is very important, as will be discussed later.

In the Buy Mode you purchase items for your Sim's house. The purchases are made from two categories, by its function or by the room it will furnish. You can also direct your Sim to add on to his existing house or build his dream house. The design, planning, and building take place in the Build Mode.

You can document your Sim's life in the Camera Mode. Here you take pictures of your Sim for their photo album. If you forget to take pictures of significant moments in your Sims' life the game will take the picture for you. All of these pictures end up in the Photo Album for viewing at any time by your Sim.

In the Options Mode, you can manage the game play. In this setting you can save your current game, change neighborhoods, choose graphics, and manage sound selections. The most important component of this mode is the free will option. Here you can give your Sim the ability to make autonomous choices. Sometimes he will take a nap, or get something to eat without direction in order to satisfy his needs. This happens because his needs score is too low. Given free will, your Sim will decide to listen to you or not depending on his mood state. Your Sim can be very temperamental and difficult to control or he can be agreeable or anywhere in between. If you decide not to give your Sim free will and then neglect the Sim's needs, the Sim can die.

The right side of the control panel contains information on the state of the Sim's needs. You can monitor mental and physical states of your Sim by clicking on the needs panel and looking at the progress bar. Green indicates that the particular need is being met, while red indicates the need must be addressed or face the consequences, literally: the grim reaper might show up. As in Maslow's hierarchy, your Sims are motivated by their needs, or in Simspeak, their motives.

The game gives the Sims eight basic motives. They include hunger, comfort, hygiene, bladder, energy, fun, social, and room. These motives drive your Sim's actions and behaviors. The rate at which these motives need to be satisfied is different for each Sim because it is linked to his personality. Those Sims who are more outgoing will have a higher need to be social and have fun. You can look at your needs grid on the control panel and then click on each need to get more information. These needs must be monitored throughout the game in order to keep balanced and healthy Sims. A "happy" Sim moves forward in life embracing new situations as they come.

In creating your Sim, you can select from a variety of personality traits. Your Sim's personality comes from selecting the degree of each quality you want your Sim to have or through their star sign. The sign's traits are either filled in by the game or taken from the personality you have given your Sim. Only the positive ones are listed and their opposites are inferred (neat/messy, outgoing/shy, active/sedentary, playful/serious, nice/irritable). You can design what type of relationship they have with other Sims. It is important to remember that your Sim's personality will be reflected in the game. Depending on the degree of the traits some activities will be harder than others. If your Sim is on the shy side then it might take more time and be more difficult to interact socially or initiate and form relationships. One of the great things about this game is that once you have created a character you can decide to edit his or her persona or delete him or her entirely and create a new Sim.

Your Sim can select from a variety of jobs or career paths in order to bring money into the household and create purchasing power. There are 10 career paths, each with 10 levels of promotion. Your Sim can choose from business, politics, law enforcement, life of crime, military, medicine, science, entertainment, athletics, and extreme sports. To find a job, your Sim can select one from the newspaper, delivered daily, or if he has a computer, from a Sim online website where he can choose from multiple job listings at a time. This can be easy or a challenge depending upon your Sim's personality and or needs state. I recommend that your Sim be in a good mood before you ask him to find a job. You can direct your Sim to find a job but because of free will, he may be happy with the first job available or might refuse or say he is too depressed. It is one story to get a job but it is quite another to keep one. There are six skill sets that correspond to all jobs. The skill sets include cooking, charisma, body, mechanical, logic, and creativity. For example, if your Sim is in entertainment he may need more charisma than mechanical skills. Your Sim can upgrade his skill set and climb the levels with promotions and raises. On the first day of work, an assigned carpool will pick him up at the chosen time and take him to work. Good ways for your Sim to get demoted or fired are having a bad attitude, not keeping up his job skills, or missing carpool twice in a row.

Sims are not immune to disasters or death. There are three types of disasters: household floods, household fires, and household robbery. These disasters can be small or catastrophic. If your Sim's house catches on fire and there is no fire alarm, the house will be destroyed and if a Sim is in the house, he could be killed. When a Sim dies, all who knew him automatically mourn for a full day. They do not need to be directed to do so.

IS SIMSPLAY SIMPLY HIGH-TECH SANDPLAY?

My bias as a play therapist is that you cannot have too many toys in your toy box. I love my sand tray and use it often; however, it is refreshing to have an alternative. Basically, I use The Sims game as a virtual sand tray for children over the ages of about 8 to 10. For my younger clients, I have found it more developmentally appropriate to use the sandtray. As Piaget described, games with rules are rarely used with children ages 4 to 7. They are most successful with those ages 7 and above (Piaget, 1962). The younger clients seem to gravitate much more toward the sand and seem to disregard the computer. Most love to get their hands, and sometimes feet, in the different textured sands. They are willing to put almost anything in the sand tray to assist them in their play.

Boik and Goodman offer that sandplay is an "imaginative activity in the sand [that is a] mirror for the individuation process" taking place in a protected and tolerant setting (2000, p. 17). The play itself is held inside a specified container. The client can choose to use water and/or objects to create a static or moving world. The results of the play are visible symbols of the unseen issues within the client's psyche. The play becomes the language in which the client communicates with himself and the therapist. Sandplay can be used with children, adults, couples, families, and groups.

I believe that Simsplay is a creative undertaking in the safe environment of cyberspace that allows for the development of self-awareness. The play takes place within the identified area of a computer screen with a variety of objects, backgrounds, and characters. The world that is created can be paused or sped up. The play is a vehicle for the unconscious to become conscious in a visible form. There is a nonverbal communication between the client and therapist that facilitates healing and growth. This video game can be used with individuals (over the age of 7) in a group, as a couple or family.

The Sims game meets most criteria set forth by Lowenfeld and Kalff. Play takes place in a fixed-size container—your computer screen. Within the container are an unlimited number of backgrounds and setting in which to play. The screen is at eye level so the child can attend to the entire image in one glance. The individual has at his disposal an almost infinite number of miniatures supplied by the game, its expansion packs, or online. The miniatures are separated from the play area until they are needed, so as not to overwhelm the player with the sheer numbers. The miniatures are from a variety of categories including people, animals, plants, household items, and transportation vehicles (Boik and Goodman, 2000). It is not the same as sand but there is the tactile sensation of typing on the keyboard and manipulating the mouse to direct the objects.

Along with The Sims (miniatures) come a myriad of choices. You create other Sims to your liking; you can choose which Sim you want to control at what time; you can choose what needs to meet or not, and you can create new Sims, or delete Sims, houses, and objects you no longer want . . . the choice is yours.

The game allows for the player's unconscious issues to be brought into awareness in a visible format that can be saved and revisited later. It provides a venue for nonverbal communication of thought, feelings, and ideas. It works in addition to psychotherapy so that therapeutic orientation is not an issue. The game provides a rich framework in which fantasies and wishes can be played out. Most of all, it is fun.

In both Sandplay and Simsplay, the play reestablishes psychological balance. In this context, James (1994) notes:

> In this mode, children give themselves exactly what they need to reduce anxieties and to resolve conflicts. Under the guise of play, they can balance power, reward themselves with fabulous riches, vanquish those who do not do their bidding, and devour their enemies. The experiences of power and invincibility enable the child to work and rework an issue until such negative feelings as fear, helplessness, and revenge are sufficiently under control to allow the child to deal with reality. (p. 53)

We have looked at the ways that The Sims simulation game is analogous to Sandplay. How is The Sims different? Besides the obvious point of being played on a computer, the biggest difference is that the player must play within the confines of the game's speed and computer memory. You must have a computer with a memory that is sufficient to run and save the games. In addition, although minimal, it takes a fixed amount of time for the game to load and set up before play can begin.

Playing the game is time consuming and may take several sessions to complete. The length of playing time depends upon the amount of time scheduled for the session and the time it takes for the player to feel finished. Leaving a game in the middle of play might be difficult.

The Sims is an interactive game. The player must be prepared for feedback from the game. At some point, your Sim will defy your commands, which can be a great challenge. It is then up to the player to address the challenge. Each player has a different approach to the defiance. This in itself can be a useful therapeutic tool.

In order to take full advantage of the game, your client must be at a certain developmental level and have an interest in playing video games. If either one is lacking, the therapy will not be as effective as it otherwise could. The Sims is not for everyone. If you are interested in using it as a therapeutic tool, I suggest you take some time to explore your Sim's world.

CASE STUDIES

When I was first introduced to The Sims, I was fascinated. I was immediately impressed with the detailed graphics and the amazing range

that was shy, neat, low in energy, playful at times, and relatively nice. She chose a modest house and furnished it so that her avatar would be comfortable. After all, Sims have a strong need for comfort. Jenny took great care in making sure that her avatar's needs were met. She never let the motive score drop more than one bar.

Although it was socially a challenge for her character (and for her), she did make some friends in order to keep her needs score from dropping. She chose to get married so that she could create a family of her own. She created her husband to have all of the personality points the same as she gave herself. She only interacted with her husband when his needs were running low. This continued for a number if sessions. Money was a need and Jenny took the first job she was offered—popcorn vender at the circus. Over the next several sessions, she began creating friends and simultaneously began verbalizing about her activities at school. Although it was apparent Jenny missed her previous school, she began to talk about people and activities at her new school. We stopped playing The Sims regularly about the time she joined the school choir. Our sessions continued for a few more months. Jenny's grades stabilized and she was eventually admitted to regular classes. Every once in a while we would revisit The Sims game in order to role play in preparation for an upcoming event in her life.

Ben

Ben was a 19-year-old college student who exhibited symptoms of anxiety and mild depression. It was his first year in college and his first time away from home. Academically, he had done very well in high school but was struggling with freshman classes. This was a completely new world for him educationally, socially, and geographically. His family and friends were states away and he was faced with creating a new support and social network. He was now responsible for himself. He shared that he had never used a washing machine, so his dirty clothes were piling up.

Ben shared that he felt overwhelmed and that it was difficult for him to follow through on anything. He did not get along with his roommate, felt isolated, and was uninterested in school activities. He had expected his college experience to be different and in his eyes it was turning out to be a disaster. In high school, Ben was popular and participated in a variety of school activities. He said that all he did now was "sit on the computer." He said he had only time for studying and preparing for classes and no time for recreation and relaxation.

Although well spoken, Ben did not want to talk about his problems. He said that talking about all that was going on with him made him more nervous. I asked if he would like to play a video game called The Sims. He had heard of the game but not played it. We set up The Sims and he created his avatar. At first he said it was a little stressful, because he did not know how to play the game. New experiences and change seemed to be the biggest challenge for Ben at that time. We processed through the setup of the game and the creation of his Sim. In Ben's case, he was very verbal during the setup and initial stages of the game. Gradually, as his comfort level increased, his verbal interactions decreased. His body language became more relaxed and he seemed to be enjoying the experience.

For Ben, the details of the play became secondary to the play itself. It was the act of playing the game that took him out of his anxious state and assisted him to enter a state of calm, relaxation, and enjoyment. It did not seem to matter what was going on with his Sims; he realized that no matter how chaotic or disorganized his Sims became, he could assist them in handling the situation by virtue of his relaxed state. This generalized to his college life. He reported sleeping better and being able to complete tasks in a timely manner. He became more aware of the feelings under his anxiety. He was able to make a few friends and said that college life was "looking up."

BEYOND SIMSPLAY

Technology is a ubiquitous force in contemporary culture. Communication devices, personal computers, and handheld games are the norm. The Sims game is one way to marry the conventional with the unconventional. In addition to using The Sims in the traditional Sandplay model, you can use the game in a more directive manner. As a role playing vehicle, individuals will be able to work out conflicts within their families, at school, at work.

I remember the lyrics from a Girl Scout song we used to sing, which went: "Make new friends, but keep the old. One is silver, the other is gold." Without a doubt, sandplay is the gold standard. The Sims game in all of its incarnations puts a new face on a time-tested methodology. As appropriate new games appear on the tech horizon, they will always be welcome in my toy box.

REFERENCES

Bradway, K. (2006). What is sandplay? *Journal of Sandplay Therapy, 15*(2), 1–3.
Bradway, K., & McCoard, B. (1997). *Sandplay: Silent workshop of the psyche.* London: Routledge.

Boik, B., & Goodwin, E. (2000). *Sandplay therapy: A step-by-step manual for psychotherapists of diverse orientations.* New York: Norton.

Electronic Arts, Inc. (2007). *Inside scoop.* Retrieved May 2, 2007, from http://simcity.ea.com/about/inside_scoop/sc_retrospective.php

Favelle, G. (1995). Therapeutic applications of commercially available computer software. *Computers in Human Services, 11*(1/2), 151–158.

Gardner, J. (1991). Can the Mario Bros. help? Nintendo games as an adjunct in psychotherapy with children. *Psychotherapy, 28*(4), 667–670.

James, L. (1994). Long-term treatment for children with severe trauma history. In M. B. Williams & J. F. Sommer (Eds.), *Handbook of post-traumatic therapy* (pp. 51–68). Westport, CT: Greenwood Press.

Maxis (2006). *Maxis—A timeline.* Retrieved May 2, 2007, from http://maxis.com/about/about_timeline1.php

Mitchell, R. R., & Friedman, H. S. (1994). *Sandplay: Past, present, and future.* New York: Routledge.

Piaget, J. (1962). *Play, dreams and imitation in childhood.* C. Gattegno & F. M. Hodgson (Trans.). New York: Norton.

Schaefer, C., & O'Connor, K. (1983). *Handbook of play therapy.* New York: Wiley.

Wells, H. G. (1911). *Floor games.* London: Frank Palmer.

Wells, H. G. (1913). *Little wars.* London: Frank Palmer.

Wells, H. G. (1895). *The time machine.* London: William Heinemann.

Wells, H. G. (1898). *The war of the worlds.* London: William Heinemann.

Wright, W. (2006). *Dream machines.* Retrieved May 15, 2007, from http:/www.wired.com/wired/archive/14.04/wright.html

CHAPTER 10

Picking Up Coins

The Use of Video Games in the Treatment of Adolescent Social Problems

George Enfield and Melonie Grosser

Upon first hearing of the use of video games in therapy, one might ask, "Can this really be therapeutic?" In an era in which clinicians are being increasingly pressured to incorporate evidence-based interventions and manualized treatments into their clinical work, how can they justify treatment that incorporates video games, particularly in light of the fact that little supportive research exists for their clinical utility and as a result, they are not yet considered best practices? While it is important for clinicians to be creative and flexible, and to develop innovative interventions, it is equally important that we continue to use tested methods.

Consideration of the use of video games in therapy requires a willingness on the part of the clinician to expand and explore alternative interventions and techniques that parallel the dynamic, fast-paced, technologically driven worlds in which our young clients live. It is often through the clues and cues provided to us in our therapeutic encounters that we can develop new, timely, relevant, and effective intervention strategies. Toward this end, video games, as a prominent fixture in both popular culture and the daily lives of many children across socioeconomic and cultural boundaries, may offer clinicians just such a resource.

VIDEO GAMES AND SOCIAL DEVELOPMENT

In the course of social development, children acquire knowledge about what is expected of them in relationships, as well as the core skills for the development of friendship, reciprocity, and cooperativeness. Competence, self-confidence, a sense of security, and prosocial attitudes facilitate the development of this complex skill set. It can be argued that the violence inherent in many popular video games works at cross purposes to social skill development, particularly in light of the fact that children learn by watching others and through vicarious rewards and punishments (Bandura, 1977). However, because of their widespread popularity and their fast-paced and dynamic nature, video games used and monitored appropriately may also be valuable tools for teaching children to get along during mutual game play and by offering social learning opportunities inherent in the actual gameplay.

Provenzo (1992) believes that the solitary nature of many video games isolates children and prevents them from experiencing the benefits of interaction with other children. Others, however, have described positive effects on children's social skill development. In this regard, Keller (1992) asserted that video games may help withdrawn children to enter social play by giving them a structured situation in which to participate and a popular topic within which to initiate discussions. Bacigalupa (2005) argues that while little research exists documenting the effective use of video games in teaching social skills to young children, there appears to be more support in doing so with children between the ages of 8 and 16 (Keller, 1992; Panelas, 1983; Sherry, 2001; Yelland & Lloyd, 2001). Further, Singer and Singer (1998, 2005) note the important role of electronic media, video games included, in the development of social behavior.

There is also research documenting the constructive impact of computer programs and interactive games (as opposed to video games) on the social development of children under the age of 8. The National Association for the Education of Young Children's position paper on technology (NAEYC, 1996) suggested that computers encourage children to work in groups, facilitate peer help-seeking behavior, and build high levels of spoken communication and cooperation. Along similar lines, Natasi and Clements (1993) report that elementary-age children learn perspective-taking and conflict resolution skills when using appropriate computer-based activities. Finally, Rebetez and Bétrancourt (2007), who use the term *edutainment*, note that in addition to providing the opportunity to learn specific cognitive skills like deductive reasoning or memorization, video games can be utilized to develop (socially) contextualized skills such as communication and cooperation.

VIOLENT VIDEO GAMES

Violent video games have historically received a great deal of negative attention. Popular opinion, particularly that of concerned parents, appears to be that children who participate in violent video games will imitate the violence based on the characters they role play in the games. Within the professional arena, the arrival of video games, especially violent ones, has rekindled the ongoing decades-old debate over whether or not exposure to violent media in general (television, movies, comics) leads to violent behavior. With the more recent advent of graphically hyper-violent games that encourage unrestrained use of weapons to fight, mutilate, and kill both bad guys and innocents, the debate has heated. Research does indeed suggest that violent video games are associated with increases in aggressive behavior, physiological arousal, and aggressive cognitions and social interactions (Anderson, 2003; Anderson & Dill, 2000; Singer & Singer, 2005). So much so, that the APA recently promulgated a *Resolution on Violence in Video Games and Interactive Media* (APA, n.d.) in which it strongly cautioned consumers and manufacturers to be aware of this association and to safeguard users of violent video games.

Video games have also come under increased scrutiny due to the increase of violence in the schools (Cesarone, 1998) and the sheer ubiquity of video games. In this context, Dill and Dill (1998) found that older children and adolescents play video games, on average, between 1.2 and 7.5 hours per week. While adolescent boys play more video games than their female counterparts, both groups play on a regular basis. Given this, how then can one justify the productive use of video games in counseling and psychotherapy?

On the other hand, and according to Gerard Jones (2002), children have an intrinsic need to feel strong and powerful. They live in a world that can be scary and unpredictable. Superheroes, video games, rappers, and movie gunmen, for better or worse, are all seen as symbols of strength for today's child. The child can then pretend to be these people, and in doing so gain vicarious mastery and strength. If a particular game, and even a violent one, provides an outlet for the fantasy expression of aggression, it may indeed have therapeutic utility under the watchful eye of the informed and intentional clinician.

VIDEO GAMES IN COUNSELING

In his recent book, *Everything Bad Is Good For You*, Steven Johnson (2005) points out that video game players spend a great deal of time not only playing the game, but on working through problems both great and small that get in the way of their ultimate goal. This mirrors life and may be beneficial for children in therapy who struggle with the complexity of social problem solving, which in essence, requires strategy, planning, implementation, and monitoring of outcome. In working on goal-setting, clients may come to realize that problems do get in the way and must be dealt with, but that is no reason to throw in the towel. If they are taught effective problem-solving and coping skills, goals can be reached. They learn not to give up as so many clients often do, thus creating a self-fulfilling prophecy. In gaming, clients often learn that they need long-term planning as well as present-focus. In this context, Gardner (1991) noted that Nintendo video games and Mario Bros.™ in particular can be excellent icebreakers, rapport builders, and setters of the stage for interaction between therapist and client. Additionally, he suggested that such games provide the opportunity for the therapist to observe clients' repertoires of problem-solving skills and frustration tolerance, as well as to provide a release for aggression and the opportunity to engage cognitively in a complex task.

In session, clinicians may include discussions about the client's day while both are engaged in (or distracted by) video game play. This venue can also be used as a vehicle for discussion of feelings, which are triggered by the video game. In this regard, play therapists are ideally positioned due to their emphasis on interactive and often creative interventions and interchanges within the playroom.

One of the greatest advantages of young clients participating in video game play is the learning process that takes place. Not only do the children need to learn about the game through the process of playing and asking for guidance, but they can create characters, build cities, and even create entire worlds, as microcosms of reality complete with political and economic structures. Further, the distance between reality and fantasy game play may provide a useful boundary or safe space in which to act out important life dramas.

A GLIMPSE INTO THE WORLD OF VIDEO GAMES

Video games are varied in content and employ different types of media. Therefore consideration should be given not only to the game but to the game system. While game systems change over time, an important consideration is whether or not the particular game allows the clinician to be active, as opposed to passive, and if one desires to use handheld decks (Gameboy™, Nintendo DS™ and PSP™), dedicated console decks (Play Station™ or Xbox™) or computers (singular versus interactive online games). If the clinician wants to have a more active role in the game play or a group process is desired, console decks and computers are the best choice.

When a clinician considers selecting games, there are a dizzying number to choose from. Computers in many respects provide the broadest base, with arcade-style games, adventure-based games, and puzzle-based games as well as numerous educational games of varying complexity. Video games can be as simple as providing basic reading or math skills, or highly complex, offering the player an opportunity to explore economics or take part in globe-hopping and time-traveling quests and adventures. Some games like Everquest™ and World of Warcraft™ can be used in counseling to provide a client with an artificial social environment in which to explore peer interactions or strengthen social problem-solving skills.

Game decks allow players to link together in a shared activity such as an adventure, but are somewhat restrictive in that both players must be in the same room at the time of play. This is in contrast to online games and MMORPG's (massively multiplayered online role-playing games) such as Warhammer™ and Dungeons and Dragons Online™. As game decks are solely dedicated to game play, as opposed to multifunction computers, play is much more fluid and the controls are simpler in design, usually limited to 10 buttons compared to an entire keyboard. When selecting a game in this medium, the therapist will have the opportunity to witness and be directly involved in the game.

Handheld decks offer the least flexibility for clinical application because the controls and the screen are housed in a single unit. While it is convenient for travel and frequently has some linking capacity so that two players can play together on one game, the therapist cannot easily observe the play and respond with questions. In essence, therapeutic dialogue is severely restricted.

Once the game medium has been decided upon, the clinician chooses the most appropriate game for the therapeutic purpose. As previously mentioned, the games can vary in complexity from the very simple "pong" game to very complex virtual worlds, including extensive nonplayer character (NPC) interactions. Clinicians should also be aware of the rating system of video games. The current rating system suggested by the Media Awareness Network (2007) is as follows:

- EC-Early childhood (age 3+). Generally there will be nothing present for most parents to find offensive.
- E-Everyone (age 6+). Minimal violence; possibly some comic mischief.

- E-Everyone (age 10+). More violence, mild language, and mild suggestive themes.
- T-Teen (13+). It has violent content, mild-to-strong language, and/or suggestive themes.
- M-Mature (17+). May contain mature sexual content, increased violence, and/or strong language.
- AO-Adults only (18+). Contains strong sexual themes and/or violence
- RP-Rating pending.

It is highly recommended that therapists review and familiarize themselves with this rating system and pay close attention to it during the initial game selection period. It is also important for the clinician to remember that the rating system, rather than being a legally codified system, is self-imposed by the gaming industry, and as such can be a flexible guideline, allowing for game selection based upon the client's developmental level rather than age per se. Clinicians should, whenever possible, play the game prior to the session to become more familiar with both the controls and to compare their perception of the rating with that of the manufacturer.

Once these considerations have been made, the field begins to narrow as the clinician can start to consider which games will accomplish the function he or she is setting out to perform. Does the clinician want to have conversation while playing? If so, then fewer control functions are called for, such as with racing and arcade games. In cases where impulse control is a focus, a game requiring more subtle control function might be more appropriate. Examples include Pit Fall™, or Flight Simulators™. Perhaps the clinician wants the client to work on problem-solving skills, so more puzzle-based games such as Mario Pincross™ or Deadly Dooms of Death™ would be the focus of consideration.

Each of these elements can be considered and mixed to match the desired treatment outcomes. In both illustrations below, console-arcade games were the medium of choice and were selected in order to allow the clinician to engage as a part of the process and yet allow for a boundary between him and the client. In both situations, the clinician was an active participant in the game at varying points in counseling.

CASE STUDIES

In this section, I (Enfield) describe the use of video games to promote social-emotional growth. David and Matt worked together, while Dakota and Jonathan were seen individually. In David and Matt's case, as well as Dakota's, video games served as a vehicle for a discussion about social problem solving, while in the case of Jonathan, social skills were addressed directly through game play. An exercise based upon these cases can be found in Exercise 10.1.

David and Matt

The first clinical example consists of two boys: 9-year-old Matt and 10-year-old David. Matt, who lived with his biological mother and younger sibling, was struggling with several issues including poor frustration tolerance, irritability, and both aggressive and destructive behaviors. Prior to beginning therapy, Matt had been the victim of physical abuse as well as a witness to domestic violence. His family was at the poverty level and in addition to receiving public assistance, the local children's protective service was regularly involved in his life. This was yet another source of anxiety for him as the threat of separation from his family constantly loomed over him. In addition, Matt's mother had a drug problem and had to constantly fend off charges of neglect. Matt had difficulty distancing himself from these domestic issues, was teased at school by peers, and often physically and verbally retaliated. Matt loved video games and derived a deep personal satisfaction from playing (and winning) them.

The other child was 10-year-old David, who was brought to counseling by his mother. The eldest of two children, David lived with both biological parents and a younger sister. David had significant problems with social interactions. His family had previously had him evaluated by a prominent developmental pediatrician, who diagnosed him with Asperger's Syndrome. When I first met him, David was in the waiting room talking to an older woman and was describing the subtle characteristics and inner workings of a CD player. His mother was sitting beside him with a stressed and embarrassed look on her face.

David required a separate entrance into the agency because at the time of his treatment, the designated smoking area was outside the front door. He would become extremely upset with smokers and would accost them with the dangers of their habit. The issue of smoking actually interfered with treatment in that David would perseverate on the topic during sessions and be incapable of addressing other issues, particularly his social difficulties.

Prior to placing Matt and David together in counseling, I had considered the work of Kline, Volkmar, and Sparrow (2000) with Asperger's Syndrome. They noted that concrete problem-solving strategies are important in teaching and building social skills. In addition, these authors linked social skill deficits with depression in clients with Asperger's.

Indeed, both Matt and David were feeling isolated, unsuccessful in social settings, sad, and lonely. The two boys were paired together so that they could learn to interact with others and begin to develop social problem-solving skills.

Initially, Matt and Dave were asked to play typical board games and to develop social stories similar to the typical interactions seen in other smaller social groups. After several sessions, it was clear that neither boy was making much progress and that they were spending a significant amount of time struggling with the complexities of direct social interactions. When the boys were addressed about the difficulty they were having with this interaction, neither had given much thought to the conflict but independently commented that this was the way many interactions with peers at school happened.

The discussion shifted to talking about movies and video games. It was quickly learned that both boys were avid video game players. While David disclosed that he did not have video games at home, Matt indicated that he had three different game systems in the home that he played on a regular basis. This opened the opportunity for them to explore video games as a way to link with each other and explore the social issues that brought them to therapy in the first place.

After this was determined, the next obstacle in the intervention process was deciding upon which game we were going to play. This became a fairly difficult obstacle as many of the games contain a significant amount of graphic violence and others pitted player against player. Because the primary function of the game was to develop peer interaction, communication, and cooperation, selection was limited to arcade-style adventure-based play, and crawler-based games. Arcade games are simply games with an arcade feel like Donkey Kong™ and Pac Man™. Crawler-based games are games in which players explore environments and make choices about the direction they go, their choices in turn having direct bearing on the characters the boys are playing as well as the outcome of the story. Myst™, Tomb Raider™, Balders Gate™, and Sherlock Holmes: Mystery of the Mummy™ are just a few examples.

Considering the purpose of the group, it was determined that a cooperative version of an arcade adventure game was the most effective way to promote interactions and positive reciprocal discussions through the natural course of play. To accomplish this, three games were initially selected and the boys played each game for one session and then made a final selection for the remainder of the group process. The initially chosen games were Sonic the Hedge Hog™ and Spyro the Dragon™. Spyro was eliminated because it was a single-player game. Sonic™ was selected because of the two-player option. When played this way, the screen was split and the boys needed to remain on the same screen in order to progress forward. Additionally, it was agreed by all that neither boy was allowed to give up.

The group process consisted of nine consecutive sessions over 2 months, and each of them followed a very consistent pattern. When the boys entered session, they asked how the previous week had gone and if there was anything they wanted to share or discuss. When the boys were finished talking with me or each other, they would begin to play the game where they left off the previous week. The objective was to work toward playing the game from start to finish, knowing that this would take ongoing effort. The final 15 minutes of the session was dedicated to a reflection of the day's activities. During this discussion, questions were asked of the boys about what worked, what was difficult, and what did not work during that day's activity.

Initially, the boys struggled with mutual and reciprocal game play. David struggled significantly with many technical areas of the game. There were several times when Matt was asked to help David as he grappled with the issues of timing and moving accurately between points. This was illustrated by difficulty jumping between locations, or from land to a moving object. While this activity was very easy for Matt, David would become very frustrated. There were several discussions about the process and how people work to engage each other in problem solving and productively interacting.

While involved in game play, the boys began discussing each other's families. This was followed by additional discussions about school and peers. By the end of the time together, the boys were helping each other solve problems they were having both at home and at school. Matt would talk with David about the difficulty he was having in math, while David would discuss difficulties with peers. It was very exciting to watch these two boys of very different backgrounds and issues working together. Matt became an expert at helping David discuss and identify his feelings related to different topics. Through this interaction a marked improvement was noted in his affect. This change, while prominent in session, was also observed by his mother and sibling in the form of reduction in bullying and negative self-talk. There were also demonstrated improvements in the school setting for Matt as his grades improved and he spent less time receiving direct intervention from the school principal.

David's changes were more subtle in nature. He continued to struggle in public situations and became easily overstimulated. What the family did report as positive change was that he was better able to self-soothe and was less inclined to act out in public. He was also observed to develop increased tolerance to change in routine.

Dakota

Fifteen-year-old Dakota was the only child of parents who divorced when he was 5 years old due to his mother's drug use. After the divorce and for the next 4 years, Dakota lived with his mother while his father lived with his own mother. At age 9, Dakota went to live with his father and grandmother while his mother attended a voluntary drug rehabilitation program. Upon her discharge, she lived on her own for a period of time and when Dakota was 12, she took him back to live with her. This created a great deal of stress and frustration for Dakota, who had become accustomed to a lack of structure or boundaries. As a result, he became highly oppositional toward his mother. In addition, Dakota's father condoned his behavior and chose not to engage in counseling. Dakota's mother was involved in her own counseling and was unable to participate in session in a consistent manner. This worked to Dakota's benefit by allowing him to more freely discuss his feelings without fear of chastisement or accusations of divided loyalty. While largely reticent and resistant to talking, Dakota did acknowledge an interest in skateboarding, movies, and video games. Game Cube™ was our therapeutic gateway.

Dakota preferred two particular games; Mario Cart™ and Naruto™. Mario is a two-person racing game in which players race each other and opponents. Naruto is a two-person combat game in which players fight each other in an arena and gain points through various hits, kicks, and throws. Over the course of six sessions, Dakota played both games equally. While I do not normally select competition-based interventions with clients, I believed that in light of Dakota's adversarial and angry relationship with both parents, and toward me, such games might prove productive in working through transference issues.

During our sessions Dakota took pride in winning and had no reluctance bragging over his victories. When challenged about this behavior, he responded, "I was only teasing." Interestingly, Dakota always had one more move up his sleeve and was able to maintain a slight advantage when playing the games, playing the different fighters and reserving enough of the information about the game to remain victorious. While he believed our session ended once he was victorious, I encouraged him to discuss his feelings both about the game and situations that were occurring around the home.

While playing Mario Cart, there was a palpably different feeling tone between us; it was a more open and relaxed time. While his competitive edge was still very sharp while playing this game, game play was frequently accompanied by discussions about how the family had let him down and how his mother had abandoned him. While his skill was great, the game did require a tremendous amount of attention and concentration, which was undermined by the anxiety that accompanied the discussions. When the discussions moved into uncomfortable realms, he was more scattered, erratic, and impulsive, and less effective in controlling the action of the characters in the game. Crashing occurred more frequently, and I was able to point out the relationship between distress over family issues and his day-to-day functioning, using his game play as an analogy. In looking back, I believe that without the social lubrication of the game as well as its use as an analogy for his real-life, day-to-day functioning, our work might not have progressed as it did.

Jonathan

Jonathan was a 13-year-old attending regular mainstream schooling and an only child living with both biological parents. While there was no reported history of abuse or neglect, Jonathan's comments suggested that his father could be verbally demeaning. His mother was a very quiet woman with limited social contacts outside of the home.

Jonathan was initially referred for counseling by his school counselor because of problematic interactions with peers. In part, because of his larger size and physical awkwardness, but more so through the use of large and unusual words and phrases in social interaction, Jonathan confused and intimidated peers. Many times those words and phrases were used out of context, which made it that much more difficult for peers to understand him, and for him to connect with them. Jonathan's mother reported that the school suspected that he had characteristics of Asperger's Syndrome, a notion that was confirmed by the family physician.

Shortly after our first meeting, it was clear that Jonathan was very interested in the use of video games and spent hours online playing adventure-based and dungeon crawler games like Diablo™, Everquest™, and World of Warcraft™. According to his mother, "He's always on the computer if he's not eating or sleeping." It seemed that Jonathan's fascination with and immersion into his cyber-adventures was related to his perception of the (real) world as a hostile place. Unlike his day-to-day interactions with peers who dismissed, ignored, or taunted him, he was powerful and respected in cyberspace.

Everquest™ published by Sony, and World of Warcraft™ published by Blizzard Entertainment, are online role-playing adventure games in which participants develop individualized skills, characteristics, and unique identities in order to interact in complex virtual fantasy adventures. In Diablo™, also by Blizzard Entertainment, players select from a class of characters and build unique identities with a wide range of skills for allying or competing with others, sometimes in violent battle, and other times in clashes of strategy en route to lofty quests.

After several sessions in which I offered traditional play opportunities including sand, art, and conversation, Jonathan and I agreed that we would attempt to use one of his favorite online games in order to develop a character through which we could explore his social difficulties. On the Blizzard™ Web site, I found a guide to "playing nice" with which I was able to develop questions and directions that might be adapted to understanding and navigating Jonathan's real world around issues of sharing, communicating, and requesting assistance from others. What was also interesting was that it was possible to estimate the number of hours Jonathan spent playing these games at home based upon the level of the character he had developed. In a sense, I was able to track therapeutic progress that occurred outside of session, particularly as Jonathan usually bragged about his online achievements at the outset of sessions.

In several sessions, I could actually witness Jonathan's online play and in doing so, was able to observe the nature of his interactional style. At one point, he was being attacked by another character in the cyber world who was clearly more skilled than he was. Jonathan was in effect feeling bullied and intimidated, and he experienced frustration and anger toward the other player. Each time that Jonathan attempted to defend himself by moving to another location or level, this cyber-bully followed and successfully attacked him. In the process, Jonathan and I shifted the discussion to his own feelings of awkwardness and powerlessness in social interactions at school, and how he intimidated others. This in turn generated a discussion of alternative strategies when he felt this way.

On another occasion Jonathan described the cyber-experience of entering an "instance." An instance is a game term used to describe a specific location in the game where players work together to achieve specific objectives. In this situation Jonathan was working through a dungeon with several other players, one of whom constantly nagged him for some of the treasure he had collected. Actually, Jonathan was unwilling to share the loot he had acquired as well as that which he had snatched from other players. Jonathan grew increasingly annoyed by this other player, commenting to me that "he was being a real pain . . . always nagging and whining. . . . Whenever I ask him for something, he ignores me, and when we're fighting the monster, he loots the chest before we can get there." Jonathan was surprisingly insightful and was able to reflect on his own feelings of frustration and disappointment in not getting his fair shake of the booty. He added, "Well, if he keeps playing like that he won't have any friends." This provided a nice entrée into further discussion about making friends and interacting with others.

While Jonathan was a relatively new client at the time of this writing, avenues for discussion have since opened in the context of his online gaming interest. Jonathan is still abrupt and has limited social insight, but is making important strides in getting along with others. He is talking with and about people outside of the game and experiencing fewer conflicts in his day-to-day interactions. He has a far way to go, but has clearly benefited from rehearsing for real life in cyberspace.

POSTSCRIPT

Children are increasingly exposed to video games and other media. Video games and computers are increasing in our culture and the culture of the clients we serve. It would serve us well to consider carefully the cost and benefit of this medium to help us work and provide a venue to explore topics and ideas that previously have met with significant resistance from clients, and in some case other clinicians. With careful consideration, video games can serve as another intervention to use with our clients to build social skills as well as promote self-esteem, increase problem-solving ability, and assist our clients in learning how to promote and live within real communities.

Exercise 10.1: Video Game Exercise

Depending upon the availability of equipment, this can be either a two- or four-person activity. The clinician's role is to function as facilitator to the discussion and to model socially appropriate responses for the group members.

Select a video game as described in this chapter on this subject. I would suggest Mario Cart™ or one of the other cartoon-based racing games. Allow each member to control a car, running the race in heats if needed. While the race is progressing, you will see the group's energy level increase and may be able to monitor this through changes in the player's body movements, language, and vocal pitch. At this point, it would be convenient to engage the client in discussion. The topic of conversation will vary and may include the experience of winning and losing, how it feels to compete and cooperate, and the experience of both gratification and frustration.

While these same objectives may be accomplished through the use of a board game, the intensity of the activity level is less, and it may not arouse the same degree of affect. Clinicians may also find that they will need more time using the slower-paced board games.

In the last 15–20 minutes of the group, I would highly recommend a reflection time. It is in this time that the clinician can ask the participants what worked and what did not, followed up by praise of all participants in one way or another. It is here that the clinician may reflect back comments made during the session. This action will make those ideas that are covert and often overlooked more concrete and relevant to the group participants.

REFERENCES

American Psychological Association. (n.d.). *Resolution on violence in video games and interactive media.* Retrieved November 6, 2007, from http://www.apa.org/releases/resolutiononvideoviolence.pdf

Anderson, C. (2003). *Violent video games: Myths, facts and unanswered questions.* Retrieved November 6, 2007, from http://www.apa.org/science/psa/sb-anderson.html

Anderson, C., & Dill, K. (2000). Video games and aggressive thoughts, feelings, and behavior in the laboratory and in life. *Journal of Personality and Social Psychology, 78*(4), 772–790.

Bacigalupa, C. (2005). The use of video games by kindergartners in a family child care setting. *Early Childhood Education Journal, 33*(1), 25–30.

Bandura, A. (1977). *Social learning theory.* Englewood Cliffs, NJ: Prentice Hall.

Cesarone, B. (1998). *Video games: research, ratings, recommendations.* ERIC Digest (EDO-PS-98-11).

Dill, K.E., & Dill, J.C. (1998). Video game violence: A review of the empirical literature. *Aggression and Violent Behavior, 3*(4), 407–428.

Gardner, J. (1991). Can the Mario Bros. help?: Nintendo games as an adjunct in psychotherapy with children. *Psychotherapy, 28*(4), 667–670.

Johnson, S. (2005). *Everything bad is good for you: How popular culture is making us smarter.* London: Penguin Books.

Jones, G. (2002). *Killing monsters: Why children need fantasy super heroes, and make-believe violence.* New York: Basic Books.

Keller, S. (1992). *Children and Nintendo.* Champaign, IL: Clearinghouse on Elementary and Early Childhood Education (ERIC Document Reproduction Service No. ED405069).

Kline, A., Volkmar, F., & Sparrow, S. (2000). *Asperger's syndrome.* New York: The Guilford Press.

Media Awareness Network. (2007). *Understanding the rating system.* Retrieved October 14, 2007, from http://www.media-awareness.ca/english/parents/video_games/ratings_videogames.cfm

Natasi, B., & Clements, D. (1993). Motivational and social outcomes of cooperative computer education environments. *Journal of Computing in Childhood Education, 4*(1), 15–43.

National Association for the Education of Young Children. (1996). *Technology and young children—ages 3 through 8.* Washington, DC: A Position Statement of the National Association for the Education of Young Children.

Panelas, T. (1983). Adolescents and video games: Consumption of leisure and the social construction of the peer group. *Youth & Society, 15*(1), 51–65.

Provenzo, E. F. (1992). The video generation. *The American School Board Journal, 179*(3), 29–32.

Rebetez, C., & Bétrancourt, M. (2007). Video game research in cognitive and educational sciences. *Cognitie, Creier, Comportament/Cognition, Brain, Behavior, 11*(1), 131–142.

Sherry, J. L. (2001). The effects of violent video games on aggression: A meta-analysis. *Human Communication Research, 27*(3), 409–431.

Singer, D. G., & Singer, J. L. (1998). Developing critical viewing skills and media literacy in children. *The Annals of the American Academy of Political and Social Sciences, 57*, 164–179.

Singer, D. G., & Singer, J. L. (2005). *Imagination and play in the electronic age.* Cambridge, MA: Harvard University Press.

Yelland, N., & Lloyd, M. (2001). Virtual kids of the 21st century: Understanding the children in schools today. *Information Technology in Childhood Education Annual, 1*, 175–192.

CHAPTER 11

Passing Go in the Game of Life

Board Games in Therapeutic Play

Harry Livesay

Board games have been, and continue to be, an entertaining and revealing reflection of American popular culture. In their work *Celebrating Board Games,* Chertoff and Kahn (2006) describe the development of American board games as a collection of societal snapshots. They observe, "[O]ur [collective] interests, our imagination, our values are all reflected in those simple boards [and the pieces] that move across them. Games have taken us through cold wars and world wars. And they've taken us through what in retrospect, seems to be the simpler time of the 1950s to the more complex times of today" (pp. 6–7).

My interest and efforts in therapeutic play using board games with children and adolescents is an outcome of my work with the clinical application of popular superheroes in therapy and the rediscovery and feelings of ownership that my clients express for cultural icons like Superman, Batman, and Spider-Man (see Exercise 11.1 for a superhero-based therapeutic exercise). At the request of many of my clients, I began to incorporate superhero-themed board games into therapeutic play. My experience with the use of board games with clients was very similar to that of psychologist Jill Bellinson, who in her book *Children's Use of Board Games in Therapy* (2002) observed:

> I was repeatedly faced with children who begged for board games, who played them in school and at home, who were not interested in the dramatic play of childhood and who could not talk out their difficulties. . . .

Their interests—in therapy and outside—were in playing structured games with rules, requirements, and winners. (p. ix)

As therapists, counselors, and other supportive adults, we often face the initial and monumental challenge of younger clients who are unable or unwilling to discuss their problems with a strange adult (Boyd-Webb, 1999). This reluctance combined with limited insight and difficulty verbalizing worries, fears, and stressors (even with the most supportive adults) compels therapists, counselors, teachers, and parents to use other means to create an environment in which children feel freer to express feelings and to communicate more effectively (Kennedy, 1989). Board games can assist in the creation of such an environment for children and adolescents because they provide two fundamental elements of play: fun and fantasy (Moyles, 1989).

For purposes of clarification, this chapter will deal specifically with three categories of board games that I utilize in my practice at a school-based clinic: traditional commercially produced board and parlor games such as Sorry!™, Candy Land™, and The Game of Life™; board games based on stories or adventures of popular culture figures such as Scooby Doo™ and Harry Potter™; and finally therapeutic board games, such as The Ungame™.

It is my hope that the therapeutic application of board games detailed in this chapter will provide fellow caring adults with helpful tools for creating an atmosphere for children and adolescents in which to share, learn, and heal by means of their natural desire to play and have fun.

CULTURAL, SOCIETAL, AND PSYCHOLOGICAL IMPACT OF BOARD GAMES

Game playing is a nearly universal human activity and, in particular, board games appear to have been a part of the human experience since the beginning of recorded history. The oldest known board game was found in Jordan and dates back to approximately 5870 B.C.E. (Board Games, 2007). Greek vases from the 12th century B.C.E. reflect representations of Trojan War heroes engaging in board games, "both for recreation and to divine the whims of the gods" (Teitel, 1998, p. 1).

According to board game historian Margaret Hofer (2003), board games serve "as cultural mirrors of our societal and technological progress [and] offer fascinating windows on the values, beliefs and aspirations of human kind" (p. 13). This belief is also shared by noted European psychology researchers Fernand Gobet, Alex de Voogt, and Jean Retschitzki. In their extensive work, *Moves in Mind: The Psychology of*

Board Games (2004), they reveal that our interest in the social and cultural impact of board games can be traced back to the latter 17th century when the "first systematic and historical studies" of board games were recorded (p. 5).

The growth and appeal of board games in 20th-century American popular culture coincided with the nation's increased urbanization and industrialization, and the transformation of the American home into a "center of education, entertainment and moral enlightenment [where] middle-class families—with expanded leisure time as well as rising income levels—embraced leisure pursuits in the home and encouraged their children to play games that would develop skills and provide moral instruction" (Hofer, 2003, pp. 13–14).

However, research on the psychological benefits of board games suggested that beyond conventional games such as chess and checkers, board games were of little interest or value to psychology in general (Gobet et al., 2004, p. 8). It has only been during the past 20 years that the therapeutic value of modern-era board games has been explored. Moreover, the limited amount of literature available has not addressed the clinical application of board games based on popular culture figures in films, television, and other forms of media.

Beginning in the 1980s, psychologists began to explore the therapeutic use of board games as a tool to identify unconscious conflicts expressed within the context of the game, and as a means to enhance client awareness and verbal expression (Schaefer & Reid, 2002). These authors also believed that communication-oriented board games allowed children and adolescents to project aspects of self, both known and unknown, during game play that involved both the presenting problem and additional areas of client functioning including self-esteem, interpersonal relations, and family dynamics. This observation was echoed by Jill Bellinson (2002), who concurred that structured games:

> can reveal a child's unconscious dynamics as well as dramatic play can for younger children and dream work can for adolescents and adults . . . we should search for the same underlying dynamics we would for these other symbolic expressions. Any method of game play can be seen and interpreted in this light. (p. 19)

Although board games can provoke competitive feelings in children, their rules require that players compete within certain limits and boundaries (Moyles, 1989). Additionally, because of their rules, requirements, and necessity of taking turns, board games may appeal to an unconscious need for "civilized communication behavior" (Teitel, 1998, p. 6). This civilizing effect of board games may explain their continued popularity.

In a 1998 *Psychology Today* article on board game play, a game developer for Hasbro, America's leading board game manufacturer, expressed the belief that play with board games actually enhances human behavior, noting that:

> probably nothing a child learns in life is more important than the need and the skill of waiting your turn. Games are perfect teachers of this skill, because if people don't take their turns, games don't work. Neither do relationships. Nor does democracy. (Tietel, 1998, p. 6)

BOARD GAMES AND CHILD DEVELOPMENT

As children age, they become more reality-oriented, and structured games become more appealing than fantasy play with dolls, action figures, and toys. Nevertheless, board games have appeal and cognitive utility to younger as well as older children. Schaefer and Reid (2002) found that while most therapists and counselors associate therapeutic play and games with sensory-motor and pretend play, few clinicians are aware of the social, cognitive, and developmental benefit of games for school-aged children and teenagers (Schaefer & Reid, 2002, in Boyd-Webb, 1999, p. 39). According to Boyd-Webb, this interest in board games occurs "when the child has achieved the level of cognitive development characterized by logical and objective thinking" (1999, p. 39). Along similar lines, and in one of her case studies, Bellinson (2002) related the example of a highly developed 4½-year-old whose interest in board games signified an "important developmental step . . . one that is often acquired during the years a child is in treatment . . . an advanced statement, an attempt to be calm, focused and mature . . . " (p. 16). She further noted that a child's progress in "accepting structure, rules and restrictions that board games provide occurs as children acquire the capacity of fair play" (p. 16).

In my own therapeutic work with children and adolescents, I have found that therapeutic play with board games provides a practice or staging area for the development and implementation of skills in the following four areas:

1. Decision Making/Strategy: In addition to helping children and adolescents improve reading and math skills, board games provide simulated situations that can teach ideas and enhance skills in dealing with complex systems such as finances, interpersonal relations, and power struggles. The effectiveness of these simulated situations in board games lies in the opportunities to teach

problem-solving and decision-making strategies in a nonjudgmental and positively reinforcing way. During game play, the therapist might explore problem-solving strategies with the child by asking, "Is this/was this a good move or bad move? Is/was there another move you can/could make? If you don't like what happened when you moved, what could you do differently the next time?" In exploring the reasoning for their decisions and choices during game play with children and adolescents, I often emphasize the significance of learning how to use one's knowledge and skills for fun and enjoyment and hopefully in making better decisions and "good moves" in real-life situations.

2. Ethical Behavior/Cheating: Through board game play, adults can promote the idea that play is fun only when the competition is fair and honest. If we think someone is cheating or not playing fairly, then the games that normally would make us happy, now make us feel sad and angry. It is normal for children to test limits and boundaries of game rules as they do in other areas of their life and this behavior should be anticipated. According to Bellinson (2002):

> Breaking rules is an expectable behavior in children in psychotherapy. Younger children are not fully able to follow rules and older children in treatment often do not have the ego strength to play within the boundaries of box-top rules. They may be struggling with the conflict over following or opposing rules imposed upon them by authorities around them and playing board games, particularly cheating at board games, allows them to work on this issue metaphorically. (p. 75)

When children and adolescents demonstrate cheating behavior, the adult player should initiate exploration as to why they are attempting to avoid or circumvent game rules. *Are they feeling threatened by our efforts? Do they feel they are not being treated fairly? Are they afraid of losing?* Upon exploration of their thoughts and feelings, therapists and counselors can explore the idea that making an honest effort and trying one's hardest every time you play is better than winning at any cost.

3. Disappointment/Acceptance: Board games are also an effective learning tool to help children deal with disappointment and to accept that losing is a part of play, not the end of the world. As children and adolescents gain a better understanding of emotions, they become more capable of emotional regulation (Joseph & Strain, 2006). Helping children cope constructively with emotions means dealing with disappointment. During board game

play, therapists can address anger and disappointment by sharing and exploring stories, thoughts, and memories of not winning a game, validating feelings of sadness and frustration, and fostering hope and anticipation for future efforts: "The next time we play this game" or "when we play another game."

As previously noted, board games do stimulate competitive feelings in children, but at the same time the rules of the game require that children compete within certain limited boundaries (Schaeffer & Reid, 2002). Although competition helps children develop problem solving and other skills, a more valuable by-product is helping children learn the difference between positive and negative competition. Negative competition occurs when a child competes for her/his self-worth and value (Black, 2007). This is most common when parents reinforce the concept that children must play to win. In therapeutic play with board games, children can learn that positive competition is better because it helps them discover their strengths and inner talents such as determination, patience, and power.

4. Impulse Control: Happiness, anger, sadness, and excitement are all emotions that children and adolescents experience in life and that may be anticipated and normalized in board game play. Learning how and when to show these emotions is the basis for impulse control. In my experience in therapeutic play with board games, children can become loud and boisterous, especially if the game is fast-paced or involves a great deal of physical activity (as with hand/eye coordination games such as Heads Up!™, or rapid-response games such as the Yes & No Game™).

Before game play, it may be necessary to normalize possible reactions: "This game is very exciting, and we need to be careful that we don't get too loud." During game play, it may be necessary to impose a "time out" if a child's emotional response impedes game play. Making positive observations about impulse control can also reinforce more appropriate behaviors; for example, "I notice when you take your time and read the cards, you do better in the game," or, "You stayed calm/you didn't get angry when I was getting ahead. I am really proud of you."

Learning impulse control is hard work and it can be especially difficult for children with ADHD (a learning disorder), family dysfunction, or trauma. Integrating cognitive behavioral techniques into board game play by teaching new skills and strategies for expressing feelings in a more constructive manner can result in better interpersonal relations with peers, parents, and teachers, improve self-esteem, and enhance classroom success (Joseph & Strain, 2006).

APPLICATIONS OF BOARD GAMES
IN THERAPEUTIC PLAY

For the purposes of therapeutic application, I have listed in this section some of the board games that I have found helpful in my school-based counseling setting. I have also included a table (see Table 11.1) with more detailed information on particular board games and suggestions for their therapeutic use as well as limitations. I do not use games that include acts of homicide such as Clue!™, and due to the time limitations within my clinical practice, I prefer not to use games that involve substantial preparation and/or offer difficulty with continuation of play during successive sessions, such as Monopoly™. Additionally, in light of the vast and ever-increasing variety of board games, I invite and encourage counselors, therapists, and other helping adults to use this information on board games and the related case studies as *starting points* in their own efforts to explore, identify, and incorporate board games in their work with children and adolescents.

TRADITIONAL/COMMERCIALLY PRODUCED
BOARD GAMES

A recent report in the trade publication *Toy Directory* (Blair, 2003) indicated that Americans currently spend approximately $870 million annually on board games, with the industry reporting a 65% increase in sales since 2001. In this age of computer-based and internet entertainment, why are board games still hot? Market researchers put forth the idea that, "When the economy is sluggish, Americans seek cost effective alternatives to having fun. Others attribute 9/11 as the catalyst to the increase in families spending more time together at home. Whatever the reason, this industry continues to be a growth sector" (Blair, 2003, p. 1).

Additionally, traditional board games such as The Game of Life™, Monopoly™, and Jenga!™, which entertained parents and grandparents as children in the 20th century, continue to appeal to children and adolescents in the 21st century by providing "an interactional experience that can be simultaneously enjoyed and analyzed and is ego-enhancing to the child" (Boyd-Webb, 1999, p. 39). These games are widely available in department and discount stores and offer therapists and counselors an ample variety of economical choices for therapeutic play. Some of these games include:

Table 11.1 A Thumbnail Guide to the Clinical Use of Board Games

Game	Manufacturer/ Availability	Activity	Clinical Applications	Limitations
Are You 4 Real? ™	Milton Bradley/ Hasbro Game not widely available in stores since 2005. New and used versions of the game available on E-Bay and Amazon.	The game tests how well you can fool your friends. Players take turns telling stories from cards that list three topics for storytelling. Examples of storytelling topics include, "*I don't like to be alone when . . .*" or "*My feelings were really hurt when . . .*" Players have to indicate if the storyteller is being "real" or "unreal" on plastic pieces that resemble beepers. When the storytelling player reveals the truth, the players who guessed correctly advance their peg on the game board path. The first to move their peg to the end of the path wins.	The game is marketed to female children and adolescents, but can be used with both genders. The game can be helpful in eliciting information on interpersonal relationships, family dynamics, and home and school related stressors. Game play can be used both in individual and family counseling. Therapeutic application of this game can include agreement with client/ family members to share the "truth" or what is "real" if the initial story presented is "unreal."	Some of the questions/ topics on the game cards are targeted more to female children and adolescents. The battery operated game board, which directs game play with an electronic voice, can slow game play. Playing the game without the electronic voice is an option. Recommended for use with older children (9 years) and adolescents. In individual sessions, storytelling play requires disclosure by therapist of their past age-specific experiences/thoughts/ beliefs (i.e., "*When I was your age . . .*").

Battleship ™	Milton Bradley-Hasbro Widely available. Variations include a standard version, an electronic version with sound, and popular-culture themed versions (Star Wars™, Pirates of the Caribbean™).	Each player places ships (of lengths varying from 2 to 5 squares) secretly on a square grid. Players try to deduce where each other's ships are and sink them. The first player who sinks the other player's ships wins the game.	The game enjoys familiarity and popularity with children and adolescents. The game is helpful in enhancing attention-sustaining skills/concentration for clients with ADHD and impulse control/behavioral challenges. The game is also useful in assisting in the development of deductive reasoning skills/process of elimination.	Game play is conducted on two square grids concurrently, which may be initially confusing for younger children and/or children with learning disorders.
Brain Quest 1–6 ™	University Games Widely available.	Players advance on a game board by answering questions for their specific grade level (1 to 6), in six topics: Math, English, Science, Social studies, and Grab Bag. The first player to reach the finish wins.	Game play can assist in reducing anxiety related to testing/exams and as a way to reinforce participation in school (i.e., making school more like a game).	Game is limited to grades 1–6. During play, adults must answer 6th grade level questions, and would seemingly have an advantage in game play.

(continued)

205

Table 11.1 A Thumbnail Guide to the Clinical Use of Board Games (*Continued*)

Game	Manufacturer/ Availability	Activity	Clinical Applications	Limitations
Candy Land™	Milton Bradley/Hasbro Widely available.	Each player advances along a colorful board with a rainbow path through candy-themed locations to the finish. The players use the plastic gingerbread man as the playing pieces.	The game can be used with children as young as three years. Candy Land™ promotes socialization, learning simple rules, following directions, and recognizing colors.	Recommended for use with younger children.
Chutes & Ladders™	Milton Bradley/ Hasbro Widely available.	Players move upwards from 1 to 100 on playing board with numbered grid squares. When landing on certain squares that contain ladders, players advance upwards. Landing on slides result in players going backward.	The game reinforces messages and images on the positive results of honesty, respect, kindness, and safety (going up the ladder), versus the negative results of rule-breaking, greed, cruelty, and hazardous behavior (sliding backward).	Recommended for use with younger children.

Clue Jr.™	Parker Brothers/ Hasbro Widely available.	This game is a nonviolent variation of its parent game, Clue, which uses deduction to solve the mystery of which pet stole "which toy."	This game can be used to assist younger children in enhancing deductive reasoning skills and learning the process of elimination in finding the answer. The game can also be used to reduce test anxiety with younger children, specifically during annual basic aptitude testing periods.	Recommended for use with younger children.
Furious Fred™	Franklin Learning Systems Available on the Internet via several retail sites.	Players move around a game board learning about important concepts and practical skills for controlling anger and avoiding violence, as they advise "Fred," a student with anger problems.	In addition to providing beneficial information on handling teasing, negative peer pressure, conflict resolution and bullying, the game is insight-building in that players take the role of peer counselor to Fred and are encouraged to share their experiences in dealing with anger and frustration.	Although the game is intended for grades 2 to 5, it can be used with middle school and junior high students.

(continued)

Table 11.1 A Thumbnail Guide to the Clinical Use of Board Games (*Continued*)

Game	Manufacturer/ Availability	Activity	Clinical Applications	Limitations
(The) **Game of Life**™	Milton Bradley/ Hasbro Widely available. Several popular character-themed versions are also available including: Star Wars™, Pirates of the Caribbean™, The Simpsons™ and Sponge Bob Squarepants™.	Players move along a game board of "life," dealing with issues and stressors of career, family, and finances. The player who has accumulated the most wealth for retirement wins the game.	The game offers children and adolescents a place to acquire practice skills for handling problems, dealing with disappointment and stress. In family counseling, the game can be an effective tool for building empathy and understanding for parents/primary caregivers who are dealing with real life issues of money, job, and providing for a family. The game can be used in enhancing attention-sustaining skills, using math skills, teaching ethical behavior, and promoting positive/hopeful cognitive progressing/hopeful perspective after experiencing a serious trauma or loss.	Recommended for use with older children, adolescents, and young adults.

Harry Potter Whomping Willow Game™	Mattel Game not widely available in stores since 2003. New and used versions of the game available on E-Bay and Amazon.	Based on the film, *Harry Potter and the Chamber of Secrets*, players get to reenact Harry's encounter with the moving and creaking Whomping Willow tree. Using plastic "car" hooks, players try to remove luggage, book satchels, and figures of Harry's pet owl from the tree.	This game is an effective icebreaker with clients of all ages. In addition to increasing the comfort and reducing anxiety, the game can also be used to augment attention-sustaining skills/on-task behavior, and in family counseling as a tool to formulate healthy alliance building, cooperative behavior, and turn-taking between siblings.	None
Jenga!™	Milton Bradley/ Hasbro Widely available. Various versions of the game include a multicolor version with a companion dice to determine which block is removed/stacked and a "truth or dare" version requiring players to tell a "truth" or do a "dare" to continue play.	A tower building game consisting of 54 wooden rectangular blocks. Each player in turn removes one block from anywhere below the highest completed tower level and places it on the top of the tower. Only one hand may be used at a time. The last player to stack a block without making the tower tumble over wins.	The game can be used with both children and adolescents to teach impulse control, turn-taking and to improve attention-sustaining behavior. The game also has a cognitive reframing benefit in that older children and adolescents are asked to visualize their selection of the wooden blocks as the "choices" they make in school and at home and their stacking efforts as the impact of their choices on themselves and others.	None

(continued)

Table 11.1 A Thumbnail Guide to the Clinical Use of Board Games (*Continued*)

Game	Manufacturer/ Availability	Activity	Clinical Applications	Limitations
Scobby Doo! Spills, and Thrills Game™	Game not widely available in stores since 2005. New and used versions of the game available on E-Bay and Amazon.	Players move along an uphill game board through a grave-yard to be the first to get to the Mystery Machine and win the game. A spinner determines how many spaces to move. If a spin results in the arrow landing on a monster or if one of the players lands on a monster space on the board, a spinning top is set loose that can knock over the figures. Any figures that are knocked down can "get back up again" and return to start.	The game can be used with children, adolescents and teens in recovery from sexual and physical abuse, family trauma and disruption, depression, anxiety, and grief and bereavement. The game helps explore and identify inner strength and resiliency when a player gets knocked down, and getting the support you need to start again.	Supervision is required for younger children in handling the spinning top mechanism.
Sorry!™	Parker Brothers/ Hasbro Widely available. Popular culture themed versions are also available including a Disney™ and Pokémon™ version.	The objective of the game is to be the first player to get all four pawns from the start to home. In order to win you have to *carefully* read and *understand* the rule cards for the game that tell you how and when to move.	The game illustrates and reinforces that idea that winning is achieved by *knowing and following* the rules, and is useful in work with children and adolescents dealing with impulse control, anger management, and behavioral problems.	Due to the reading level of the game cards, younger children (ages 5–7) may require assistance/ clarification in reading and understanding game rules.

The Ungame™	Talicor Widely available. The game is available in age-targeted versions for teens, children and families.	Game play involves movement of pawns on a playing board by answering questions from two stacks of cards: one with lighthearted topics and the other with more serious topics. Other spaces on the board encourage players to exchange thoughts and feelings or describe how they've been affected by recent emotions.	The game provides a way to elicit and explore thoughts, beliefs, stressors, and family dynamics in a non-intrusive manner.	Due to the reading level of the game cards, the game may be more appropriate for older children (above age 8), adolescents and young adults.
Topple!™	Pressman Toy Company Widely available.	The game involves stacking colored disks on the topple tower at different levels as directed by roll of a dice. The more pieces that are stacked on the tower, the more the tower can turn, sway, and tip! Players get points for each piece stacked on the tower. The winner is the player with the most points, who doesn't cause the pieces to topple.	Like Jenga!™, this game can be used with both children and adolescents to teach impulse control, turn-taking, and to improve attention-sustaining behavior. Tracking points during the game can also enhance addition skills. Cognitive reframing with this game can include exploration of thoughts and beliefs on dealing with disappointment or adversity and 'starting over'.	None. Game rules can be altered to accommodate younger children with limited math/calculation skills.

(continued)

Table 11.1 A Thumbnail Guide to the Clinical Use of Board Games (*Continued*)

Game	Manufacturer/ Availability	Activity	Clinical Applications	Limitations
Worst Case Scenario-Survival Game™	University Games Widely available. The game is available in a junior version for younger children. A revised version of the game, The Worst Case Scenario Surviving Life™, is also available. This version offers some interesting reframing possibilities in that *wrong* answers result in loss of body parts of the playing pieces!	Game play involves moving forward from start by determining the best solution from a list of three to a particular challenge, (e.g., Do you know how to escape from the trunk of a car? How to survive a shark attack.) The first player to reach the finish is the winning survivor.	This game can be played with adolescents and older teens to build trust, foster self-confidence, explore decision-making styles, identify and validate coping skills and provoke discussion on feelings/thoughts that occur when a solution to a challenge is one you don't agree with or don't like.	Due to the reading level of the game cards, the game is recommended for use with older children, adolescents and young adults.

Yes & No Game™	Pressman Toy Company	Play involves reading a card with a list of rapid-fire questions to your opponent. If the opponent answers yes or no to any question, the asking player keeps the card. If the other player gets to the end of the questions without saying yes or no they keep the card.	This game can be used to enhance impulse control skills in a fun and fast-paced way.	Due to the reading level of the game cards, the game may be more appropriate for older children (above age 8), adolescents and young adults.
	Widely available.		The game can also be used to stimulate exploration and discussion on the benefits of thinking before you speak with parents, teachers, and authority figures.	
		The player with the most cards at the end of the game is the winner.		

Candy Land™ (Milton Bradley)

Developed in the 1940s by a person in recovery from polio, the game has become a cultural icon due to its status for many as the first board game they played as children (Candy Land™, 2007). The game is very useful for therapeutic play with younger children because it requires no reading ability and only minimal counting skills. Therapeutically, I have used the game to establish trust with younger children (ages 4–7 years) who often don't have the interpersonal communication skills or comfort level to be engaged in more interactive or complex therapeutic play. Additionally, I have used the game to positively reinforce attention-sustaining behavior of children with ADHD. Interestingly, Candy Land™ was a favorite game of one my clients who was dealing with multiple family losses and the aftermath of Hurricane Katrina. Through play with Candy Land™, the client shared compelling memories of playing the board game with her grandmother prior to the storm. During repeated play with the game, she began to reveal feelings of sadness and grief as she relieved the experiences of the events. In this way, Candy Land™ served as a catalyst for adaptive grieving.

The Game of Life™ (Milton Bradley)

One of the oldest "modern" board games still in use was originally developed in 1860 and provided Americans with relief and diversion during the Civil War (Hofer, 2003). Although the game is very capitalistic in nature (the more money and property you have the better), the game provides an opportunity to identify and discuss decision-making skills, problem solving, disappointment and stress, and even building empathy and understanding for parents/primary caregivers who are often dealing with real-life issues of money, job, and providing for a family. I have used this game with older children and adolescents in order to increase attention-sustaining skills, and for building hope for the future after the experience of serious trauma and loss.

The Worst Case Scenario Survival Game™ (University Games)

This game invites players to "use their survival instincts and skills to outlast their opponents" (Board Game Geek, 2007) by determining the *best* answer to a particular challenge with three possible answers. Although the challenges presented can be of a scary nature (how to cross a piranha-infested river), they also contain practical and even humorous situations (how to scratch an itch in a cast). I use this game with adolescents and older teens to build trust, foster self-confidence, explore decision-making styles, and as a basis for identifying and validating coping skills. This game also has the cognitive benefit of exploring feelings and thoughts when even the best answer to a challenge is one you don't agree with or don't like.

Sorry!™ (Parker Brothers)

Another universally popular board game, the slide pursuit game of Sorry!™ is based on the Indian game of Parchisi (Sorry, 2007). Played by multiple generations of Americans during the last 75 years, the objective of the game is to be the first player to get all four pawns from the start to home. In order to win, players must carefully read and understand the rule cards for the game that tell you how and when to move. Sorry!™ illustrates and reinforces in a nonjudgmental manner that winning is achieved by knowing and following the rules. During game play, I explore the client's thoughts and beliefs about using and adapting this process outside of therapy. In this application, Sorry!™ mirrors Virginia Satir's notion of the *family microcosm* (Laign, 1988). Just as Satir believed that "by knowing how to heal the family, I know how to heal the world" (Laign, 1988, p. 20), the child or adolescent client, through game play, can began to believe, "If I can win by playing by the rules in this game, then I can play by the rules and win at home and school."

BOARD GAMES BASED ON A POPULAR CULTURE FIGURE

This category of board games can include those developed for a particular pop culture figure or event, or traditional board games themed or marketed in conjunction with a popular character found in a movie, television show, or book, such as Clue: The Simpsons™, or Game of Life: Disney™. These games appeal to children and adolescents on two levels: through their knowledge and familiarity with the game itself and their interest and enthusiasm for a popular cultural figure or media. Conversely, this is also one of limitations of popular culture themed games, in that the shelf life of these games is limited as movies, television, and other manifestations of popular culture move from popularity to obscurity rather quickly. Therefore, the selection of pop-culture themed games for therapeutic play should include more well-known characters in popular culture. Examples would include games featuring Superman, Batman, Disney and Looney Tunes characters, Scooby Doo, and other cultural icons that have stood the test of time and continue to be rediscovered by successive generations. Two board games from this genre that I have found useful in my practice with children and adolescents include:

Scooby Doo! Thrills and Spills Game™ (Pressman)

Using one of four plastic figures of the Scooby Doo gang (Velma, Daphne, Shaggy, and Fred) and a color-coordinating Scooby Doo figure, players move their team uphill through a graveyard to be the first to get to the Mystery Machine. A spinner determines how many spaces to move. If the spin results in landing on *monster space* on the dial or the game board, a spinning top is set loose that can knock the figures over. Any figures that are knocked down can get back up again and return to start. In addition to being a great deal of fun, this game is a cornucopia of reframing possibilities and symbolism. I have used the game with children, adolescents, and teens dealing with recovery from sexual and physical abuse, family trauma and disruption, depression, anxiety, grief, and bereavement. It provides a nonthreatening platform for exploring feelings of fear, pain, anger, isolation, and hopelessness, and can assist clients in identifying the members of their own real-life team (their social support system) who can help overcome the scary places and monsters that they encounter. The game is also about finding inner strength and resiliency when you get knocked down, and getting the support you need to start again.

Harry Potter Whomping Willow Game™ (Mattel)

Based on the second installment of the Harry Potter film series, *Harry Potter and the Chamber of Secrets* (Columbus, 2002), players reenact the scene in which Harry and Ron use a flying car to return to Hogwarts and crash into the anthropormorphic and frightening Whomping Willow tree. Using plastic "car" hooks, players try to remove luggage, book satchels, and figures of Harry's pet owl from the tree. This game can be an effective icebreaker with clients of all ages. In addition to increasing the comfort level and reducing anxiety during the initial therapy visit, the game can also be used to augment attention-sustaining skills/on-task behavior. I have also used the game in conjunction with family therapy to formulate healthy alliance building (Robbins & Szapocznik, 2000), cooperative behavior, and turn-taking between siblings. Additionally, this game can be used for reframing perspective and instilling hope for children who have felt marginalized or isolated by poor academic performance, in that the skills used for successful achievement against the Whomping Willow (staying focused, believing in yourself, not giving up) can be adapted for successful achievement in the classroom.

THERAPEUTIC BOARD GAMES

These games are designed to elicit information from children and adolescents by having them respond to or describe "some aspect of their lives or fantasies, and allowing the therapist to respond" (Bellinson, 2002, p. 34). The appeal of these games is twofold: for clients, they resemble and follow patterns of other structured board games; for therapists they provide opportunities to hear thoughts and beliefs and to "learn some aspect of a child's current or past life, directly or metaphorically" (p. 35).

The growth and popularity of therapeutic board games in the past 20 years has been phenomenal, and even commercial toy and game manufacturers such as Milton Bradley (Are You 4 Real™) and Cardinal (Chicken Soup for the Family Soul™) are developing games about sharing, caring, and feelings. Therapeutic board games may be broad in scope, with an emphasis on exploring client experiences and enhancing client response (The Ungame™, Exploring My World™). They can also target specific problems and issues such as anger management (Furious Fred™ Anger Solution Board Game™), self-esteem (The Self Esteem Game™), stress and anxiety (Dr. Play Well's Coping With Stress Card Game™), and impulse control (Look Before You Leap™).

Generally, I have found therapeutic games to be more effective tools with older children (above age 8) and adolescents who are more open to guided exploration and discussion, and are better able to verbalize, identify, and associate feelings and behaviors. A therapeutic themed game that I find very useful is The Ungame™. Created in 1972 by therapist Rhea Zacich, The Ungame is a noncompetitive game that explores thoughts, feelings, and experiences by fostering "listening skills as well as self-expression" (Board Game Geek, 2007). The Ungame™, which is available in age-targeted versions for teens, children, and families, asks players to move pawns on a playing board by answering questions from two stacks of cards, one with lighthearted topics and the other with more serious ones. Other spaces on the board encourage players to exchange thoughts and feelings or describe how they've been affected by recent emotions (The Ungame™, 2007).

CASE STUDIES

Bradley: Clinical Application of Traditional/ Commercially Produced Board Games

Bradley, an 8-year old White male, was referred for counseling services by his mother in response to recent incidents of lying and defiant behavior with teachers. During his first visit, Bradley demonstrated avoidant behavior and resistance to any efforts to test his understanding for the reason of the visit.

In an effort to elicit participation, I allowed Bradley to select a board game from the game cupboard. Bradley selected Sorry!™, expressing "really liking this game," and disclosing that, "I beat my cousins at this game all the time." During initial game play, Bradley demonstrated challenges with compliance to game rules and poor impulse control, requiring cessation of game play several times during the session to request his cooperation and to review and clarify rules for game play.

At the beginning of his second session, I explored his interest in continuing our game of Sorry!™ and contracted with Bradley an agreement to play by the rules of the game with the promise of allowing him to stop the game when "it's not fun anymore."

After some initial regressive behavior, Bradley and I continued the game. He demonstrated increased attention-sustaining behavior as he began to display greater success in moving his pawns from start to home. This session included some directive feedback with Bradley on taking his time to read the instructions on the playing cards, such as moving *backward* four spaces instead of *forward* and identifying the cards that offered him a choice to make a strategic move, such as moving 11 spaces versus changing places with an opponent or splitting a move of 7 spaces between two pawns. As game play progressed, Bradley demonstrated marked recall of game strategies and used these effectively to his advantage. The session concluded with Bradley's successful efforts in winning the game and exploration of his thoughts and feelings about winning by playing by the rules.

In two successive sessions, Bradley was allowed to choose other games to play in session. These included Jenga!™ and Battleship™. With Jenga!™, Bradley initially demonstrated regressive behavior—removing wood pieces haphazardly, not waiting his turn, prompting directive feedback from the therapist on his past successful efforts in winning by the rules at the previous session. With Battleship™, Bradley demonstrated cheating behavior during the first round of play, moving boats on his concealed game board to avoid being hit. During the second round of play, I emulated Bradley's cheating behavior, eliciting from him an angry response, "You're cheating!" This session concluded with exploring

Bradley's thoughts and feelings on cheating and reinforcing his prior successful effort in winning by the rules with Sorry!™. Other interventions included securing the cooperation of Bradley's mother and teacher in reinforcing the message of winning by the rules, and when possible, offering Bradley choices that resulted in a positive outcome in whatever he decided to do (allowing him to play his video games for a specified time after he finished his math or his spelling homework).

Through board game play, I was also able to reinforce with Bradley other positive behaviors of seeking clarification and asking for help to learn the rules in order to win at home and at school. By his fifth session, Bradley disclosed his ongoing challenges of keeping up with homework assignments and his resultant feelings of shame and embarrassment when "I can't do the work." Additionally, he admitted that his lying to teachers was prompted by his challenges in understanding the work covered in class and his fear that "they (other students and siblings) call me dumb if I tell them I don't get it." Further work with Bradley included validation of his feelings, confronting disorganized negative messages from peers and siblings, emphasizing his successful abilities in board game play and video games, and having him identify, via reframing, efforts he uses in game play that he could apply in the classroom—"paying attention," "asking questions," "taking my time," and "being excited." Bradley's mother and teacher also agreed to include the use of math flash cards, word games, and puzzles to augment classroom instruction, making it more competitive (and like a game), and close monitoring and intervention when derogatory words like dumb and stupid were used by peers and siblings. Additional therapeutic play efforts included use of Brain-Quest™, a grade-specific question-and-answer board game allowing Bradley to choose questions from scholastic categories of Math, Social Studies, Science, English, and Grab Bag.

Miguela: Clinical Application of Therapeutic and Popular Culture Board Games

Miguela was a 13-year-old Hispanic female who was referred for counseling services due to an episode of severe emotional distress following a male school peer's unpleasant and highly upsetting behavior. Upon initial assessment with the client and her mother, it was disclosed that Miguela was also the victim of 5-year-long sexual abuse by her stepfather. During the initial intervention by law enforcement and children's protective service personnel, Miguela and her family had received only short-term crisis counseling with neither follow-up counseling nor extended family therapy. Additionally, during an individual assessment session, Miguela disclosed that her mother and other family members discouraged discussion of the abuse due to shared feelings of guilt, shame, and sadness, stating, "It makes them feel bad to talk about it."

To begin the process of addressing her mother's avoidance in discussing the abuse and to foster feelings of trust, I initiated with both Miguela and her mother therapeutic play with *The Worst Case Scenario Survival Game*™ during their second session. In this session, Miguela and her mother played in opposition to each other with the therapist providing assistance in reviewing game rules and providing clarification of the challenges and choices of the game cards they selected. During game play, both Miguela and her mother expressed great enjoyment for the game and demonstrated mutually supportive behavior in advancing on the game board. At the end of play, I initiated limited exploration and discussion with both of them on shared feelings related to the challenges selected and discussed during game play. Discussion included exploration of thoughts and beliefs of being able to survive the hostile and scary situations described. I also shared my observations of the mutually supportive interaction witnessed between parent and child, and elicited from them current examples of cooperative and supportive interaction.

Successive sessions with Miguela and her mother included a combination of bibliotherapy with discussion of selected readings from Maya Angelou's poem *Life Doesn't Frighten Me* (1993), and a nonconfrontational case scenario from the book by Amy Bahr, *Sometimes It's O.K. To Tell Secrets* (1988). During a subsequent session, I initiated play with The Ungame.™ In preparation for game play, I reviewed the game's rules and disclosed that the game cards may request disclosure of memories and/or experiences that could trigger painful feelings. Both agreed to continue game play with the caveat of terminating play immediately if they wished to do so. During play, Miguela selected a card asking, "If you could relive one year of your life, what year would it be?" Miguela disclosed that she would relive the year that she and her mother spent the summer with extended family members out-of-state, away from her stepfather. Miguela disclosed feeling "happy and safe" during that time. Miguela's revelation elicited an emotional response from her mother, who expressed feelings of sorrow for "not being able to make it like that for you all the time." With mutual agreement, game play was stopped, and Miguela's mother disclosed additional unprocessed feelings of guilt, shame, and anger during the remainder of the session. This began the process of Miguela and her mother finally being able to openly discuss the abuse with each other.

During a subsequent individual session, I initiated play with the popular culture-themed game, *Scooby Doo! Spills and Thrills*™. Miguela had previously disclosed her childhood enjoyment of Scooby Doo cartoons and the recent Scooby Doo live action movies. During game play, we discussed unique aspects of the game such as the uphill design of the board, the graveyard setting, and the conflicting feelings of excitement and fear that occur when the monsters come out via the spinning top. Upon exploration of other times in her life when she had experienced conflicting emotions, Miguela revealed feelings of guilt and shame of being both frightened and sexually aroused during the abuse by her stepfather. In acknowledging and validating her conflicting emotions as a result of the game play, Miguela was now able to begin replacing the guilt and confusion with understanding and acceptance that her body acted in a natural way to what happened and that she was not a bad person, but a survivor.

Other efforts with Miguela and her mother included postplay discussion on specific topics illustrated via a particular board game: sharing secrets and nurturing understanding (Are U For Real?™), and fostering hope for the future (The Game of Life™). Through the therapeutic use of board games, Miguela and her mother were able to remove the obstacle of fear to come to terms with their anger, sadness, and guilt to begin the process of healing.

CONCLUSION

Board games, because of their cross-cultural and generational appeal, as well as their seemingly permanent place in popular culture, can offer counselors, therapists, and other adults an enjoyable, entertaining, and nonintimidating method for exploring thoughts, feelings, and beliefs of children and adolescents. As demonstrated in the above case studies, therapeutic play with board games can also provide a comfort zone for care professionals to observe social skills and interpersonal communication, explore family dynamics and functioning, and provide a means to assist younger clients and family members in resolving conflicts, and in coming to terms with unprocessed feelings, building understanding, and moving forward.

It should be noted that the selection of appropriate board games in therapy should always correspond with the age, interests, reading level, and cognitive abilities of the client. Moreover, board games should be used in conjunction with a variety of clinical tools (drawing/therapeutic art activities, role play/storytelling with action figures/puppets, bibliotherapy), to enhance therapy with children and adolescents by serving "as a means to refine diagnosis, as an opportunity to enhance ego function and as a natural route to improving a child's socialization skills" (Schaefer & Reid, 2002, p. 39).

Finally, board game play combined with cognitive reframing, insight building, and empowerment can instill awareness that overcoming life's challenges does not have to be an overwhelming endeavor, nor a process that has to be faced alone. Board game play can provide a staging ground where adults can assist children and adolescents in learning that winning and losing are all a part of the game of life.

Exercise 11.1: My Favorite Superhero

My favorite superhero is _____.

Draw a picture of your favorite superhero:

I like _____ (name of superhero) the most because she/he is:
_____ **1st reason** (Pick from the words listed below)
_____ **2nd reason** (Pick from the words listed below)
_____ **3rd reason** (Pick from the words listed below)
_____ **4th reason** (Pick from the words listed below)

Angry	Big	Brave	Fast	Friendly
Funny	Good	Helpful	Honest	Powerful
Quick	Scary	Smart	Sneaky	Strong

Superheroes have special powers, and my favorite superhero has the power

to _____
and to _____
and to _____.

If I had these powers too, the FIRST thing I would like to do would be:

_____.

The *My Favorite Superhero* questionnaire provides a fun and non-threatening way to explore a child's experience/thoughts/beliefs via their preference for a favorite superhero. This brief questionnaire can be very revealing in the client's identification and ranking of specific characteristics that they associate with their favorite hero. Additionally, the client's responses to the symbolization question related to their application of the hero's powers can provide a foundation to identify and deal with stressors and challenges within the home and school environments.

Colored pencils, markers, or crayons should be incorporated in the administration of this questionnaire, allowing the client to creatively interrupt, via drawing her/his favorite superhero. The questionnaire can be self-administered with older children and adolescents, or it can be completed together by the client and the therapist.

REFERENCES

Angelou, M. (1993). *Life doesn't frighten me.* New York: Stewart, Tabori and Chang.

Bahr, A. (1988). *Sometimes it's o.k. to tell secrets.* New York: Putnam Publishing.

Bellinson, J. (2002). *Children's use of board games in psychotherapy.* New York: Jason Aronson.

Black, B. (2007). *Winning at all costs: It's not worth it.* Retrieved August 2, 2007, from http://healthgate.partners.org

Blair, P. (2003). *Board games: $870 million dollar industry saw a 65% surge in sales.* Retrieved July 14, 2007, from http://www.toydirectory.com

Board Games. (2007). *Board game: History.* Retrieved July 18, 2007, from http://en.wikipedia.org/wiki/Boardgames

Board Game Geek. (2007). *The Ungame.* Retrieved July 20, 2007, from http://www.boardgamegeek.com

Boyd-Webb, N. (1999). *Play therapy with children in crisis* (2nd ed.). New York: Guilford Press.

Candy Land. (2007). *Candy Land.* Retrieved July 18, 2007, from http://en.wikipedia.org/wiki/Candy_Land

Chertoff, N., & Kahn, S. (2006). *Celebrating board games.* New York: Sterling.

Columbus, C. (Director). (2002). *Harry Potter and the chamber of secrets* [Motion picture]. United States: 1492 Pictures.

Gobet, F., de Voogt, A., & Retschitzki, J. (2004). *Moves in mind: The psychology of board games.* Hove and New York: Psychology Press.

Hofer, M. (2003). *The games we played: The golden age of board and table games.* New York: Princeton Architectural Press.

Joseph, G., & Strain, P. (2006). *Helping young children control anger and handle disappointment.* University of Illinois at Urbana-Champaign: The Center for Emotional and Social Foundations for Early Learning. Retrieved July 29, 2007, from http://www.uwex.edu

Kennedy, E. (1989). *Crisis counseling with children and adolescents.* New York: Continuum.

Laign, J. (1988, October/November). Healing human spirits, creating joy in living: Interview with Virginia Satir. *Focus on Chemically Dependent Families, 11*, 20–21, 28–32.

Moyles, J. (1989). *Just playing?* Philadelphia: Open University Press.

Robbins, M., & Szapocznik, J. (2000, April). Brief strategic family therapy. *Office of Juvenile Justice Bulletin,* 1–12. Retrieved August 2, 2007, from http://www.ncjrs.gov/pdffiles1/ojjdp/179285.pdf

Schaefer, C., & Reid, S. (Eds.). (2002). *Game play: Therapeutic use of childhood games* (2nd ed.). New York: Wiley.

Sorry. (2007). *Sorry* (game). Retrieved July 18, 2007, from http://en.wikipedia.org/wiki/Sorry

Teitel, J. (1998). Wanna play? *Psychology Today*. Retrieved June 15, 2007, from http://psychologytoday.com/articles

The Ungame. (2007). *The Ungame*. Retrieved July 18, 2007, from http://en.wikipedia.org/wiki/The_Ungame

PART V

Television

CHAPTER 12

Big Heroes on the Small Screen

Naruto and the Struggle Within

Lawrence C. Rubin

CARTOONS, CARTOONS EVERYWHERE

Saturday mornings, if you were lucky enough to be a kid with a TV, no homework, a cooperative sibling, and tolerant-enough parents beginning in the early 1960s, could mean only one thing—cartoons! While they inhabited the diminutive universe of the small screen, the colorful, larger-than-life characters of cartoondom thrilled, shocked, entertained, and most of all engaged generations of children. They played, fought, flew, and romanced their way into the lives and imaginations of young viewers who tuned in week after week to be part of a seemingly inexhaustible range of adventures, follies, and fantasies. They had sufficient appeal and market power to make the quantum jump from the prime time slots of the major networks, and the magical power to leap from our television screens onto our clothing, lunchboxes, vitamins, board games, sleeping bags, furniture, jewelry, wallpaper, and every imaginable staple of our diets.

To name but a few in relative chronological order from the 1960s through the 1980s; *Casper the Friendly Ghost, Magilla Gorilla, Beany and Cecil, Rocky and Bullwinkle, The Jetsons, Flintstones, Sky Hawks, Quickdraw McGraw, George of the Jungle, Top Cat, Atom Ant, Secret Squirrel, Space Ghost, Penelope Pittstop and Sweet Penelope Purebread, Underdog, Dudley Do-Right of the Northwest Canadian Mounties, Heckle and Jeckle, Lancelot Link, Sabrina and the Groovy Goolies, The Pink*

Panther, Johnny Quest, Deputy Dawg, The Houndcats, Fantastic Four, Yogi's Gang, Hong Kong Phooey, Fat Albert and the Cosby Kids, Jabbeyjaw, Super 6, Super President and Spyshadow, McDuffy the Talking Dog, Superfriends, Fangface, Tom and Jerry, Alvin and the Chipmunks, Banana Splits, Scooby Doo, The Archies, Bugs Bunny and the Roadrunner, The Drak Pack, Popeye and Olive Oyl, Richie Rich, The Smurfs, Berenstain Bears, Herculoids, Teenage Mutant Ninja Turtles, Josie and the Pussycats, Dynomutt, The Funky Phantom, Care Bears and Turbo Teens, and of course Zazoo U, Garfield, and *The Space Cats.*[1]

The fact is that this list represents only a portion of the total number of cartoons aired between 1960 and 1989 in the 8:30 to 11:30 A.M. Saturday time slot. It does not even begin to approximate what would follow in the next two decades and be dubbed the "toon boom" (Kellogg, 1992). Beginning with the airing of *The Simpsons* on Fox TV in 1990, which was the most successful animated character family since Fred Flintstone's three decades earlier (Mitchell, 1995), the medium of the television cartoon was poised for a revolution. In 1992, media mogul Ted Turner created the cable Cartoon Network (CN), a 24/7 animation oasis for the young and young at heart. Beginning with Looney Tunes, CN features such animated favorites as *Dexter's Laboratory, Johnny Bravo, Ed, Edd n Eddy, Ben Ten, The Land Before Time, The Life and Times of Juniper Lee, Teen Titans,* and perennial favorite *Scooby Doo.*[2] In 1991, Nickelodeon TV, another cable channel that had aired over a decade earlier, created Nicktoons, which was dedicated to innovative cartoon programming. Some of their popular programs include *Doug, Rugrats, Ren and Stimpy, Rocko's Modern Life, Hey Arnold!, Jimmy Neutron—Boy Genius, Cat Dog,* and *Sponge Bob.*[3]

As have their predecessors, the cartoons of the "toon boom" generation have been wildly popular, and in addition to the characters finding their way onto merchandise of all kinds, full-length multimillion-dollar movie adaptations of favorite television cartoon characters have ensured both their popularity and longevity. Additionally, as its name implies, the Cartoon Network as well as Nickelodeon have broken free of the Saturday morning time slot and offer cartoon programming virtually around the clock. With the advent of electronic recording devices such as Tivo, and other cable networks such as TV Land, which airs vintage and syndicated cartoons, children of all ages are never more than a remote-click away from their favorite animated characters.

With all of the various forms of video entertainment available today including the Internet, video games, and iPods, one would think that television in general, and television cartoons in particular, might have lost their popularity. This is simply not the case, as cartoons seem to be timeless in their appeal. In spite of the competing forms of entertainment, children between ages 2 and 18 watch between 2–3 hours of television daily, and 54% of children in this demographic watch so-called children's entertainment, foremost among which is cartoons (Roberts, Foehr, Rideout, & Brodie, 1999). Cartoons often rank highly in Nielsen ratings among television-watching teens.[4]

Interestingly, but perhaps not surprisingly, "Saturday morning has long served as a shorthand epithet for culture judged to be juvenile, low-quality, moronic, mind-numbing, or cut rate" (Burke & Burke, 1999, p. 1). It has been argued that cartoons are a diminutive and debased form of entertainment that perpetuate gender stereotyping, racism, and violence (Abel, 1995; Levinson, 1975; McCauley, Woods, Coolidge, & Kulick, 1983; Swan, 1995; Thompson & Zerbino, 1995); make it difficult for younger audiences to separate reality from fantasy (Middelton & Vanderpool, 1999); distort children's moral development by modeling demonization of the "other" (Fouts, Callan, & Piasentin, 2006); and sow the seeds for stigmatization of the mentally ill through negative vocabulary and character depictions (Wilson, Nairn, Coverdale, & Panapa, 2000). Additionally, cartoons have been redressed for their poor quality, particularly in the case of what is called limited animation, which makes use of recycled scenes and minimization of action, repetitive and monotonous plotlines, endless efforts to sell children something, and reinforcement of the viewer's passivity (Burke & Burke, 1999).

In contrast to the above, however, equally strong arguments prevail suggesting that they also contain prosocial messages, provide an opportunity for shared narratives, and tap into timeless truths often found in myth and folklore (Anderson, 1984; Mitchell, 1995; Wilson et al., 2000). In this latter regard, Anderson (1984) conceptualized children's cartoons, particularly science fiction-themed tales, as modern-day [techno] mythology in which "a complete and convincing microcosm can be created, a vivid fantasy world which purports to teach practical lessons about real world issues" (p. 160). Among these real-world issues, he identified nuclear annihilation fears, the emerging threat to humanity by machines, and the toxic impact of the corporate mentality. This was particularly prescient, considering it was written over two decades ago, before the contemporary, but not necessarily novel societal nightmares of genocide, terrorism, and global warming consumed our daily attention.

ANIME

As noted above, Western cartoons, the kind Americans have grown up with over the last five decades, have been criticized on the grounds that they are silly, sentimental, and sanitized, particularly Disney animation, where with few exceptions endings are notoriously happy. With the advent of superhero comics in the 1930s,[5] and the slew of subsequent animation on both the big and small screens, characters, contexts, and plots grew darker and more painfully human. While the implementation of the Comics Code in the mid-1950s slowed the so-called moral decline of the medium, and by association our youth, the industry rebounded during the subsequent years to produce a host of very edgy comic book characters that were then adapted to cartoon form. However, it took an Eastern influence, that of Japanese popular culture, to turn the tide on soft-core sensibilities.

Manga, or Japanese comic art (literally translated as "whimsical pictures"), dates to antiquity and consists of caricature, cartoon, editorial pictures, syndicated panels, and daily humor strips (Clements & McCarthy, 2006). As an art form, it "is immersed in a particular social environment that includes history, language, culture, politics, economy, family, religion, sex and gender . . . reflecting the reality of Japanese society along with myths, beliefs, rituals, traditions, fantasies and Japanese way of life [which also] depicts other social phenomena such as social order and hierarchy, sexism, racism, ageism, classism and so on" (Ito, 2005, p. 456). Unlike Western cartoons, which are often exclusively character and plot driven, Manga reflects Japanese communication patterns and worldview and in so doing, "relies more on contextual cues such as facial expression, gestures, eye glances, length of timing of silence, tone of voice and grunts" (p. 457). Manga is not isolated to the wide-eyed action figures that Westerners have become familiar with, such as Pokémon or Yu-Gi-Oh, but encompasses a broad range of subgenres including characters and stories about politics, history, and sexuality, that may be disturbingly graphic.[6]

Just as Western comic book and magazine figures have crossed into animated form, so too has Manga been transformed into the medium known as anime. Described as possibly Japan's chief cultural export (Napier, 2001), anime, unlike the precise, often real-life and heavily orchestrated Western cartoon, relies on nonfluid movement and stagnant posing of characters to build tension, the use of sounds that are symbolically tied to Japanese culture, and the incorporation of fantasy motifs for expressing important issues and struggles that are often sexual and violent. Additionally, unlike its Western counterpart, which relies on constant movement and quick dialogue provided by famous actors and comedians, anime makes use of big eyes and dramatic facial features to convey intense emotion, wild and vibrant hair colors to express the character's individuality, and exotic, artistically rendered settings that are often fantastical and surreal (Price, 2001). And unlike Western cartoons, which often provide certainty, resolution, and more than a fair share of sanitization, particularly those aired on broadcast and mainstream cable TV networks, anime deals more openly, graphically, and directly with uncertainty, death, social messages, the clash between traditional and contemporary issues, mortality, morality, gender, and inequality.

Anime has many genres and subgenres,[7] some of which are similar to Western counterparts, and others quite different. To name a few, they include action/adventure (*Ninja Scroll* and *Naruto*), horror (*Wicked City*), progressive or stylized (*Voices of a Distant Star*), Shojo or "young lady" (*Mermaid Melody Pichi Pichi Pitch*), Shonen or "young boy" (*Dragon Ball Z* or *Pokémon*), Seinen or "young man" (*Cowboy Bebop*), Josei or "young woman" (*Gokusen*), Bishojo or "beautiful girl" (*Magic Knight Rayearth*), Bishonen or "beautiful boy" (*Fushigi Yugi*), robot/mecha (*Mobile Suit Gandam*), postapolcalyptic (*Neon Genesis*), Maho Shojo or "magical girl" (*Sailor Moon*), Maho Shonen or "magical boy"' (*D. N. Angel*), Moe or "cutesy" (*A Little Snow Fairy Sugar*), Komodo or "child" (*Hello Kitty*), and finally a number of romantic genres that include the sexualized and explicitly sexual (Clements & McCarthy, 2006). American cartoon viewers of the last several decades are probably most familiar with anime that has crossed the globe, including *Speed Racer, Kimba the White Tiger, Voltron,* and *G Force*.

This range of provocative subjects along with the unique visual style of anime may explain, at least in part, anime's popularity outside of Japan, and particularly in the United States (Grigsby, 1998). Adding to the appeal of anime is the incredibly diverse range of themes available to the viewer. Within the medium of Japanese animation, one can find:

> wrenching dramas, cheesy romances, storybook adventures, spooky thrillers, historical fantasies, robot shows, gothic fairy tales, slapstick parodies, futuristic dystopias, sports dramas, sci-fi series, gimmicky sci-fi series, sexy cyberpunk technomythologies, misogynistic violent pornography, sword and sorcery stories, spoofs of sword and sorcery stories, epic environmental cautionary tales, Norse goddess romances, not to mention your normal, everyday life family soap operas. (Price, 2001, pp. 153–154)

And like its counterpart, manga, anime is "deeply embedded in all aspects of Japanese society: folklore, legends, history, religion, moral assumptions and aesthetic standards, to name a few" (Price, 2001, p. 256). Providing a glimpse into the exotic, other-worldly Japanese culture as it does for the not-so-worldly American viewer may also account for the popularity of anime.

NARUTO

The anime character of interest in this current discussion is known to viewers simply as Naruto. His full name is Naruto Uzumaki. Children and teens, both in the United States and Japan, not to mention other industrialized nations, who have helped elevate him to the status of anime superstar are also likely to be familiar with related anime action characters such as Pokémon, the pocket monsters, Dragon Ball Z, Yu-Gi-Oh, and Cowboy Be Bop, all of which have appeared on trading cards, video games, and in the movies, not to mention on either Nickelodeon or Cartoon Network. However, Naruto is currently in a league of its (his) own. Created by Masashi Kishimoto, originally appearing in 1999 as a manga in the 43rd issue of Japan's *Shonen Jump* magazine, Naruto soon made the transition to anime under the auspices of VIZ Media, featuring as one of Cartoon Network's blockbuster "toonamis." In 2002, a Naruto-based feature-length film won the Academy Award for best animated feature, followed in 2006 by being ranked in the top 20 animated properties by retail watchdog ICv2, in the top 25 of *USA Today*'s Best Sellers, and winning the Quill Award ("Viz Media," 2007a, 2007b, 2007c, 2007d, 2007e).

The story of Naruto[8] is appealing on a number of levels; as a coming-of-age story, a superhero tale, and a fast-moving action drama featuring a rich cast of ever-evolving characters. The story begins in Japan's mythical Leaf Village, Konohagakure, where a powerful entity called the Nine-Tailed Demon Fox, who is purportedly powerful enough to cause cataclysmic damage with the swipe of any of its tails, goes on a rampage of destruction and human devastation. The leader of the village, Yondaime, who is called the Fourth Hokage (a ninja warrior of great power), sacrifices his own life to seal the demon inside the newborn orphan Naruto Uzumaki. The Hokage's wish was to both contain the destructive energy of the fox and to elevate and empower the orphaned infant in the eyes of the village.

The Nine-Tailed Fox or Demon Fox[9] is an entity of great sadistic and malevolent power who also has a deep sense of honor and respect for Naruto. This sets the stage for ever-present tension between the two characters. As a result of being the container of this great energy force, Naruto has accelerated healing power, incredible stamina, and the strength and ability to use the Multiple Shadow Clone Technique to duplicate himself or other characters. As a young child, Naruto was at the mercy of the malevolent force within him, striking out at anything and anyone near him during intense emotional states. As he undergoes training, Naruto learns to harness the energy, or *chakra*, of the demon fox, calling on only as much power he needs at the time, rather than succumbing to it. However, as he draws upon more and more of the fox's power, he surrenders a proportionate amount of his own will, to the point that he puts friends and himself at risk.

As noted above, the Fourth Hokage hoped that by implanting the demon fox within the orphan Naruto, that he would gain the admiration and respect of the members of his village. However, the opposite occurred as they shunned him, and in futile attempts to attain acceptance, Naruto became an impulsive, hyperactive, attention-seeking, and troublesome trickster. The very first episode of the series finds him defacing the village monuments of the first three hokages, much to the dismay of all. Naruto manages to graduate from the ninja academy, upon which he learns of the demon fox within him and also learns that there are indeed people both inside and outside of the academy who care for him.

Naruto leaves the academy as part of *Team 7* with his two close friends Sasuke Uchiha[10] and Sakura Hurano[11] on a series of adventures and perils, with the ultimate goal of returning to the village and becoming a hokage. Sasuke struggles to step out from the shadows of and seek revenge on his powerful older brother Itachi, who murders the clan, as well as to find his parents, who were lost in the carnage. He, like Naruto, is an orphan who in the beginning of his quest is alienated from the team, but who learns to value membership and others. Sakura Hurano, whose name translates as "the spring of cherry blossoms," is a shy and self-conscious fellow student at the ninja academy, where she develops an infatuation with Sasuke. She is a highly intelligent member of the team with great powers of memory and medical abilities, who learns to harness the power of her chakra and who ultimately becomes a great warrior.

Naruto as a Clinical Resource

In a previous book (Rubin, 2006), I demonstrated the clinical utility of the superhero genre. By tapping into the various facets of the superhero metaphor, including the origin story, secret identities, transformative journeys, the clash between the hero and the villain, and even the ever-present sidekick, the clinician could expand and deepen the therapeutic narrative with children, teens, and adults. From the above overview of the plot and characters of the Naruto, the clinician once again has at her disposal a wealth of narrative material with which to connect with clients of all ages struggling with a range of clinical and developmental issues. To name a few, there is the story of parental loss and accompanying search for connection and identity that ultimately leads Naruto and Team 7 beyond the safe confines of their village into the world of peril. The presence of the demonic fox within him and his struggle to harness its potential destructive power provides for a wonderfully rich metaphor for the struggle to contain and channel intense and often negative emotion. Socialization and the search for acceptance both by others and of himself is a primary motivational element in Naruto's journeys, both within and outside of himself. The vanquishing of enemies in order to bring peace to his village is a powerful redemptive and ultimately transformative act that helps Naruto to become a powerful ninja, as well as a complete and mature person. There is also the ever-present temptation to use personal power for gain at the expense of others' needs.

In many ways, Naruto's story is consistent with the epic journey of the classical hero, who according to Joseph Campbell (1956) ventures forth from the safety of an imperiled homeland on a physically and mentally challenging journey of self-discovery, ultimately returning enlightened. Naruto's tale also contains elements of the story of the modern American superhero (Lawrence & Jewett, 2002), who by accident or legacy is transformed into a larger-than-life figure, and who battles forces both within and outside of himself in order to achieve redemption and to restore peace to a society into which (s)he never quite fits. As we shall see in the case to follow, Naruto was a valuable clinical resource for a struggling 9-year-old boy.

CASE DISCUSSION

Intake Information

At the time of referral, Kiko, an otherwise friendly and affectionate 10-year-old, was one pink slip away from expulsion from his third-grade placement in a local parochial school. While not typically aggressive, Kiko, according to his increasingly exasperated teachers, had temper tantrums, was manipulative, would shut down and sulk when disciplined, and was highly attention-seeking. Kiko had complained to both his parents and teachers that other children did not like him, refused to choose him for games, and made fun of him for reasons that were unclear to the adults in his life. Historically, Kiko had been similarly disruptive in earlier grades and struggled with reading, for which he had received tutoring and which caused him to "feel dumb."

Within the home, Kiko was the only child to parents who had co-raised the father's daughter from a previous relationship. Kiko's parents were both very involved in his life; however, his mother, who was very protective of him and had been raised in an alcoholic family, had very little tolerance for displays of anger, and made it quite clear that such emotion was unacceptable. In contrast, Kiko's father, a blustery yet benevolent patriarch who came from a broken home, often lost his temper, particularly toward his grown daughter who lived sporadically with the family. Kiko's parents argued frequently over discipline, argued in front of him, and often found themselves on opposing sides composed of mother and son against father and daughter.

Documentation

From an academic standpoint, Kiko had obtained satisfactory grades since kindergarten, and achieved in the median percentiles on national standardized testing; however, his classroom performance never quite rose to the level of the potential his testing suggested or his parents and teachers expected. Standardized perceptual and visual perception evaluations suggested some visual motor and language deficits, which were thought to be related to his reading difficulty, and as a result, Kiko underwent a series of visual therapy trainings with no clear improvement in his performance. A private psychological evaluation suggested intellectual functioning within the high average range with even greater potential and no apparent learning deficits. In short, there was no clear and compelling psychometric basis for Kiko's reading difficulties, which, in conjunction with his difficulties in self-control, continually frustrated both his parents and teachers. Surprisingly, Kiko never received a formal personality or emotional assessment; however, several drawings were available, which were militaristic.

Assessment

During this next phase, Kiko visited the playroom for several sessions during which he was allowed to use whatever media he chose while the therapist served as participant/observer. Kiko drew, played in the sandbox, with the dollhouse, and with puppets, as well as constructing stories. His parents joined him for one of these sessions during which the therapist invited them to engage in family drawing and construction as well as storytelling.

Kiko was an animated, expressive, energetic, and engaging boy who during the first meeting spontaneously described and acted out his passion for Naruto. Kiko seemed particularly interested in the Nine-Tailed Demon Fox that "comes out and he can use it to attack people who hurt him." Kiko also seemed particularly aware that Naruto was an orphan who used his power to protect friends and offered that "people have powers that they don't know they have until they come out." Kiko was familiar with the notion of chakra, and described it as "my own natural power."

Interestingly, when I reflected on Kiko's imagination during that first session, he immediately and angrily responded, "Hey, that means I imagine things and make things up like my friends say." In this regard, Kiko noted that it had been hard for him to make friends at school and that the other boys in his grade were into sports rather than the fantasy play that he enjoyed. During the second assessment session, Kiko outlined the various subnarratives of Naruto, focusing on the special relationship between the members of Team 7 and how his own behavior at times alienated him from the other children in his class. Kiko seemed to be a particularly intuitive and insightful boy who clearly identified with the Naruto narratives, and in doing so, was able to express some of the difficulties he was having. During the latter part of the session, I constructed a Naruto sentence completion task with item stems such as "If I were Naruto," "The thing that makes Naruto sad," "What Naruto wants to know the most about it is," "What Naruto was most afraid of," and "If I were Naruto, I would . . ." While Kiko seemed to understand my intention to use this task to side-handedly ask him questions about himself, he played along, indicating that he would like to have the power of a ninja who could control his chakra, that he worried about losing power, and at times wanted to be invisible, particularly at the ninja academy (the equivalent of his school).

In puppet play, vulnerable animals were victimized by the stronger predatory beasts that nevertheless apologized for their aggressive behavior and ultimately helped their victims back to recovery. Kiko was initially sheepish about such play, noting, "This is sort of kiddish," suggesting that he was very sensitive to being perceived as a little boy. Kiko also seemed very interested in the lava lamps that I had in my office, querying about how they worked and appreciating the manner in which the lava moved upwards toward the top when heated and returned to the bottom when cooled, and even drew the connection between this kinetic relationship and the way feelings, particularly anger, moved through his body on their way toward expression.

In the last of the three sessions, Kiko spent most of his time in the sand tray constructing an elaborate military scene pitting cowboys and Indians. He spent a considerable amount of time building the fortresses, fences, and areas of protection so that by the time the hour drew to a close, he had time for but one volley, and even then, engaged hesitantly in the skirmish. Kiko asked his mother to view his construction, and almost immediately offered "Sorry about the violence" to her in seeming anticipation that she would disapprove of the martial nature of the scene.

During the following visit, Kiko was joined by his parents. The family created a play genogram that shed light on the dynamic of anger within the family as the father was variously depicted through the miniatures as large, overbearing, and aggressive. All family members agreed that the mother, from the various animal personages, was the fun-loving problem solver who could stand up to the bellowing father. Kiko was alternately described as quick and devious, playful, and as a snake who could "bite you when you weren't looking." During the "build-a-house" portion of the session, Kiko's father was intent on creating a strong foundation, which coincided with his powerful presence in the family; however, he was not particularly successful at delegating tasks to Kiko and his mother. Kiko and his mother resisted and built interesting appendages to the house, which suggested that they were a team unto themselves rather than cohesively connected to the father.

During the subsequent review of the assessment with the parents, all parties agreed that play therapy in conjunction with parent counseling would be the most effective way to assist the family, and that Kiko's parents would also work on their own marital issues with an outside therapist with whom I would work in conjunction.

Treatment

Over the course of treatment, several themes emerged and wove themselves through Kiko's various play activities. It was clear that he struggled most intensely to control his own intense feelings, but was otherwise able to express fear of his father's anger. Kiko once again drew on the story of the powerful Nine-Tailed Demon Fox that had been implanted in Naruto, through which we were able to draw out examples of situations that happened both at home and at school in which he was angry, and explore how to give words to his feelings both at the time of their occurrence as well as in the counseling session. Here, Kiko recognized that the Nine-Tailed Fox, or the metaphor for his own sealed-in anger, was something that everyone had inside them, particularly his father. During one point in treatment, Kiko play-acted the overthrowing of the powerful and aggressive king by his subjects, at the end of which he tearfully admitted that his father's anger scared him, and that he often worried his parents would divorce. With his permission, this information was shared with the parents, who initiated marital counseling.

During the course of counseling, Kiko surprisingly confronted his parents about the relationship with his stepsister, who he had figured out must have come from a previous relationship. He was able to tie this awareness into Naruto's story, particularly as it related to the fragmentation of Team 7, and their ability to pull together. In this context, Kiko's parents were able to work together to make a place for his stepsister and address the rift in the family that had been created by this child of the father's previous relationship. Additionally, Kiko discussed the relationship between Naruto, Sasuki, and Sakura, who like members of his family battled, but ultimately reconciled for the benefit of the team.

One of Kiko's favorite play activities was clay modeling, and he chose to reproduce several versions of the office lava lamp, even taking a hardened Play-Doh version home as an amulet. Several discussions about the relationship between the motion of the hot lava and the rising tide of his own emotions helped Kiko to develop a more effective means of emotional expression and self-regulation. Like Naruto, Kiko enjoyed a sense of strength and power, which toward the end of our work together, he channeled through the creation of a variety of colorful superheroes using a Web-based program called Hero Machine.[12]

Outcome

As the end of the school year approached, Kiko had found a small group of friends at school who enjoyed fantasy play, and particularly Naruto and other animated characters. His parents had progressed nicely in their marital work and were communicating better, particularly around child-rearing issues. The family was planning a cross-country trip, and while Kiko was no longer at imminent risk for expulsion, they decided that his intellectual, educational, and social needs could be better met through public school attendance. In this regard, he received a full psychoeducational evaluation by the local school board, and was looking forward to the fourth grade. Kiko had entered counseling with the animated ally of Naruto, but left as a ninja in his own right, who like Naruto had developed a deeper appreciation for his own power, plus a better ability to channel it, and to reach out to others. His parents were willing participants in both his and their own ninja training and the Nine-Tailed Demon Fox was no longer an immediate threat, but instead a force to be understood, acknowledged, and respected. While therapeutic happy endings are nice when they occur, Kiko and his family clearly had a ways to go; however, they had taken sizeable strides.

CONCLUSION

Children are drawn to television cartoons for innumerable reasons. Cartoons are colorful, fast-moving, intriguing, confusing, and at times, shocking. They challenge the viewer to anticipate, problem solve, vicariously engage in adventures, and stimulate fantasy development as well as provide shared social narratives, symbols, and icons that build cultural awareness and social connection.

Anime, with roots in Japanese antiquity, is a relative newcomer on the American small screen. In addition to providing viewers with all of the above benefits, anime is exotic and other-worldly, edgy and unique in its visual and cinematic style. Mass marketing, merchandising, and advertising hype notwithstanding, anime in general, and Naruto in particular, can be engaging at the sensory, fantasy, and social level, and particularly well suited as a therapeutic resource.

Creative clinicians who recognize the value of popular culture, and in particular television and more specifically cartoons, have at their disposal a virtually limitless trove of resources for engagement, fantasy, and metaphor development, as well as shared narrative with young clients of all ages. The tale of Naruto, the Nine-Tailed Demon Fox, the adventures of Team 7, and all of the colorful characters of this particular slice of anime contain clear and numerous therapeutic elements, including parent loss, social ostracism, the search for identity and connection, the perennial battle between good and evil, and others awaiting the eager clinician. This search is not limited to Naruto, or even the other action-packed anime adventures that are available on television. Jimmy Neutron, boy genius, Chucky Finster of the Rug Rats, Ben Ten and his miraculous shape-shifting amulet, Dora the Explorer, Hi Hi Puffy Ami Yumi, and Kim Possible are also emulative models and characters who, each in their own way, can take both client and viewer on important therapeutic adventures.

Kiko was one such traveler, enamored by the world of Naruto for reasons that were both obvious and yet not clear to him as he struggled in his own personal quest for self-regulation, esteem, connection, and a secure place within his own family. As with Kiko, clinicians may utilize specific components of particular cartoon narratives, a child's identification with a certain character, or even visual elements of that character as a means for developing personal iconography. However, the very first step is for the interested clinician to butter up some popcorn and set aside time to become familiar with the numerous cartoons available to today's viewer. The clinician must think encompassingly as a child, adult, and particularly as a therapist, always asking, "How can this cartoon help therapeutically?" but more importantly, being attentive to those cartoons and little pieces of popular culture that clients bring with them to counseling.

Kiko was already poised to utilize Naruto in his therapeutic work; however, others, even those who enjoy cartoons, may not be similarly prepared to utilize their favorite characters metaphorically or even descriptively in treatment. In such cases, the clinician is urged not to impose a cartoon theme on their client or into therapy, but perhaps to instead query at the outset what cartoons a client is interested in, and then to engage that client in a discussion over what elements of that cartoon are particularly engaging and why. Clinicians must also be careful to consider the match between their client's developmental level and that of the nature of the cartoon character and story. Interested clinicians are also advised to pepper their play rooms with a variety of cartoon action figures, just as they might include puppets and superhero figures.

In the final analysis, cartoon character, client, and clinician become members of a team, poised to venture into the mysterious, often painful, but potentially rewarding and liberating land of counseling and play therapy.

NOTES

1. See http://en.wikipedia.org/wiki/Saturday_morning_cartoon for a full listing of all Saturday morning television cartoons from the 1960s through the present.
2. See http://www.cartoonnetwork.com for a full listing of animated television programming.
3. See http://www.nickelodeon.com for a full listing of animated television programming.
4. For the 2007 survey entitled "Top TV Ratings," see http://www.nielsenmedia. com/nc/portal/site/Public/menuitem.43afce2fac27e890311ba0a347a062a0/ ?show=%2FFilters%2FPublic%2Ftop_tv_ratings%2Fcable_tv&selOneInd ex=1&vgnextoid=9e4df9669fa14010VgnVCM100000880a260aRCRD; for the 2007 survey titled "Teens Tune into Local TV," see http://www.nielsenmedia. com/nc/portal/site/Public/menuitem.55dc65b4a7d5adff3f65936147a062a0/ ?allRmCB=on&newSearch=yes&vgnextoid=b0694664875c5010VgnVCM 100000880a260aRCRD&searchBox=LPMs.
5. The release of DC's Action Comics #1, which introduced Superman, is considered the beginning of the Golden Age of comics and superheroes.
6. See http://en.wikipedia.org/wiki/Manga for a comprehensive listing of Manga characters and plots, both past and present.
7. For an additional and comprehensive description of the genres and subgenres of anime, see http:en.wikipedia.org/wiki/Anime.
8. For a complete description of Naruto, see http://en.wikipedia.org/wiki/Naruto; and for a complete description of the various Naruto story arcs, see http:// en.wikipedia.org/wiki/List_of_Naruto_story_arcs.
9. For a complete description of the Nine Tailed Fox, including history, see http://en.wikipedia.org/wiki/Tailed_beasts#Nine-Tailed_Demon_Fox.
10. For a complete description of Sasuke Uchiha, see http://en.wikipedia.org/ wiki/Sasuke_Uchiha.
11. For a complete description of Sakura Hurano, see http://en.wikipedia.org/ wiki/Sakura_Haruno.
12. See http://www.ugo.com/channels/comics/heroMachine2/heromachine2.asp.

REFERENCES

Abel, S. (1995). The rabbit in drag: Camp and gender construction in the American animated cartoon. *Journal of Popular Culture, 29*(3), 183–2002.

Anderson, C. C. (1984). The Saturday morning survival kit. *Journal of Popular Culture, 17*(4), 155–161.

Burke, T., & Burke, K. (1999). *Saturday morning fever: Growing up with cartoon culture.* New York: St. Martin's Press.

Campbell, J. (1956). *The hero with a thousand faces.* New York: Meridian Press.

Clements, J., & McCarthy, H. (2006). *The anime encyclopedia: A guide to Japanese animation since 1917.* Berkeley, CA: Stone Bridge Press.

Fouts, G., Callan, M., & Piasentin, K. (2006). Demonizing in children's television cartoons and Disney animated films. *Child Psychiatry and Human Development, 37,* 15–23.

Grigsby, M. (1998). *Sailormoon: Manga* (comics) and *anime (*cartoon) superheroine meets Barbie: Global entertainment commodity comes to the United States. *The Journal of Popular Culture, 32*(1), 59–80.

Ito, K. (2005). A history of manga in the context of Japanese culture and society. *The Journal of Popular Culture, 38*(5), 456–475.

Kellogg, M. A. (1992, December 19). The toon boom. *TV Guide, 41,* 6–8.

Lawrence, J. S., & Jewett, R. (2002). *The myth of the American super hero.* Cambridge, England: Eerdmans.

Levinson, R. (1975). From Olive Oyl to Sweet Polly Purebread: Sex role stereotypes and televised cartoons. *Journal of Popular Culture, 9*(3), 561–572.

McCauley, C., Woods, K., Coolidge, C., & Kulick, W. (1983). More aggressive cartoons are funnier. *Journal of Personality and Social Psychology, 44*(4), 817–823.

Middleton, Y., & Vanderpool, S. (1999). *TV cartoons: Do children think they are real.* (Report No. PS 028201) (ERIC Document Reproduction Service No. ED437207).

Mitchell, T. (1995). *Kid's stuff: Television cartoons as mirrors of the American mind.* (Report No. CS 509 035). Canyon, TX: West Texas A & M University (ERIC Document Reproduction Service No. ED386771).

Napier, S. (2001). *Anime from Akira to Princess Mononoke: Experiencing contemporary Japanese animation.* New York: Palgrave.

Price, S. (2001). Cartoons from another planet: Japanese animation as cross-cultural communication. *Journal of American and Comparative Cultures, 24*(1/2), 153–169.

Roberts, D., Foehr, U., Rideout, V., & Brodie, M. (1999). *Kids and the media at the new millennium: A comprehensive national analysis of children's media use.* Retrieved August 10, 2007, from http://www.kff.org/entmedia/upload/Kids-Media-The-New-Millenniu-Report.pdf

Rubin, L. (Ed.) (2006). *Using superheroes in counseling and play therapy.* New York: Springer Publishing.

Swan, K. (1995). *Saturday morning cartoons and children's perceptions of social reality.* (Report No. PS 023908). San Francisco, CA: Paper Presented at the

Annual Meeting of the American Educational Research Association (ERIC Document Reproduction Service No. ED390579).

Thompson, T., & Zerbinos, E. (1995). Gender roles in animated cartoons: Has the picture changed in 20 years? *Sex Roles, 32(9/10)*, 651–673.

Viz Media announces next stop on national road tour for Shonen Jump Naruto. (2007a). Retrieved August 6, 2007, from http://www.vizmedia.com/news/newsroom/2006/11_roadshow.php

Viz Media expands Naruto momentum with new DVD releases of Naruto the Lost Story and latest Naruto uncut boxed set. (2007b). Retrieved August 6, 2007, from http://www.vizmedia.com/news/newsroom/2007/05_expandnaruto.php

Viz Media launches Naruto nation campaign to dramatically increase release rate of hit manga series Naruto and pave the way for part 2. (2007c). Retrieved August 6, 2007, from http://www.vizmedia.com/news/newsroom/2007/04_narutonation.php

Viz Media's manga Shonen Jump Naruto named winner of 2006 Quill Award. (2007d). Retrieved August 6, 2007, from http://www.viz.com/news/newsroom/2006/10_narutoquill.php

Viz Media's Naruto does it again! Manga at number 25 on USA Today's Top 150 Best Seller list. (2007e). Retrieved August 6, 2007, from http://www.vizmedia.com/news/newsroom/2007/03_narusatoday.php

Wilson, C., Nairn, R., Coverdale, J., & Panapa, A. (2000). How mental illness is portrayed in children's television: A prospective study. *British Journal of Psychiatry, 176*, 440–443.

CHAPTER 13

Marcia, Marcia, Marcia

The Use and Impact of Television Themes, Characters, and Images in Psychotherapy

Loretta Gallo-Lopez

It has been called "a vast wasteland" (Minow, 1961) and is often referred to in such negative terms as "the boob tube" or "the idiot box" (Kaufman, 2007). The American Academy of Pediatrics (2001) warns that television negatively impacts the thoughts, perceptions, and behavior of children and adolescents, who are especially vulnerable to its influence. Others extol the beneficial aspects of television, such as its ability to teach values and expose its viewers to other cultures (Good Things, n.d.). Whatever one's view of television, most people would agree with Minow's (1961) assertion that television is "an instrument of overwhelming impact on the American people." And like it or not, television is an integral part of our everyday life; its characters, images, and themes are a reflection of our society and our culture. What we see and hear on television influences the way we dress, the way we speak, and the way we view ourselves and the world. We identify on different levels with the characters, images, and themes that are beamed into our homes, and now onto our computers and MP3 players on a weekly and sometimes daily basis.

This chapter will explore the means by which the themes, characters, and images we see on television can be used as agents of psychotherapeutic change. Television's impact on the self-view and perceived roles of its audience members will be examined within the context of its significance to psychotherapy. The relationship between psychotherapy and television will be critiqued by identifying the ways in which psychotherapy and psychotherapy patients have been presented on television and the subsequent impact of this presentation on the television viewing public. Next a thorough analysis of the iconic 1960s/1970s family comedy series, *The Brady Bunch* (Schwartz, 1969–1974), will be offered as the foundation for the case presentation to follow. Finally, the case presentation will demonstrate how the use of television themes, characters, and images provided a terminally ill child the means with which to address and explore significant and profound issues of life and death.

TELEVISION'S IMPACT ON ROLE AND SELF-IDENTITY

Each of us plays a series of different roles in our lives and in our relationships to others. We are at various times throughout our lives mother, daughter, father, son, husband, wife, friend, employee, consumer, caretaker, and so on, depending on the given situation and the person or people with whom we are interacting. Landy (2005) explains the significance and the purpose of those roles via an understanding of the dramatic nature of human life, indicating that "people take on and play out roles in order to express particular needs" (p. xxiii). These roles are elements of our self-identity and are continually impacted and changed as a result of our life experiences and our exposure to the world. These experiences are many and varied, and television's "overwhelming impact" (Minow, 1961) on the roles that we play and the way that we play them cannot be ignored. Ott (2003) asserts that "television both shapes the nature of identity by providing identity models and provides the symbolic resources for enactment" (p. 58). As audience members view television from their own unique perspectives, their interpretation and understanding of what they see will be unique to their lives and specific sets of life circumstances. Rose (1995) argues that television's "narratives have become playgrounds for children's depictions of their needs and struggles. Some of the stories presented have such wide appeal, that when they are filtered through the minds of individual children, they become laden with metaphoric significance" (p. 60). It is this filtering that makes each individual's experience, understanding, and interpretation of the material unique. And it is the use of this material in psychotherapy that gives it new meaning and greater significance.

Ekstein (1983) espouses the notion that in order to understand what children are expressing and communicating through their play, drawings, and stories, one must become familiar with the myths, stories, and language that comprise each child's "private mythology." That "private mythology" comprises the secret language that the child has chosen in order to communicate his thoughts and feelings. Ekstein declares that a child's play is "a myth, an image of his inner life and, of course it has truth in it" (p. 416). Today, much of what represents the private mythology of children is gleaned from the stories, characters, and heroes that they connect with each day through television. It is what Rose (1995) refers to as the metaphorical significance of these characters, heroes, and stories, that when recognized in the play of children allows us entry into their world.

Rose echoes Ekstein's assertion that essential to the success of the therapeutic process is the therapist's awareness of the forces that influence children's understanding of the world. Rose recognizes television as being one of the most influential of those forces and advises clinicians that

> to become familiar with the characters and plots of television programs that play such a central part in so many children's lives is to learn the language of their culture and experience. To utilize this in some form as part of the therapeutic process is to reach out to children in a new and potentially powerful manner. (p. 62)

PSYCHOTHERAPY IN OUR LIVING ROOMS: I'M NOT A THERAPIST BUT I PLAY ONE ON TV

Psychotherapy-Related Themes, Images, and Characters on Television

By examining television shows, characters, and themes involving psychotherapy, we can gain an understanding of the impact of television on society's views and perceptions of psychotherapy. Television and psychotherapy have had a strange but interesting relationship. Many people have little knowledge or understanding about the process of psychotherapy other than through the images and characters they have seen on TV. These images have likely influenced people to seek or to avoid therapy depending on how those images are processed. One of the earliest television depictions of psychotherapy was CBS's *The Bob Newhart Show* (Zinberg, 1972–1978), a comedic vehicle for Newhart's Dr. Bob Hartley. Many of the show's comedic moments involved the eccentricities of Dr. Hartley's patients. These patients included nervous and amoral Elliot Carlin, and Mr. Peterson, the quintessential henpecked husband who attends Dr. Hartley's group therapy sessions in order to learn how to stand up to his wife. While it is doubtful that these characters influenced many people to seek psychological services, they might have otherwise inspired identification and empathy in the audience.

The Sopranos (Chase, 1999–2007), the HBO television series about anxiety-ridden organized crime boss Tony Soprano, presents a more serious view of psychotherapy. Over the series' six seasons, Tony Soprano and his psychiatrist, Dr. Jennifer Melfi, delved into the sources of his anxiety, and explored issues ranging from his early family history to his relationship with his mother and his struggles with his son. In contrast to the glib and sarcastic persona of Dr. Hartley, Dr. Melfi's role was a professional and respectable one. In fact, some therapists have considered the therapeutic relationship between Tony Soprano and Dr. Melfi to be one of the best and most realistic ever portrayed in popular media.

Beyond this view is the impact of this relationship on the general viewers. Several of my young adult male clients have jokingly referred to me as their own private Dr. Melfi, and during therapy sessions would comment about Tony Soprano's therapy process, making comparisons and pointing out similar symptoms. It is doubtful that these young men relate to Tony Soprano as a cold-blooded killer. It is more likely that they relate to the multidimensional nature of his persona—a man who projected a strong tough guy image, while inwardly experiencing intense emotional pain and stress. Tony's willingness to seek help for his problems appeared to give these young men permission to do the same without seeing themselves as weak and vulnerable. Comparing their therapist to Dr. Melfi was one way of reinforcing that connection.

Psychotherapy and psychotherapy patients have been prominent themes in many other shows. *Degrassi Junior High* (Schuyler, 1987–1991), a show whose target audience is teenagers, depicts the lives of a group of teenagers, many of whom have emotional problems. Craig is a musician with bipolar disorder and a substance abuse problem. Emma has bulimia, Ellie is depressed and self-mutilates, and Darcy has attempted suicide. Several of the episodes depict characters involved in group therapy sessions. This show seems to have had both a negative and positive impact upon its audience members depending upon how the particular issues resonate with their individual life experiences. Several of my female adolescent clients who watch the show consistently admitted that they were much less resistant to coming to therapy because of the therapy experiences of the teens in Degrassi. Others, however, seemed to emulate some of the problems of the characters, looking for similar traits within themselves and even self-diagnosing significant problems.

Sometimes, psychotherapy shows up on television in unusual places and in unexpected ways. In my initial session with Max, a 10-year-old boy with attention deficit disorder, I presented a box of figures with characters from cartoons and television shows. Max grabbed a figure of Bart Simpson, the mischievous, wisecracking son on the long-running animated show *The Simpsons* (Brooks, 1989–2007). Max told me that he knew about what happens in therapy because he saw a Simpsons episode where Bart went to therapy. Max told me that when his mom told him he would be coming to therapy he remembered seeing Bart in therapy and thought it would be fun. Max was referring to a particular episode of the Simpsons called *Yokel Chords* (Price & Dietter, 2007). In this episode, Bart gets into trouble at school for teasing and scaring the other kids by telling them a fabricated story about a cannibal cafeteria worker named Dark Stanley. Bart tells the other kids that Dark Stanley had killed students in the past and put them in his stew. Bart's story sends all the other kids running and screaming from the cafeteria after he pretends to find a body part in a bowl of stew. Bart successfully achieves his goal, which was to eat everyone else's lunch. As part of his punishment, Bart is referred for five therapy sessions, which are to be paid for by the school. Bart quickly bonds with his psychiatrist, Dr. Stacey Swanson, who uses violent video games (rated "Bad for Everyone") and a fill-in-the-blank game—Sad Libs—to help Bart to open up and express his feelings. After completing his five sessions Bart becomes depressed and misses his therapist. He uses an empty chair to pretend to talk to his therapist about his problems. Bart's mother Marge becomes concerned and pays for her son to have one final session with Dr. Swanson. Bart achieves a sense of closure as a result. Bart's experience inspired Max and instilled in him a positive perception of therapy that allowed him to quickly establish a trusting relationship with his therapist.

TELEVISION THEMES, CHARACTERS, AND IMAGES IN PSYCHOTHERAPY

Icky Vicky is a baby-sitter on the Nickelodeon animated cartoon show *The Fairly Odd Parents* (Hartman, 2001–2007). At first glance Vicky looks like a typical 16-year-old baby-sitter with her pony-tailed red hair, green midriff shirt, and sweet disposition. However, when left alone with her charge, 10-year-old Timmy Turner, Vicky becomes a cruel and sadistic tyrant. Vicky even has her very own theme song, written and performed on the show by singer Missy Elliott, who chants "Hey, Vicky. won't you please explain, why you get so much enjoyment out of causing kids pain" (www.lyricsandsongs.com). The dichotomy between Vicky's personality, sweet and kind in front of adults and pure evil when in her baby-sitter role, makes this character especially suited for therapeutic exploration of issues related to abuse and conflictual feelings. This was the case with Jenna, an 11-year-old girl who had been the victim of physical abuse by her adoptive mother. Jenna had been adopted at the age of 10 after spending many years in foster care. To the outside world Jenna's mother appeared to be a kind and compassionate woman who loved her adoptive daughter very much. However, one day Jenna arrived at school with a limp, and when questioned, admitted that her mother had hit her in the back of her legs with a baseball bat. When children's services was called, they discovered that Jenna had many bruises and she reluctantly disclosed that her adoptive mother had been routinely beating her. Jenna was placed in foster care and referred for counseling. In her therapy sessions, Jenna used the Icky Vicky character to process her abuse experience and to explore her feelings related to her adoptive mother. Jenna enjoyed drawing, so we used the TV Show Storyboard Technique (Gallo-Lopez, 2001) to provide her with the opportunity to create a story based on the Icky Vicky character. The TV Show Storyboard technique utilizes a storyboard format in order to allow children to draw stories frame by frame. Jenna's storyboard detailed Vicky's abusive behavior toward the children in her care. Jenna's story ended with Icky Vicky getting arrested and then apologizing and begging forgiveness from the children she had harmed. Through this exercise and the Icky Vicky character Jenna was able to begin to process her abuse experience and to acknowledge the conflictual feelings she had about her adoptive mother.

THE BRADY BUNCH

The Brady Bunch (Schwartz, 1969–1974) is a television series about a blended family comprised of a woman with three daughters and a man with three sons and their housekeeper named Alice. Although *The Brady Bunch* was never a critical or ratings success during its original airing, it became quite popular in syndication, which in turn transformed it into a cultural phenomenon (Marinucci, 2005). *The Brady Bunch* began airing in syndication in September 1975 and since that time at least one episode of the show has been broadcast in some United States location, every day of every year through 2007. Syndication allowed the show to be seen by generations of young people, many of whom were not yet born when the show first aired. Part of the show's enormous popularity with children and teens was based on the fact that episodes were presented from the children's perspective. The Bradys were an idealized, happy family and many viewers longed to be part of a Brady-type family. As a matter of fact, the show's producers sent a special form letter to children who wrote to the show expressing the desire to run away from their homes and families and move in with the Bradys.

Marcia Brady, the eldest of the Brady daughters, was portrayed in the series by actress Maureen McCormick. Marcia is a popular, attractive, successful high school student with long blonde hair and stylish clothes. In the book *Who's Your TV Alter Ego?*, Lusky (2007) presents a questionnaire that asks, "Which sibling from the Brady Bunch are you?" After responding to questions such as, "If you were a room in a house which room would you be?" readers tally their responses and are then given a profile of their Brady alter ego. The Marcia profile points out Marcia's many friends, active social life, and quest for perfection.

Jan Brady is the middle sister and in the series was portrayed by Eve Plumb. Jan is not as popular as Marcia and is often awkward and insecure. Her jealousy of Marcia is a theme that runs throughout the series. In one episode, Jan expresses frustration that she never wins anything while her sister Marcia seems to win award after award. Jan's exasperation leads her to shout what has since become the show's famous catchphrase, "Marcia, Marcia, Marcia!"

The Brady Bunch characters, themes, and images became the primary focus of the play therapy sessions of the terminally ill child described in the case presentation below. Through the filter of this child's own personal experience, the characters of Marcia and Jan Brady took on a special supportive connection. The themes of family life and teen experiences evolved into future adventures and the journey toward adulthood. The stereotypical images of the idealized family and the perfection that is Marcia became the medium for exploring significant and difficult issues.

CASE PRESENTATION

Professionals who work with terminally ill children, whether doctors, nurses, therapists, or clergy, often describe these children as possessing an enlightened understanding of their world and their lives, and an almost other-worldly perception of the future.

Mia was a child who clearly possessed an enlightened view of herself and her world. She was a 6-year-old girl with Wilms tumor, a form of cancer that attacks the kidneys and often, as in Mia's case, metastasizes to other areas such as the lungs (Medline Plus, n.d.). I refer to Mia in the past tense because this case involves a child who did not survive her illness, a child who lived only 6 years. And it was Mia's acceptance of her imminent death that led to the therapy sessions that are described here.

Mia was the only biological child of older parents. An adult half sister, Tara, from her mother's previous marriage, had moved out of state and Mia rarely saw her. Mia's parents had always competed for her love and affection and Mia's illness served to intensify their battle. In response to their daughter's diagnosis and repeated unsuccessful attempts at treatment, Mia's parents had also become obsessed with finding a cure and with protecting her from anything that might lead to a decline in her condition. The parents hovered over Mia, doing for her things she could easily have done herself. They worried about infection, so they kept her isolated, especially from other children. In their search for a cure, Mia's parents also micromanaged her diet and as a result many of Mia's favorite foods were eliminated from her meals. Since her diagnosis, Mia had spent much of her life in hospitals and medical centers, often in isolation due to concerns about her vulnerability to infection. She craved and feared social interaction, just as she craved and feared independence and separation from her parents.

When I first observed Mia involved in free play in the hospital play room, I was struck by her physical appearance. Mia was a slight child, with pale skin and a festive hat covering her bald head. Her arms were marked with the familiar scars of child cancer sufferers, who endure so many needles in their arms from blood being drawn, fluids being replaced, and medication being administered, that their veins eventually collapse. Mia, like many young cancer patients, had ultimately been fitted with a catheter in her chest. Her gait was slow and unsteady, making her at times resemble an old woman more than the young child that she was.

It was hard to miss the domineering and intrusive presence of Mia's mother. As if trying to envelop her child in a protective cocoon, Mia's mother was always at her side, directing her play, protecting her from any play experience that could result in physical harm. Mia's mother also limited her interactions with other children by interfering in any group play experiences. Observation of Mia with her father revealed similar patterns of interaction.

Mia's play at this point had taken on a repetitive quality. She used large rectangular cardboard blocks to build a house around herself, essentially barricading herself in and everyone else out. One of her parents, most often her mother, would sit on the outside giving instructions as to how to construct the walls and where to place the furniture. Eventually, Mia would orchestrate a disaster such as a car crash or a hurricane that would destroy the house, sending all of the blocks tumbling down. The walls that represented Mia's attempts to separate and begin to establish an identity distinct from her parents had to be destroyed by forces beyond Mia's control—metaphoric, I believed, of the impending destruction her cancer presented. Mia was ultimately ambiguous about separating from her parents, desiring independence but still longing for the safety they represented.

Mia had been referred for individual play therapy in order to give her the opportunity to explore issues related to her illness and treatment, and to help her to find a means of expressing the myriad of feelings she kept locked so tightly behind the façade of the sweet, compliant little girl. Mia needed the opportunity to explore her inner world without her mother's interference, but as therapy was about to begin, neither of them was ready to separate. The first play therapy session was conducted with Mia's mother present.

Mia chose to begin the initial session in the play kitchen where she created a house complete with the essential dramatic fourth wall, built from the cardboard blocks that had been her fortress during the free play sessions. She indicated that she was to be Marcia and assigned me the role of Jan, her younger sister. I immediately recognized these characters as two of the sisters from the *Brady Bunch* show. Mia's character choice was an interesting one. From a merely physical perspective, Mia's identification with Marcia was an obvious choice. Marcia, like the other Brady sisters, "had hair of gold like their mother" (Brady Bunch Shrine, n.d.). Mia had hair of gold before the cancer, and the endless, agonizing treatment took it from her. Beyond the physical, Marcia was also part of a large, cheerful, idealized television family. With two sisters, three brothers, and a dog, Marcia was never lonely. And, as a product of Mia's private mythology, Marcia Brady was a superstar, popular and beautiful, with her whole, perfect life ahead of her.

My understanding of the significance of Mia's character choice allowed me entry into her inner world and strengthened her trust in me, establishing the foundation of our therapeutic relationship. I asked Mia about our parents, Carol and Mike Brady, and wondered aloud how old our characters of Marcia and Jan were. Mia indicated that our parents were dead but had left Alice, the housekeeper, "to spy on us." Mia cast her mother in the role of Alice and directed her to do her spying from outside of our newly built house.

Marcia and Jan were the roles Mia and I would enact throughout our many sessions together. The roles would evolve and expand depending on Mia's needs. Mia's strong identity with the role of Marcia formed the basis of her incredible ability to project her wishes, fears, and emotions onto this character.

Mia's mother accompanied her to the second session and she was again cast in the role of Alice, the housekeeper spy. However, at the end of this session Alice was eliminated, as "Marcia" loudly proclaimed, "We don't need her anymore, we can take care of ourselves." And before the start of the next session, Mia told her mother to stay behind, she would enter the play room alone.

Over the weeks that followed, prominent themes in the lives of Marcia and Jan included dates with boyfriends, abandoned babies left on the doorstep, housekeeping, and the performance of a variety of other adult household tasks. These themes were incorporated into our dramas in a variety of different ways and provided opportunities for Mia to explore the difficult issues of separation and her growing sense of individuation.

Subsequent sessions involved the quest for mastery and control. Marcia and Jan explored various career choices, from secretaries to flight attendants to models. The sisters would often win awards for being the best at their jobs and were always the most beautiful and popular of anyone in their chosen fields.

It is interesting to note the symbiotic relationship of the two sisters that Mia had created. In the actual *Brady Bunch* television show, the relationship between Marcia and Jan was fraught with conflict, jealousy, and competition. But the relationship between Mia's Marcia and Jan was supportive and loving. They experienced life together. Mia's longing for her half sister Tara and the constant loneliness she felt as an only child became the fabric of Marcia and Jan's relationship. Many of the sisters' adventures were based on Tara's life. They traveled to cities where Tara had lived and worked at places where Tara had been employed. In many of the sessions, Marcia's boyfriend's name was Ben, Tara's boyfriend's name.

As Mia's therapy progressed, the predominant themes continued to evolve. Caretaking and the preparation of food became a central focus. The babies that had been abandoned on Marcia and Jan's doorstep in previous sessions were nurtured and lovingly cared for. They were bathed and fed, their diapers were changed, and they were tenderly rocked to sleep. Food became a consistent theme as well, as the sisters prepared, served, and dined on elaborate meals with their boyfriends. By creating these wonderful dinners which our invisible boyfriends praised and devoured, Mia was endowed with feelings of mastery and pride. Entwined in these themes of food and eating were issues of control. Mia as Marcia could eat and enjoy all of the foods that were forbidden by her highly restrictive diet, allowing her to exert control over this essential aspect of her existence.

The role of Marcia allowed Mia to engage in activities and events she was beginning to realize she might never experience in life. As Marcia, Mia could experience romance, child rearing, careers, and independence. She ate what she wanted, went where she wanted to, with whomever she wanted. She was in control of her life.

Issues related to death and dying began to surface when Mia was forced to endure an extended period of isolation due to a worsening of her condition and the perilously fragile condition of her immune system. Sessions were conducted in Mia's hospital room, where both she and I wore masks to guard against her possible infection. During one of these sessions Marcia and Jan reprised their roles as flight attendants. We diligently served food and distributed blankets and pillows to the passengers. Mia as Marcia excitedly turned to me, yelling that the plane was about to crash. We instructed the passengers to fasten their seatbelts and then carefully fastened ourselves into our seats. Upon Mia's direction the plane crashed and she and I were thrown to the ground. Mia indicated that although we had been injured, we were still able to help the passengers, many of whom were injured and several of whom were dead. Together, Mia and I as Marcia and Jan carried the dead bodies of the passengers off of the plane and covered them with the crisp white hospital sheets we had borrowed from the hospital cart in the hallway. As Jan, I expressed fear and sadness and pretended to cry. Mia told me that since none of our friends had died, we didn't have to cry and didn't need to be sad. Stepping out of the role of Jan, I told Mia that death always made me feel sad, no matter whose death it was. Mia at first expressed surprise but then joined me in mourning and together we held funeral services for the dead passengers.

In a later session, Mia, again in the role of Marcia, enacted a telephone call that brought the news that Marcia and Jan's brother Bobby, the youngest of the Brady brothers, had been killed in a car accident. Mia laughed after she told me the news, and then looked at me, as if awaiting my response. In the role of Jan, I cried and grieved, and spoke of how much I would miss our brother. After a few moments, Mia was able to join me in mourning our brother's death. We shared some of the wonderful memories we had of him and how very important he was in our lives. I believed that through Bobby's death, Mia was exploring possible reactions to her own death. She was looking for reassurance that she would be missed and remembered.

As she explored themes of death and dying, Mia edged progressively closer to examining her own mortality. She moved from scenes that involved the death of strangers, to a scene that involved the death of a family member, and finally to a scene in which she enacted her own death. The scene began with Marcia and Jan having dinner together in a restaurant. As in earlier sessions, food was again a prominent issue. An imaginary waitress took our order and served us our food. Mia, in the role of Marcia, tasted the food and grabbed her throat, choking. "It's poison, this food is poison!" she screamed, and dropped her head to the table, her arms hanging limp at her side. As Jan, I tried to wake her, shaking her and trying to lift her body from the table. Each time she collapsed back down onto the table, limp and still. Finally she turned her head toward me and whispered, "I'm dead, make believe I'm dead." I cried and grieved, "My sister is dead. I'm so sad, I will miss her so much." After a few moments, Mia again turned to me and whispered, "Make believe my boyfriend comes and kisses my hand." Mia slowly lifted her hand to be kissed by her imaginary boyfriend. She then slowly and dramatically awoke and rose up. She laughed and said, "See I'm not dead anymore, I'm alive again!" We then laughed and celebrated, making toasts to Marcia's life with glasses of water.

Through this enactment, Mia found a way to accept and prepare for her own death. The cancer that filled her body was replaced by a poison that would kill her in much the same way. But as Marcia, she would die as she imagined, but it would not be forever. As in the fairy tale of Sleeping Beauty, Mia would be awakened by her prince and together they would live happily ever after.

This session was the last in which Marcia and Jan were present. Mia had utilized these themes and characters to work through incredibly profound issues and upon achieving a sense of resolution was ready to move on. In subsequent sessions, Mia became more interested in group play and often requested to play board games or to do puzzles. Within a few weeks Mia and her parents left the country to try yet another experimental treatment. Two months later, she was dead.

In the progression of therapy, Marcia had become a vehicle for Mia to travel into a fantasy world, and to enact life events she neither could nor would experience in reality. Eventually, her travels as Marcia afforded Mia the distance she needed to explore such profound issues as the death of a loved one and ultimately her own death. Through her fairy-tale ending, Mia created a means of accepting her death and through that acceptance to move forward and affirm her life.

CONCLUSION

Through this discussion, I do not seek to elevate television to the status of a profound art form or an agent of therapeutic change. Rather I have sought to identify the connection that we as a society have to the characters, themes, and images that television imports into our world and our consciousness, and to understand how through that connection our clients might better communicate their thoughts and their pain. Through the emotional distance afforded by projecting their issues onto a television character, children can express without censoring and allow hidden issues to surface.

Whether it is the young men who vicariously receive permission to honestly and openly express their own emotions through Tony Soprano's work with Dr. Melfi, or the children who learn that therapy can be a good thing by watching Bart Simpson find answers and solace, television has had and continues to have a profound and lasting impact on the way we see ourselves. As clinicians, if we were to ignore this fact, we would likely miss the wealth of information that our clients are seeking to communicate. As Mia grappled with issues that no 6-year-old should ever have to consider, she sought understanding via the familiarity and normalcy that Marcia Brady represented. Marcia afforded Mia the emotional distance that enabled her to explore topics too frightening to address directly. Marcia also provided an opportunity for Mia to free herself from the role of a child cancer patient and to venture out into the world beyond.

REFERENCES

American Academy of Pediatrics: Committee on Public Education. (2001). Children, adolescents and television. *Pediatrics, 107*(2), 423–426.

Brady Bunch Shrine. (n.d.). Retrieved September 26, 2007, from http://www.bradybunchshrine.com

Brooks, J. (Producers). (1989–2007). *The Simpsons* [Television series]. Los Angeles: 20th Century Fox Television.

Chase, D. (Producer). (1999–2007). *The Sopranos* [Television series]. New York: HBO.

Ekstein, R. (1983). Play therapy for borderline children. In C. E. Schaefer & K. J. O'Connor (Eds.), *Handbook of play therapy* (pp. 412–418). New York: Wiley.

Gallo-Lopez, L. (2001). TV show storyboard. In H. Kaduson & C. Schaefer (Eds.), *101 more favorite play therapy techniques* (pp. 8–10). Northvale, NJ: Jason Aronson.

Good things about television. (n.d.). Media Awareness Network. Retrieved October 10, 2007, from http://www.mediaawareness.ca/english/parents/television/good_things_tv.cfm

Hartman, B. (Producer). (2001–2007). *The fairly odd parents* [Television series]. Orlando, FL: Nickelodeon Network.

Kaufman, R. (2007). *A nation of morons: Is television making us stupid?* Retrieved October 2, 2007, from http://www.turnoffyourtv.com/commentary/morons/stupid.html

Landy, R. (2005). Introduction. In A. M. Weber & C. Haen (Eds.), *Clinical applications of drama therapy in child and adolescent treatment* (pp. xxi–xxvii). New York: Brunner-Routledge.

Lusky, N. (2007). *Who's your television alter ego? The ultimate television character personality test.* New York: Simon Spotlight Entertainment.

Marinucci, M. (2005). Television, generation X and third wave feminism: A contextual analysis of The Brady Bunch. *The Journal of Popular Culture, 38*(3), 505–524.

Medline Plus Medical Encyclopedia: U.S. National Library of Medicine and the National Institutes of Health. (n.d.). *Wilms tumor.* Retrieved October 19, 2007, from http://www.nlm.nih.gov/medlineplus/ency/article/001575.htm#symptoms

Minow, N. *Television and the public interest.* (Speech delivered May 9, 1961, Washington, D.C.—Federal Communication Commission). Retrieved October 10, 2007, from http://www.americanrhetoric.com/speeches/newtonminow.htm

Price, M. (Writer), & Dietter, S. (Director). (2007). Yokel chords. [Television series episode]. In A. Jean, J. L. Brooks, M. Groening, & S. Simon (Producers), *The Simpsons.* Los Angeles: Fox Broadcasting Company.

Ott, B. (2003). "I'm Bart Simpson, who the hell are you?" A study in postmodern identity reconstruction. *The Journal of Popular Culture, 37*(1), 56–82.

Rose, A. (1995). Metaphor with an attitude: The use of The Mighty Morphin Power Rangers television series as a therapeutic metaphor. *International Journal of Play Therapy, 4*(2), 59–72.

Schuyler, L. (Producer). (1987–1991). *Degrassi junior high* [Television series]. Playing With Time.

Schwartz, S. (Producer). (1969–1974). *The Brady bunch* [Television series]. American Broadcasting Company.

Zinberg, N. (Producer). (1972–1978). *The Bob Newhart show* [Television series]. CBS.

CHAPTER 14

The Sopranos and a Client's Hope for Justice

Thelma Duffey and Heather Trepal

People who feel wounded often yearn for justice, for some retribution for their suffering. Indeed, there can be few experiences more troubling than feeling wronged, particularly when the perpetrator appears to be dismissive of and unaffected by the offense. In some cases, even acknowledgment of wrongdoing by the perpetrator is not enough. The pain remains too great. No doubt, life can feel excruciatingly unfair, and at times, it is.

Some clients come to therapy with the hope of resolving painful injuries. They retell their stories, reframe their experiences, attempt to heal, and still remain in pain. We often see, at the core of their hurt, two things: denial, or a fantasy wish that time could be reversed (Kübler-Ross, 1969), and in other cases, a desire for retribution (Enright, 2001). Indeed, when we live with the reality of an unbearable loss, we may feel a need to *do* something: fix it, or "make it go away" (Duffey, 2005a). When this is not possible and we are impotent to correct a wrong, some of us experience a desire for payback.

In this chapter, we will briefly discuss principles of grief, loss, and acceptance/forgiveness and how they relate to hurt, betrayal, and a person's hope for justice. We will also discuss ways in which the cinema can be used in counseling as a catalyst for this work. Finally, we will use a case study to illustrate how *The Sopranos* (Chase, Grey, Winter, Landress, & Weiner, 1999–2007), a popular Home Box Office (HBO) series, was used in counseling by a therapist and her clients. Implicit in this discussion is the understanding that bad things happen to good people

(Kushner, 1981), and there are no guarantees that doing our best will net the results we want (Kushner). Still, to live freely, we work through our injuries as best we can and free our hearts to move forward.

GRIEF, LOSS, AND FORGIVENESS

Relational injuries are discussed in the literature (Jordan, 2000, 2001; Miller, 1986; Miller & Stiver, 1993, 1995, 1997; Walker, 1999) and depicted in the media. These relational injuries often result in abstract losses in the form of a dream's death (Duffey, 2005b). Feelings of hurt, betrayal, and related injuries can result in the phenomenon of despair, many times resulting in feelings of profound grief and loss. Not uncommonly, these relational losses also lead to feelings of impotency, disbelief, anger, and hopelessness (Duffey, 2005a, 2005b; Worden, 1991). Anger and resentment are often directed toward others, and all too often, toward the self (Duffey, 2005a, 2005b; Fitzgibbons, Enright, & O'Brien, 2004; Worden, 1991). Indeed, how does one come to terms with these acute feelings following unjust treatment? How can we give context to the unforgivable? And further, how do we move past our own struggles with self-forgiveness when we feel duped, betrayed, and hurt? Clearly, depression and acute anger following experiences of injustice can often be traced to our own belief that we could have done better, protected ourselves or others more carefully, or perhaps, avoided the situation. Simply put, living with these messages can be excruciatingly painful.

We will not attempt to fully explore the extensive literature on grief and loss in this chapter, but rather, we will highlight relevant principles of these issues as they relate to the experiences of hurt and betrayal. According to Elizabeth Kübler-Ross (1969), there are five stages that injured parties experience when in grief: shock/denial, anger, depression, bargaining, and acceptance. Although current literature describes how we move in and out of these experiences as we negotiate our pain, most agree that acceptance, or coming to terms with our experiences, is critical for resolution. Duffey describes the hurt, anger, disbelief, confusion, and ultimate resolve involved in "releasing a dream" (2005b, p. 1). In cases of relational injury, the injured party must come to terms with the fact that the injury—and a new reality—exist. Until then, the injured party will experience any number of feelings, including resentment, hurt, anger, and rumination (Duffey, 2005a, 2005b; Worden, 1991). Sadly, chronic rumination results in a loss of control; that is, when we ruminate, our thoughts control us. Worthington & Scherer (2004) consider each of these issues as breeding grounds for unforgiveness. Unforgiveness comes when we are unable to accept painful realities and hold feelings of anger and resentment toward the perpetrator and/or ourselves (Baumeister, Exline, & Sommer, 1998). Indeed, painful injuries by a perpetrator can become so profound that a person's freedom to live, love, and grow can become compromised. In cases such as these, some people come to terms with these injuries through grief and loss work.

Acceptance, the final stage in the grief process (Kübler-Ross, 1969), is sometimes achieved through the experience of forgiveness. Nonetheless, one issue in the forgiveness discussion involves a belief that to forgive is to condone. For many, taking such a position could feel like a betrayal to the self. However, according to Enright (2001), the act of forgiveness is not one of condoning, but rather, an act of release. In fact, researchers posit that when unjustly injured, we forgive by acknowledging that the perpetrator has no right to our forgiveness, and thus acknowledge the unjustness of the damage as legitimate and real.

Increasing our capacity for resolve following an injury through acceptance and forgiveness is one means of coping with perceived transgressions and injustices (Worthington & Scherer, 2004). Working through these issues has resulted in decreased angry feelings, hostile behaviors, and aggressive, obsessive thoughts (Fitzgibbons et al., 2004). Further, as we are able to reach resolve through the processes of acceptance and forgiveness, some experience greater hope and self-esteem, and a decrease in feelings of anger, anxiety, and depression (Al-Mabuk, Enright, & Cardis, 1995; Coyle & Enright, 1997; Freedman & Enright, 1996). Indeed, the process of forgiveness is not only formidable, but also elusive, for many. However, engaging in such a quest can be equally fruitful.

CINEMATHERAPY

One intervention used by therapists and clients toward this end is cinematherapy (Dole & McMahon, 2005; Duncan, Beck, & Granum, 1986; Hesley, 2000, 2001; Lampropoulos & Spengler, 2005; Newton, 1995; Sharp, Smith, & Cole, 2002; Tyson, Foster, & Jones, 2000). Although the cinema is most often used to entertain us, it also provides a context for people to introspect and relate to the characters' struggles and adventures (Dole & McMahon, 2005; Hesley, 2000, 2001; Sharp et al., 2002; Tyson et al., 2000). In fact, many people socialize around cinema-viewing experiences and bond through related discussions. In therapy, these discussions can be particularly illuminating, as the client identifies with the experiences depicted in film, and projects the thoughts, feelings, needs, and wants of an illustrated character (Dole & McMahon, 2005; Hesley, 2000, 2001; Lampropoulos & Spengler, 2005; Sharp et al., 2002; Tyson et al., 2000).

Struggles depicted in the cinema can take on a life of their own when we see pertinent qualities from our own situations depicted onscreen. "Tessa" watched a movie about Pocahontas and Captain John Smith (Malick, 2005) with her passionate, yet elusive, significant other. In the film, Pocahontas fell deeply in love with Smith, who appeared to reciprocate her affection. In spite of his persistent declarations of love, he expressed even greater ambivalence, going so far as to make Pocahontas believe he had died. Grief-stricken to the core, she could not release him or her memories of their time together.

In time, Pocahontas married, but her heart remained in reserve. Although she cared for and appreciated her husband, her sadness and loss following Smith's absence remained palpable, restricting her capacity to freely give or receive love. Still, the two created a mutually supportive and respectful relationship. And, they both loved and cared for their young son. Pocahontas grew to become an internationally recognized and acclaimed figure. She even traveled to England, where she was publicly acknowledged. It was there she discovered that John Smith was alive and well. They met face to face, and with poise and grace, she acknowledged the good she saw in him and expressed her hopes that his dreams would come true. At the same time, Tessa could see that Pocahontas saw Smith in a different light, with all his human foibles and relational limitations. She also saw how little he offered and how he did not have Pocahontas's best interest at heart. Interestingly, at one point in the movie, Tessa's partner said just that, "He does not have her best interest at heart," which touched Tessa to the core.

It had become regretfully clear that Tessa's best interests were not a concern to her partner, a reality she deeply grieved. That evening, she looked over at him as he sat next to her on the couch, and the expression in his eyes was not unlike that of John Smith's. He cared, but he cared more about himself. He was passionately, rather than personally, connected. In a nutshell, he was not the man she had thought him to be, and their relationship was poignantly lacking in mutual respect or regard. With tenderness and a deep sense of loss, she took the facts in.

Like Tessa, clients frequently identify with characters in film. They vicariously experience the adventures, losses, and loves depicted in the cinema (Dole & McMahon, 2005; Duncan, Beck, & Granum, 1986; Hesley, 2000, 2001; Lampropoulos & Spengler, 2005; Sharp, et al., 2002; Tyson et al., 2000). Through film, they are able to see semblances of their experiences on-screen, and from a detached perspective, "see" the nuances of the experience with greater clarity (Hesley, 2000, 2001; Sharp et al., 2002; Tyson et al., 2000). From this, many are able to discern its viability and ultimate quality.

Additionally, clients are able to see, through film, alternate endings to stories similar to theirs. They are able to "try on" different possibilities, and experience, through the characters in the film, the associated feelings each path brings (Hesley, 2000, 2001; Sharp et al., 2002; Tyson et al., 2000). For example, in the film, Pocahontas finally discovered who John Smith really was and what he had actually given in the relationship (Malick, 2005). She also came to terms with her genuine love for and commitment to her husband. She had long carried a torch for Smith. And tragically, soon after becoming free of her feelings of idealization, she was struck with a deadly illness. The movie was highly motivating for Tessa. She loved her partner in much the same way that Pocahontas loved John Smith. She had invested greatly. And like Pocahontas, her investment had been far from fruitful. Tessa knew what it was like to give her heart to an ambivalent love. She became acutely aware of the separation she would need to initiate if she were to free her heart and reclaim her dignity and self-respect.

Like Tessa, clients are able to project feelings onto characters that symbolically parallel their own. Sometimes these parallels are exaggerated, and through that experience, clients can work through current relational challenges and existential landscapes. Such was the case of one couple, "Kelly" and "Nate," who attended therapy following Kelly's discovery of Nate's affair. With the dramatic series, *The Sopranos* as a catalyst, they faced their struggles with betrayal, loss, heartache, and the ultimate hope for justice.

THE SOPRANOS

The HBO critically acclaimed television series *The Sopranos* officially ended its run in the spring of 2007. The mob family drama began in 1999 and unfolded over 86 episodes. Although the series finale was widely debated, many fans were left with unresolved feelings about the fate of the main characters (Carter, 2007). While covering a synopsis of the entire six-season show is beyond the scope of this chapter, we would like to highlight several of the main characters and events from the final season, as viewers are often left with final impressions. For a complete synopsis of the series and more detailed information about the characters, please visit the official HBO Web site: http://www.hbo.com/sopranos

Tony Soprano

Mob boss, husband, sociopath, lover, uncle, father, murderer. These are all words that can be used to capture the many identities of the Italian-American icon, Tony Soprano. Presented as a hard-working mob boss and family man, viewers watched Tony's story unfold over the course of the show and were privy to the daily workings of his life. He was portrayed as a complex (or simple, depending on the lens through which one viewed the show) and contrasting study in character. Sometimes, viewers were given glimpses of his sensitive side, and this was sharply contrasted with moments when his dark nature emerged.

As a husband, Tony was loving and gentle with his wife, and at the same time involved with an endless string of mistresses or *goomars,* as the mobsters call them. His wife, Carmela, was at times aware of his indiscretions, and although they would fight vehemently, she always took him back. As a father, Tony wanted what was best for his family, and would go to any length to protect them. He struggled with some aspects of his position that were necessary evils, such as needing to kill his cousin and a close associate. According to the story line, both betrayed him in different ways, so letting them live would have caused bigger problems in the long run. In addition, complicated family issues often invaded his business dealings, as the two were sometimes intertwined. For example, Tony cared for his ailing Uncle Junior, who accidentally shot him, and he supported his sister by taking care of the body when, out of veiled self-defense, she killed her lover.

> TONY: What was your mother like? She ever let you down, do anything to hurt your feelings?
>
> DR. MELFI: Of course she did. She was controlling, manipulative at times. She also never tried to kill me. (Winter & Van Patten, 2006)

Given all of these complicated factors, it is no wonder that Tony experienced stress. Interestingly, he spent time in therapy with a psychoanalytic therapist named Dr. Melfi, trying to deal with his anxiety and panic attacks and inadvertently delving into the issues of his past. The therapeutic relationship between them runs the gamut, and most of the time, Tony seems to know something, but not enough. What little awareness he does have, he uses to meet his own needs. In fact, even his investment in therapy appears to be self-serving, as his insights breed grounds for his rationalization. Still, rooted in the turbulent and complicated relationships of his youth, Tony spends some of his most illuminated moments in the past. He struggles with issues of loss and psychological abandonment, particularly stemming from his mother Livia, a complicated and manipulative woman, who tried to have a "hit" taken out on him. Livia exists in stark contrast to Tony's wife, Carmela.

Carmela Soprano

As the dutiful wife of mob boss Tony Soprano, Carmela serves many purposes as a character in the story. As a housewife and budding entrepreneur, she finds comfort in cooking, and has a need to offer food during times of stress. She also tends to the children's issues with school and relationships, and looks to Tony to assist with discipline. Theirs is a "don't ask, don't tell" marriage where Tony shares little with his wife about his daily happenings. Instead, they connect on issues of family and the social network in their extended mob family.

Carmela has strong relationships with the other mobster's wives and is a queen bee, of sorts, in this network. In brief moments, when she is disgruntled with her marriage and particularly discontented with the kind of man Tony has become, Carmela toys with the idea of gaining her own independence. She does this through business ventures, or once, through an attraction to one of Tony's associates. During one of the later seasons, Carmela and Tony briefly separated, but in the end, they struck a deal and she took him back.

A. J. and Meadow Soprano

> Meadow was sharper, but I remember the same thing with her. It's like watching an angel fall. They're perfect and then they become like us. (Tony Soprano in Kalem & Garcia, 2004)

During the final season, Tony and Carmela's children A.J. (Anthony Junior) and Meadow, in some sense, grow into their familial roles. A.J. experimented with a more adult relationship with an older woman, fell in love, and suffered a broken heart. Prone to his father's depression and anxiety, A.J. fell into despair, and at Tony's urging, began to socialize with kids his age that turned out to be involved with small-scale gangster business. In one sense, the final episodes presented a prelude of life to come as A.J. entered therapy. Once passive, he later tasted the life of criminal behavior, including feeling an adrenaline rush from watching another human being get hurt. Meadow was not attracted to the violent aspects of her father's occupation, but was instead more attracted to social justice. At the end of the series, she indicated that she was finally settled on a future occupation, law.

The Final Season

During the final season, a feud with a fellow mob family escalated, as did Tony's irritation with a member of his own family, his nephew, Christopher. Although he had been under pressure to have Christopher killed in the past for his drug abuse, Tony advocated for him to try rehab. As the series came to a close, he wound up killing him with his own hands after a drug-induced car wreck. In addition, tension mounted with the other mob family and culminated in the death of the group's leader.

In essence, the final eight episodes built up to nothing. In the last scene, Tony, Carmela, and A. J. were sitting in a diner eating onion rings listening to *Journey* on the jukebox. A variety of characters were coming in and out of the diner, and Meadow was on her way in. Tony looked up, and the scene turned black (Chase, 2007). This ending, open to interpretation, left many viewers wanting more, and various contrasting outcomes have been debated (Carter, 2007).

CASE STUDY

Cinematherapy can have a powerful effect on clients and assist them to be less defensive and more receptive to therapeutic intervention (Sharp et al., 2002). To illustrate the use of cinematherapy with clients, we offer the case of a heterosexual couple reeling from the aftermath of an affair. *The Sopranos* is utilized as a medium to assist these clients in coming to terms with challenging life circumstances around issues of fairness, ambiguity, and resolve.

Kelly and Nate

Kelly and Nate were a married couple in their mid-30s who sought counseling to filter through their relationship in the aftermath of an affair. The couple had been married for just over 8 years, although they had been together for nearly 10. The couple was deciding if they wanted to remain married. Nate had an affair with a coworker, and although the affair had ended, Kelly could not seem to forgive him. By both accounts, she continued to punish him in other aspects of their relationship. Nate indicated that her punishment caused him to withdraw from the relationship even further and consider separating. He also reported that he had attempted to "meet Kelly's demands" by ending the affair and make her feel safe by asking his boss to assure that his work and travel assignments did not coincide with the other woman's. Kelly reported that she was still "willing to try and make it work," although she also admitted conflicting and lingering feelings surrounding the betrayal.

The therapeutic process was making little headway when the counselor asked the couple what activities they enjoyed. They looked at each other and quickly responded *"The Sopranos!"* Kelly and Nate shared that the television series had a very special meaning for them, as they had watched it during the entire course of their relationship. In fact, at the time they entered therapy, the series was in its final season, and the couple reported they were filled with anticipation for the outcome.

Sensing the connection that existed for them regarding the show, and understanding that talk therapy was at a standstill, the therapist asked Kelly and Nate if they would do some homework that involved their relationship and *The Sopranos*. She asked them to sit down together and watch the series finale. She also asked them to specifically spend some time contemplating the characters in the show, perhaps even discussing and processing these reflections with one another, before the next session.

When they met again, the therapist asked them to consider the character with whom they most identified, and she asked a series of questions. This is consistent with cinematherapy recommendations outlined by Sharp et al. (2002), where clients are asked not only to view the medium but also to process the material, perhaps through indirect and metaphorical connection(s) with a character(s). The therapist asked them to choose a character and to then talk for a while about this person's thoughts, feelings, relationships to others, and alternative solutions to their actions (Sharp et al., 2002).

As an Italian American, Kelly had a strong sense of identification with some of the cultural constructs displayed on the show. For example, simple things like the importance of food and religion reminded her of her extended family. Moreover, she was also Catholic and resonated with Carmela's struggles with her faith. Despite some identification with Carmela, Kelly rebelled against the character's seemingly forgiving history with respect to her husband's series of infidelities. She chose to discuss the character of Tony.

KELLY: Here is how we connected through this show. When we were dating and through the early years of our marriage, we would always reserve Sunday as our special night to open a bottle of wine and watch the show, always planning on at least one hour of postepisode discussion, debate, and commentary. It was evident to me, from the beginning, that Nate and I had different views of life, based on how we talked about the show, even down to what we honed in on with the characters, especially Tony.

She added:

For example, I think I am a hopeful person. I really believe in it and want to see redemption. As an undergrad literature major, I also want there to be a moral to the story, with actions resulting in some form of consequence. What I really liked about this show, from the beginning, was the sense that Tony was presented with two sides: good and evil, if that's what you want to call it. What I struggled with was the idea that he was never held responsible, in reality or emotionally, for his crimes.

Nate saw things a little differently. He affirmed, "I used to think I saw things as more black and white where Kel sees the shades of gray." He never bought into the idea that any of the characters, Tony in particular, would be able to change. When asked to identify a character, Nate also chose Tony.

NATE: Tony is tough, fat, childish, intelligent, and charismatic. He knows how far he can push and not go beyond . . . but he can't see past his own face. He's self-centered, and he was born to be self-centered, taught to be self-centered. It was a learned behavior. He wasn't strong enough to follow his heart. He saw other people as his main problem and he resolved his issues by blaming them. He used bullying, violence, and extortion to get what he wanted. Fear was what brought Carmela back after he was unfaithful. But he did love his family and tried to do what he thought was best for them, at least in his own mind. I never felt like he needed to get punished, though. He just was who he was; he wasn't going to change.

The Betrayal

Nate's characterization of Tony was especially compelling, given the discovery of his own affair and betrayal during what Kelly described as the most stressful time in their marriage. According to Kelly, she was almost due with their first baby when she learned that Nate had been having the affair with his coworker. The stress of the disclosure caused strain in the marriage and the couple drifted further apart. Kelly reported that a significant moment occurred when, 2 days after having the baby, she came home from the hospital and the final *Sopranos* season was starting. She and Nate sat down on the same couch, on Sunday night, to watch it together once again. She thought, "*Maybe* there is hope for this marriage, maybe things will return to normal."

Like many couples in similar situations, Kelly and Nate attempted to recover from the betrayal. And in so doing, they discovered the powerful nature of ambiguity. During these times, people ask themselves such questions as: "How is trust restored? How can I know that this won't happen again? What does it take to recover from the hurt that comes with being disregarded and disrespected by someone we love?" These and many other questions arise at times of such ambiguity.

The Sopranos accentuated these points. Indeed, how do we reconcile our losses, in this case, the loss of trust in a relationship, when we are reminded that people *seemingly* get away with murder and continue to behave as they please, regardless of the impact on their loved ones? How do we live with the reality that people can hurt others and experience no consequence for their actions? By all appearances, Tony didn't skip a beat. Our last glimpse of him had him sitting at a diner, eating onion rings, surrounded by the people he loved most. Audiences everywhere struggled with their expectations for the series finale. Still, there were others who thought Tony was living his own hell, one profoundly influenced by his internal conflicts, unresolved losses, transparent vulnerabilities, undeniable immaturity, and defiant and obstinate insecurities. Discussions of justice versus injustice were rampant, no doubt.

In the end, both Nate and Kelly were struck by their opposing feelings with respect to the ending of the series. These feelings paralleled, in great part, their perspectives on their own relationship. Nate, in identifying with and rebelling against his identification with Tony, "was who he was" and didn't know any better. There was no need for atonement. He tried to do what was best for his family. Kelly, on the other hand, felt she needed the atonement and struggled to forgive him. Thinking back at Nate's previous profession to "meet her demands," his seeming lack of empathy for her feelings and his apparently low understanding of the impact of his behavior on others became clearer. When we are fully aware of the pain we cause people we profess to love, we take measures to do right by them. Nate ultimately, in fact, ceased his hurtful behaviors, but he may not have had the language or communication skills to express his heartfelt sorrow. This could have fed Kelly's feelings of impotence.

With *The Sopranos* as a catalyst, Nate is learning to put words to his behaviors so he, too, can forgive himself for betraying his wife and family. It was easy enough to blame Kelly for her lack of forgiveness. At the end of the day, as Nate is truly able to recognize the damage his behaviors caused, and the pain he inflicted, he can more compassionately forgive himself and express his genuine remorse without defensiveness. As Nate sees that "Tony is who he is" but also recognizes that Tony is not the model he aspires to emulate, he can more easily see that, although we are who we are, we can also become inspired to grow in our capacities to love and make amends.

On the other hand, Kelly has her own challenges. Life is not a fairy tale, even though many of us want the happy ending. Just as Kelly wanted the idyllic, and in her mind, fair and just ending where Tony would somehow pay for his crimes, both concrete and crimes of the heart, she was left with feelings of ambiguity and emptiness. By not knowing how Tony's issues were resolved, Kelly was reminded of life's unfairness and experienced less hope for the future of her marriage. Moreover, although Kelly wanted the fairy-tale happily-ever-after marriage and family, what she had, instead, was a real relationship with betrayal currently at the fore.

Not unlike Tony Soprano, Nate at times makes decisions based on his emotions, or those emotions in the moment. He also uses his awareness of his emotions to meet his own needs, consistent with the affair. Can Kelly comfortably remain in the marriage knowing that Nate might not truly understand what impact his behaviors have on her? Can she live with the ambiguity that the future might hold? How can she reconcile the loss of trust with her hopes for the future?

As the person in the relationship who strayed, Nate felt a lot of pressure to repent or make things right for Kelly. He recounted how originally, when they had watched the show together, he and Kelly had long discussions about Tony's nature and how she had thought that he was "morally corrupt" and should "get what is coming to him." When that didn't happen in the final episode, Nate was struck by how life isn't all black and white and how justice doesn't always triumph over evil or wrongdoing. Rather, life sometimes just continues on. At the same time, he finds comfort in seeing that when people are committed to make things right, that may be enough to sustain them.

Leading to these insights and taking into account both of their observations and perspectives on the show, the therapist asked them to consider their own relationship and the way they were dealing with the affair, and their thoughts about the future.

THERAPIST: Kelly, it is important to you that justice is served, so to speak. It was difficult to know that Tony didn't pay for his crimes, in any concrete way, at the end of the show. Can you see how this may relate to your feelings about Nate and the affair? What would justice look like in this case? Could you consider living with the ambiguity of what the future might hold for your relationship, knowing what happened in the past?

KELLY: (Turning to Nate). You had the affair *and* want to keep the marriage. What is the moral of the story or the lesson learned in that? I have to live with what happened and the fear that you'll do it again.

NATE: Is that how you think it works? I learned my lesson. I have to live with what I did in my own mind every day. It's not like when Tony Soprano totally lacked awareness of the effects of his actions on other people. I am consumed by them. I see how you've changed since I hurt you, and I have to live with that, knowing that I am responsible.

In this case, Nate was becoming accountable for his actions, naming the damage he had created. He didn't shrug his shoulders and say, "I am who I am." He didn't continue to do what he had been doing to hurt her. He chose to be accountable and to cease his hurtful actions. He loved her and he chose to stay. For Kelly, the journey toward healing involved releasing the dream of life as they had hoped it would be. It also involved accepting that what had happened was wrong and that she had been hurt. In addition, her work involved trusting that Nate was genuinely sorry for his actions, and in finding that trust, she could continue on.

By metaphorically using *The Sopranos* and juxtaposing the themes of fairness (i.e., betrayal at the hands of someone who purportedly loves you) and ambiguity (i.e., what will the future bring?) with the relationship issues Nate and Kelly were facing, the therapist helped them to see that they each had a role to play with respect to the future.

CONCLUSION

Clients bring issues of hurt and betrayal to their therapy experiences with the hope that they can work through these and lay the past to rest. This is a difficult feat, as these issues can strike with a vengeance, leaving people helpless to resolve them and move forward. Cinematherapy is one tool used by counselors toward this end. In this chapter, *The Sopranos* was implemented to help an estranged couple use the experiences of a fictive family to negotiate their way back to each other. Both Nate and Kelly were able to reassess their positions on how to treat people they profess to love. They were also able to reassess their positions on how to communicate remorse and forgiveness in ways that the other could hear. Moreover, through the series, both people had a bird's-eye view on how lonely it can ultimately be to exploit and injure others without remorse, and how ultimately weak a person becomes who uses power in destructive ways.

We may not always see justice served in this lifetime. Still, through fictive dramas like *The Sopranos*, we can see that, at the end of the day, the best justice can come in knowing we can't escape from ourselves. In the case of Kelly and her search for justice, and Nate's resolve to make amends, they discovered that living a life of reckless disregard for others has its costs, while becoming accountable to the people we hurt, and ultimately to ourselves, provides promise for redemption. As researchers Tsang, McCullough, and Fincham (2004) discuss, forgiveness following interpersonal transgressions can generate deepened connection within close relationships. Counselors can use cinematherapy and artistic means such as *The Sopranos* to help clients like Kelly and Nate transcend their difficulties and transform their views on love, loving, and humanity.

REFERENCES

Al-Mabuk, R. H., Enright, R. D., & Cardis, P. A. (1995). Forgiveness education with parentally love-deprived late adolescents. *Journal of Moral Education, 24,* 427–444.

Baumeister, R. F., Exline, J., & Sommer, K. L. (1998). The victim role, grudge theory, and two dimensions of forgiveness. In E. L. Worthington, Jr. (Ed.), *Dimensions of forgiveness: Psychological research and theological forgiveness* (pp. 79–104). Philadelphia: Templeton.

Carter, B. (2007, June 17). Fans online sift for clues in the "Sopranos" finale. *New York Times.* Retrieved September 20, 2007, from http://www.nytimes.com/2007/06/16/arts/television/16sopr.html?_r = 1&ref = television&oref = slogin

Chase, D. (Writer/Director). (2007). Made in America [Television series episode]. In D. Chase (Executive Producer), *The Sopranos* [Television series]. New York: HBO.

Chase, D., Grey, B., Winter, T., Landress, I. S., & Weiner, M. (Executive producers). (1999–2007). *The Sopranos* [Television series]. New York: HBO.

Coyle, C. T., & Enright, R. D. (1997). Forgiveness intervention with postabortion men. *Journal of Consulting and Clinical Psychology, 65,* 1042–1046.

Dole, S., & McMahan, J. (2005). Using videotherapy to help adolescents cope with social and emotional problems. *Intervention in School and Clinic, 40,* 151–155.

Duffey, T. (2005a). Grief, loss, and death. In D. Comstock (Ed.), *Critical contexts in human development* (pp. 253–268). Pacific Grove, CA: Brooks/Cole–Thompson Learning.

Duffey, T. (2005b). Releasing the dream. In T. Duffey (Ed.), *Creative interventions in grief and loss therapy: When the music stops, a dream dies.* New York: The Haworth Press.

Duncan, K., Beck, D., & Granum, R. (1986). Ordinary people: Using a popular film in group therapy. *Journal of Counseling and Development, 65,* 50–51.

Enright, R. D. (2001). *Forgiveness is a choice: A step-by-step process for resolving anger and restoring hope.* Washington, DC: American Psychological Association.

Fitzgibbons, R., Enright, R., & O'Brien, T. (2004). Learning to forgive. *American School Board Journal, 191*(7), 24–26.

Freedman, S. R., & Enright, R. D. (1996). Forgiveness as an intervention goal with incest survivors. *Journal of Consulting and Clinical Psychology, 64,* 983–992.

Hesley, J. W. (2000). Reel therapy. *Psychology Today, 33*(1), 54–58.

Hesley, J. W. (2001). Using popular movies in psychotherapy. *USA Today Magazine, 129*(2668), 52–55.

Jordan, J. (2000). The role of mutual empathy in relational/cultural therapy. *Journal of Clinical Psychology, 56,* 1005–1016.

Jordan, J. (2001). A relational-cultural model: Healing through mutual empathy. *Bulletin of the Menninger Clinic, 65,* 92–103.

Kalem, T. (Writer), & Garcia, R. (Director). (2004). All happy families . . . [Television series episode]. In D. Chase (Executive producer), *The Sopranos*. New York: HBO.

Kübler-Ross, E. (1969). *On death and dying*. New York: Springer Publishing.

Kushner, H. S. (1981). *When bad things happen to good people*. New York: HarperCollins.

Lampropoulos, G. K., & Spengler, P. M. (2005). Helping and change without traditional therapy: Commonalities and opportunities. *Counselling Psychology Quarterly, 18,* 47–59.

Malick, T. (Writer/Director). (2005). *The new world* [Motion picture]. United States: New Line Cinema.

Miller, J. B. (1986). What do we mean by relationships? *Work in Progress, No. 22.* Wellesley, MA: Stone Center Working Paper Series.

Miller, J. B., & Stiver, I. P. (1993). A relational approach to understanding women's lives and problems. *Psychiatric Annals, 23,* 424–431.

Miller, J. B., & Stiver, I. P. (1995). Relational images and their meanings in psychotherapy. *Work in Progress, No. 74.* Wellesley, MA: Stone Center Working Paper Series.

Miller, J. B., & Stiver, I. P. (1997). *The healing connection: How women form relationships in therapy and in life*. Boston: Beacon.

Newton, A. K. (1995). Silver screens and silver linings: Using theatre to explore feelings and issues. *Gifted Child Today, 18,* 14–19.

Sharp, C., Smith, J. V., & Cole, A. (2002). Cinematherapy: Metaphorically promoting therapeutic change. *Counselling Psychology Quarterly, 15,* 269–276.

Tsang, J. A., McCullough, M. E., & Fincham, F. D. (2004). The longitudinal association between forgiveness and relationship closeness and commitment. *Journal of Social and Clinical Psychology, 25,* 448–478.

Tyson, L., Foster, L., & Jones, C. (2000). The process of cinematherapy as a therapeutic intervention. *The Alabama Counseling Association Journal, 26*(1), 35–41.

Walker, M. (1999). Race, self, and society: Relational challenges in a culture of disconnection. *Work in Progress, No. 85.* Wellesley, MA: Stone Center Working Paper Series.

Winter, T. (Writer), & Van Patten, T. (Director). (2006). Members only [Television series episode]. In D. Chase (Executive producer), *The Sopranos*. New York: HBO.

Worden, W. J. (1991). *Grief counseling and grief therapy*. New York: Springer Publishing.

Worthington, E. L., Jr., & Scherer, M. (2004). Forgiveness is an emotion-focused coping strategy that can reduce health risks and promote health resilience: Theory, review, and hypotheses. *Psychology and Health, 19,* 385–405.

PART VI

Sports

CHAPTER 15

Using the Popularity of Sports Culture in Psychotherapy

Jan M. Burte

SPORTS CULTURE

The sports culture consists of a subgroup of individuals who identify strongly with sports as either an athletic participant or a nonparticipant in sports. The sports culture has its own idiosyncratic mores, rules, icons, traditions, beliefs, and behaviors. It has rules of conduct for athletes, nonathletes, spectators, and fans. It has dress codes ranging from looking like a jock, to wearing a team logo, cap, or shirt. It has its icons (Babe Ruth and Tiger Woods), traditions and holidays (the Super Bowl and Super Bowl Party), beliefs (fairness in sports), behaviors (training regimes), and unique idioms (the Boston Chopper). In some respects, it can be a unifying common denominator that spans ethnic boundaries, age, and gender. It can also create division within a culture (Yankee vs. Red Sox fans regardless of ethnicity or religious beliefs). Finally, it is present in most aspects of daily life for those who function within the culture.

If we examine sports culture within almost any society, we find a unique subset of beliefs and behaviors that are unique to, and in many ways define, that society (Guest, 2007). The expression and manifestations of sports culture may also significantly vary from individual to individual and change over time within a single individual or the larger society (Overman, 1997). The psychological meaning of sports also changes within the cultural context (Guest, 2007) including the different ways in which athletes prioritize achievement motives (Kolt et al., 1994) and develop team affiliation (Rees, Brettshneider, & Brandle-Bredenbeck, 1998).

Gender, culture, and activity level may also play a significant role in the motivation for young athletes and nonathletes to participate in sports (Weinberg et al., 2000).

For the purposes of this chapter, we are going to examine those individuals who, although they may strongly identify with other cultural, ethnic, gender, or age variables, also identify themselves within the mainstream of the sports culture. Cultural identification represents a choice made by an individual. It is malleable and rarely identical to that of other individuals even within the same cultural group. This holds equally true within the sports culture.

In examining the sports culture, I have found that there are numerous categories in which individuals place themselves, some of which frequently overlap. These categories include Athlete, Nonathlete, Recreational, Elite, Participant, Spectator, Casual, and Avid. From a psychotherapeutic perspective, these delineations help to direct therapeutic intervention and often guide understanding of the individual's expectations, needs, motivation, and accessibility as well as guiding the clinician in addressing issues such as perfectionism (Stirling & Kerr, 2007) and locus of control (Murphy, 2005).

THE ATHLETE VERSUS THE NONATHLETE

You gotta be a man to play baseball for a living, but you gotta have a lot of little boy in you too.

—Roy Campanella

Creating a Self-Definition

Individuals who define themselves as athletes often have a clear sense of their athletic ability relative to their peers. The very nature of athletic competition creates an opportunity for constant feedback relative to others. Young or old, it is often the passion for competition, the pleasure of playing, the drive and desire to win that makes athletes successful. Martina Navratilova was recently quoted as saying, "Whoever said 'it's not whether you win or lose that counts' probably lost." For some athletes, this can enhance performance, but for others it impedes success. Young athletes' actual performance relative to their peers can exist in a conflicted manner relative to their fantasized future achievements. For example, ask many Little League players (whether in a top "A" or lower "B" league) and they will describe in detail their expectations and dreams of being a major leaguer. Good for them! However, a time often arrives, when a reassessment of their future career, scholarship, or employment goals needs to be addressed, even if it is "just in case you do not make it to the bigs."

For an elite child athlete, pressures and expectations can become overwhelming. Performance issues can weigh heavily on a young elite athlete. The opposing priorities to fit academic, family, and social demands around vigorous workout and competition schedules can be overwhelming. Truly elite athletes (junior Olympians) at times have to choose between the benefits of competing on a school team and virtual schooling in order to meet the challenges of national competitions. However, the majority of young athletes I have worked with remain in academic programs and juggle academic, social, and sports demands. For teens, playing at the high school level is critical for college scholarships and school selection. All of these pressures are unique to this group of elite athletes and often become the focus of their therapy.

Demanding workout schedules and competitions leading to burnout are not uncommon and in some ways are the "organic chemistry" and SAT equivalent of the academically oriented. The common denominator for both the athlete and nonathlete is whether or not they can do well under continuous pressure. Often, the sports psychologist is called upon in this scenario to help young athletes see beyond the immediate situation. Parents can be problematic at this juncture, particularly if they are too enamored with their own dreams and aspirations for their child attaining a college scholarship or pursuing a career in amateur or professional sports.

Needless to say, athletes share in common many similarities with nonathletes. However, for athletes their self-identification often impacts upon their reaction to events and their response becomes more visibly quantifiable as it is evident during competition. Often significant family sacrifices need to be made, therefore the pressure to remain dedicated and maintain a peak level of performance is always present. At times these pressures are expressed in emotions that run counter-productively to peak performances and adversely influence the athlete's self-perceptions.

CASE STUDY 1

Stoke play is a better test of golf, but match play is a better test of character.

—Joe Carr

Tommy was a 14-year-old junior PGA golfer, whose anger and low frustration tolerance began to have a serious impact on his scores. If he bogied a hole, Tommy would become self-critical and self-denigrating. Frequently he would then rush or misplay subsequent shots. Upon observation during a tournament, it became clear that his internalized anger would manifest itself physically. His grip would change, his forearms would tighten, his shoulders would shift, and he would be frowning. Even his exit from the green would change. At these times, Tommy would become so angry that he would drop significantly in the standing.

Intervention for this young golfer involved visualization, relaxation, and self-talk techniques, focused upon creating positive appraisals of himself regardless of any individual, shot, or hole. Therapy focused upon utilizing rational emotive approaches such as "de-awfulizing" specific events, refocusing on a bigger picture (inclusive of viewing the tournament as a learning experience, rather than an end result), reducing his self-imposed anger and negative self-talk, and reiterating positive self-statements. Internalized encouragement had to be learned. In addition, he needed to learn to pursue his own personal goals and achieve peak performances and not view his performance as a means of gaining parental approval.

CASE STUDY 2

When I go out on the ice, I just think about my skating. I forget it is a competition.

—Katarina Witt

Tim, a high school tennis player, though technically sound, had not yet developed the necessary motivational and instructional self-talk necessary to sustain him as he moved to increasingly higher levels of competition. Although he had learned self-talk phrases such as "focus," "breathe," "relax," and "explode," he had not learned how to successfully implement these phrases in a competitive stressful situation in which he was behind in games. In fact, in some situations his physiological state was so elevated that he was distracted, and his breathing became shallow and tense to the point where positive self-statements felt too incongruent to be employed. To develop his ability to physiologically respond to these and additional self-statements, Ericksonian hypnosis techniques were employed to mirror, pace, and direct his physiological state to the point where the self-statements could be accepted and employed. Through the use of imagery and hypnosis, Tim was able to recreate his physiological states in the office and in practice situations.

Based upon Araoz's *The New Hypnosis* (1985), FIDEL (Focused Internally Directed Experiential Learning) is a form of nondirective hypnosis I developed and have employed effectively with athletes to enhance the communication of cognitive self-talk and self-appraisal with sensory motor input and output (Burte, 2004). Its goal is to promote peak performance by eliminating negative internal neuro-cognitive imagery and experiences.

Utilizing the FIDEL approach, Tim was able to practice self-talk during covert imaginary tournament conditions. Interestingly, for Tim and most if not all young athletes (including those at minor league and professional entry levels of play), a large proportion of self-talk training is aimed at teaching them to dismiss negative self-talk more so than to merely initiate positive self-talk. Young athletes must learn not to fear a mistake or loss. Elite adult athletes with years of experience, coaching, and training expect to execute tasks successfully most of the time and view errors or losing as a natural consequence of their job. However, for young athletes who are learning new skills and facing increasing competition, "failing up" is common. As soon as they achieve one level they move up to the next, where facing stiffer competition and the need to learn new skills are commonplace.

Baseball is 90% mental—the other half is physical. (Yogi Berra)

For example, I have witnessed average hitters maintain their composure and batting averages as they began to face curve balls for the first time at about the age of 11 years old. I have also observed the big hitters with overly high expectations fall apart when they are literally and figuratively thrown a curve ball. The average hitter expects to fail and embraces it, whereas the big hitter becomes confused and angered by the change in outside events and must first learn a new dialogue of positive self-talk associated with these changes. Adult elite athletes benefit by opening up clear pathways for subconsciously driven pure peak performance behaviors (i.e., maximization of "in the zone" responding.)

For these athletes doubting their confidence, discouragement and fatigue can lead to negative demotivational self-talk, and negative instructional self-talk (i.e., "I can't do it," over-thinking and anxious thoughts, mental errors). Learning to uncover and eliminate negative self-talk (Burte, 2002a, 2002b), and implementing positive self-talk, can result in a multitude of improvements in attitude, motivation, and performance (Zinsser, Bunker, & Williams, 2001).

Self-talk represents a crucial skill that can significantly enhance performance. Motivational self-talk can assist athletes to build self-confidence, increase effort, and control anger, arousal, and anxiety. Instructional self-talk has been shown to enhance different aspects of performance through attentional, focus, and technical and tactical self-instruction (Landin & Hebert, 1999).

In addition, temper tantrums are rarely tolerated in sports and often ejection or penalties are the result. Athletes must learn to remain calm and focused when they feel violated in some way by either an opponent or a referee/umpire. The ability to refocus is much more critical in athletic performance than in almost any other endeavor. Dismissing a bad call is essential to success. For the athlete, it is a part of his or her culture. Ruminating is a luxury left to the nonathlete. When a teacher marks an answer on a test wrong when in fact it is correct, the student or the parent can usually rectify the problem with a phone call. However, in sports the athlete can rarely argue a call, even though on occasion an appeal may be possible.

> Slump? I ain't in no slump. I just ain't hitting. (Yogi Berra)

Any batter in a slump or golfer with the "yips" can in some way describe how ruminating is supplanting their muscle memory, resulting in impaired performance. Learning to relax physiologically is a critical skill that all individuals within the sports culture must learn. Therapists should focus on techniques such as hypnosis, biofeedback, neurofeedback, and reframing when helping these individuals. This is, however, not at all limited to the athlete. Sports fans, spectators, and noncombatants often report experiencing the same difficulties to the detriment of their happiness, work, or daily functioning. One need only observe an international soccer match to see the patterns of behavior that have resulted in injuries and even deaths of fans and referees.

> I never blame myself when I'm not hitting. I just blame the bat and if it keeps up, I change bats. After all, if I know it isn't my fault that I am not hitting, how can I get mad at myself? (Yogi Berra)

Abrams and Hale (2004) suggest that key components of controlling anger for athletes are to address their heightened physiological arousal by teaching progressive muscle relaxation, employing imagery, and learning to "quiet themselves down" (p. 106). They also suggest athletes must learn how to reevaluate their thinking by talking it out with coaches, communicating, learning to respond positively to constructive criticism, not using anger as a tool to create distance or intimidation within a team setting, taking a time out, engaging in problem solving, and learning to evaluate and modify their behaviors. These then are the additional tasks of the therapist working with the hot-headed athlete or fan whose thinking and behaviors are negatively impacting his or her performance or functioning. Even at the level of professional sports, hot-headed athletes find themselves traded to other teams because of their destructive impact upon the team. Coaches are not immune to this behavior. Who can forget Billy Martin or Pete Rose, who were known to occasionally kick up more than a little infield dirt? Young athletes need to learn levels of emotional control under stressful physiologically arousing conditions, while being scrutinized by others in order to succeed.

MAINTAINING A POSITIVE ATTITUDE
REGARDLESS OF PERFORMANCE

The price of success is hard work, dedication to the job at hand, and the determination that whether we win or lose, we have applied the best of ourselves to the task at hand.

—Vince Lombardi

Maintaining a positive attitude regardless of performance is a basic skill that also must be taught to all athletes and is in some ways inconsistent with much of what they are taught in other areas of functioning.

As a coach of a youth baseball team, I have watched how parents' reactions can alter the mood and attitude of their children on the field. As a wise professional coach with over 30 years of experience once explained to me, "A positive attitude is important to achieving success but seeing failure as an acceptable outcome is critical to sustaining peak performance." He described that it is not uncommon for a middle school or high school player to misfield a ball or make an error. After making an error, a young fielder often drops his head or eyes and looks to the stands only to see his parents upset, hushed, or embarrassed. At that moment that player is no longer in the game but rather is in his head. He has lost track of the fact that in most sports competitions, errors are as much a part of the event as are great plays and that mistakes need to be embraced as a natural consequence of playing and enjoying the game.

CASE STUDY 3

Show me a guy who's afraid to look bad and I'll show you a guy you can beat every time.

—Lou Brock

David was an 11-year-old travel team baseball second basemen. He had played baseball since he was 6 years old. He had been fed critical negative statements of never being good enough throughout that entire time. He was more often anxious than relaxed during games, but was otherwise capable of extraordinary performances during practices and in the batting cages. He had struggled with self-esteem issues. His family dynamics included a father who "almost made it to the minor leagues." This father believed that if he pushed his son hard enough, the son could make it. Therapy for this young man took place on the field during practice and during games. Repetition of positive self-talk was critical in keeping him focused and maintaining an accurate level of self-assessment of his expectations.

An example of David's response style was demonstrated when during a game, he misplayed a difficult chopper. Let us compare two subsequent sets of thoughts. The first set contains the ones David went through before he walked off the field: "I cannot believe I missed that ball. Everybody saw me blow it. Even my parents are upset. I hope I don't get benched. Please don't let another ball get hit to me." The second set of thoughts are the ones he received from the bench coach: "Okay, you can't make them all. That's what makes the game fun. You'll get it next time. Let's go. Head up. Let's turn two (perform a double play). Think the ball into the glove." As a side note, a few instructive words had to be said to his dad in the stands, who was reacting with groans to every misplay of the ball rather than giving encouragement and enjoying the opportunity of watching his son play ball with the other great kids.

Unlike schoolwork, homework, or exams, failure in sports needs to be embraced and enjoyed in order for success to be sustained in a sport. Too often I have met athletes whose internalized mind-set was locked on nonathletic ways of thinking that create unattainable expectations by definition. No one bats 1,000, scores every three-point shot, lands every double toe loop, or eagles every hole. A technique I often use to challenge my young patients' thinking is to apply a series of tests to help point out the errors in their thought processing. I suggest we have a competitive door handle turning contest. We will see who can open a door successfully, 100 times in a row. After they have become bored, some time before they reach the 100th time, I point out to them the principle that if they can do it perfectly every time, it is not much of a sport. Athletes are trained to walk differently and stand differently (athletic stance) when in a competition. Their mental processes must also reflect this alternative cultural stance.

THE FAMILY

Within the sports culture, a young athlete's parents are critical members of his team but not in the fashion they think. I have witnessed occasions when parents harass the umpire or referee. Consequently, when there is a close call to be made in whose favor, do you think the umpire will make that call? I have even stood astonished when parents shout out to their kids things such as, "It is not your fault, the rest of the team is letting you down," or, "Do not listen to the coach, he does not know what he is doing." The sports culture is full of examples like this. Treatment often involves family therapy where we as therapist need to instruct parents on how to behave and accept team and individual poor performances or defeat (yes, even their own perfect player makes mistakes) and offer encouragement whether the team is winning or losing. I guarantee that you do not need to know the score of the game to know which team is winning or losing, if you listen for one minute to the parents in the two opposing bleachers.

Rarely do I see these behaviors displayed by parents in any other area of the child's functioning. The oxymoron is this: In order for most children to be able to compete at any significant level of organized competition, parental support is necessary in the form of organizing schedules, paying coaches, and providing transportation. Yet, after going through all that effort, they still undermine the child's enjoyment and performance through their negative or critical responses during competition. I call this "deconstructive support." It is up to us as sports psychologists, therapists, or coaches to stop parents at these times and rectify the situation.

Deconstructive Support

Deconstructive support can be recognized and needs to be treated in therapy. It is usually first identified by the child, who states, "I don't like it when my parents come to the game because I always play worse." For example, Joey, a good starting pitcher and a better-than-average hitter, turns to his father and mother after each pitch or swing. After each pitch they provide him with a critical commentary. On his way back to the dugout from the batter's box, they tell him why he struck out—or even worse, yell things like, "What the hell were you thinking, swinging at that pitch? Get your head in the game!" They even continue to yell at him in the dugout. Yet, since he plays well and is being successful at times, these same parents assume their behavior is working. Soon, Joey begins to lose interest in the sport for his own enjoyment and begins to play for their extrinsic approval. Eventually, to the shock of his parents, Joey decides to quit the baseball team and leaves the sport. The cause is the critical perfectionist manner in which his parents have applied their values and needs within the context of a sports culture that uniquely embraces defeat as a natural possible consequence within any competition. When he no longer wants to meet their expectations, he is forced to step out of the culture and finds alternative cultures with which to identify. This can lead to disastrous results.

The sports culture in many ways is a culture unto itself with a language of its own, guided by rules of conduct that are either self-imposed or imposed by others. Athletes and families need to embrace these concepts and understand that losing is as much a part of competition as is winning while all the while remaining driven to succeed. Athletes almost by definition must be competitive, and it is the drive to win that inspires increased performance. Therapy, which uses this mind-set by setting challenges for the athlete, may at times be more effective than other forms of intervention. Therapy might focus upon helping athletes differentiate between adaptive and maladaptive perfectionism. Enns, Cox, Sareen, and Williams (2001) describe adaptive perfectionism as a positive pursuit of achievement while maladaptive perfectionism is associated with fear of failure resulting from negative evaluation by self and others.

Perfectionist thinking inflicted by parents upon their children is not an uncommon problem and is not much different on the surface from academic pressure. However, the critical issue is that for young athletes, sports participation is supposed to be fun. As therapists, we need to help athletes such as Joey successfully remove themselves from their parent issues and their unfortunate intrusive deconstructive support. Family therapy is a modality that works best. Helping Joey talk about the impact that their behaviors have upon specific skill execution and helping the parents to be encouraging or remain quiet in critical situations is essential. For many athletes, it is also embarrassing or distracting when parents feel the need to instruct them during a game. Often even coaches will not give instruction until after a game is complete.

These behaviors, which parents see as appropriate and acceptable to express within the sports culture, would hardly be welcomed in a classroom setting. Imagine if in a sixth grade math class Joey's mother and father were permitted to insult the teacher (the umpire), harangue their child (the player), and denigrate the other students (his teammates). Counselors need to work within the competitive model and understand the nonspecific quality of athletic sportsmanship. One needs a big ego to believe he or she is able to successfully more times than not hit a round ball with a round stick (today almost nobody consistently bats over .400), perform a perfect double toe loop, or sink every putt or basket. At times, as a therapist it is necessary to remind parents and athletes about their purpose and intent in engaging in sports, whether as a participant or as an observer.

DRUGS, ALCOHOL, AND FOOD

If you don't do what's best for your body, you're the one who comes up on the short end.

—Julius Erving

For the athlete, drugs take on a very different meaning than for the nonathlete. Ask an athlete the question, "Do you take drugs?" and a typical response might be, "You mean like steroids?" I do not mean to imply that athletes do not use recreational drugs. However, recent data suggests that they are less likely than nonathletes to do so. It may be due to the closer monitoring or to a different set of values. A different self-definition based upon a different set of values or a difference in the culture within which they define themselves may account for this. Terms like goth, gangster, geek, and jock often describe patterns of behaviors, dress codes, and self-definitions that dictate a lifestyle and choices. It is no different for those who identify themselves as athletes.

Pritchard, Milligan, Elgin, Rush, and Shea (2007) found that 80% of NCAA athletes drink alcohol and 25% binge at least once weekly. While Koss and Gaines (1993) suggested that college athletes may be drinking less in general, findings are mixed as to whether athletes drink more than nonathletes (Wechsler & Davenport, 1997). Along related lines, recent studies suggest that being involved in athletics may decrease the likelihood of smoking (Pritchard et al., 2007; Rigotti, Regan, Majchrzak, Knight, & Wechsler, 2002). Pritchard's research also indicated that disordered eating was more common amongst athletes than nonathletes, and that female athletes had greater body image dissatisfaction than did nonathletes, while male nonathletes had greater body dissatisfaction than did male athletes. However, it remains unclear if there is a difference in the frequency of eating disorders in athletes versus nonathletes (Reinking & Alexander, 2005). Overall these studies clearly point out that athletes versus nonathletes demonstrate significant differences in self-perception, values, and behaviors, particularly as these impact on their use of drugs and alcohol.

In the context of the above, I would like to direct our focus to the medications and drugs, both legal and illegal, that are more commonly utilized by athletes within the context of the sports culture. The list of drugs used and abused by athletes may surprise many individuals, especially when we consider the role of parents in obtaining some of these medications. Drugs utilized to enhance performance or speed recovery may include anabolic adrenergic steroids, psychostimulants, ergonomic aids, narcotic analgesics, beta-adrenergic blockers, diuretics, diet pills, and weight enhancers. Although more commonly found at higher levels of performance, at least some of these drugs do appear at almost all levels within the competitive sports culture and may reflect the pressures experienced by individuals who are immersed within the sports culture. Often the philosophy of "whatever it takes" overrides good judgment. For this reason therapists should perform initial paper-and-pencil drug screenings, and when necessary refer for medical drug testing. Children are given painkillers in order to suppress pain, which should be a huge "stop sign" to stop training in young athletes. Overuse and overtraining injuries are common in developing bodies.

Athletes utilize psychostimulants to enhance focus and concentration during long workouts and superstitiously become dependent on them for competition. I have known parents to plead a case for psychostimulants for their children, reportedly for ADD but actually in order to allow the child to meet both their academic pressures and enhance their athletic performance. College athletes report higher levels of stress than nonathletes due to the combined academic and athletic demands (Kimball & Freysinger, 2003). The increasing prevalence of commercials espousing the dangers of steroid use is obviously not directed toward professional athletes. I have encountered numerous situations in which young men and women illicitly utilize steroids obtained from other athletes or steroid dealers. The rationale was to get a competitive edge despite the risk or consequences inherent in their action. Parents often are unaware of illicit steroid use, or even more unfortunately conveniently fail to notice (or acknowledge) the rapid muscular development in their teen. All too often, I have heard of young athletes and families who have lost their perspective and have endangered themselves with drug utilization.

Often family therapy is a critical element in treating young athletes and their families in order to understand the true dynamics underlying these inappropriate behaviors and mixed messages. Other drugs may be used to regulate weight, sleep, and anxiety. Travel team, school team, and tournament-level competitions can be very demanding upon the physiology of both young and adult athletes. I am no longer surprised when I hear that medications such as benzodiazapines (Atavan and Xanax) to reduce anxiety, somnambulistic drugs (Lunesta, Tylenol PM) for sleep, and beta blockers (propananol and inderol) to reduce tremors and lower heart rate are being utilized by young and adult athletes to enhance performance. Stimulants and diet aids are also used to keep young athletes at specified weights when weight classes are an issue or appearance is a factor, such as in the case of wrestling, football, or figure stating. Treatment in these situations is twofold: First, a close analysis needs to be done wherein both parents and athletes need to readdress their agendas and priorities. Second, an alternative solution needs to be presented.

For some athletes, the drive to perform at optimum levels motivates them enough to engage a potentially harmful career ending and even illegal behavior in order to succeed. However, therapy can provide healthier, more appropriate, and legal alternative strategies to maintain motivation and enhance performance. John Eliot (2004) suggests solid motivational strategies to foster autonomy, competence, and correctness in athletic performance. He identifies key elements, which include learning to *push the edge, experience success, change one's thinking, get involved, praise others, vary training, put oneself first, think positively* and *remember one's dreams*. Though presented as motivational aides, they also reflect strategies necessary for avoiding drugs along the road to success. Therapists should focus on these important elements in addressing athletes who are struggling emotionally. In addition the therapist should stress that having fun is a critical element in maintaining involvement within the sports culture.

INJURY

You learn you can do your best even when it's hard, even when you are tired and may be hurting a little bit. It feels good to show some courage.
—Joe Namath

To an individual invested in the sports culture, injury can be psychologically traumatic. It is imperative that a therapist working with a self-defined athlete appreciate this reality. A temporarily disabling knee or neck injury to the average person is frightening or inconvenient and our cognitive training as therapists teaches us to help that person put the injury into perspective. However, for young and adult athletes, it can be devastating. For many, their self-definition, their dreams (whether realistic, premature, or unrealistic), are gone. Depression is common. Rapid deterioration in other areas of functioning, such as school and social life, are not unusual. Depending on the timing of the event, it can be career-ending, as I see with many of the young athletes with whom I work. You are off the scout list. For young athletes, scholarships and dreams can be lost in the blink of an eye.

Recently, I learned of a young diver who had a previous eye injury resulting from a childhood accident. By high school however, he had become a state and regional champion diver and was on his way to college with a full scholarship. Then in a competition, just a few weeks before the start of college, he misjudged a dive and "belly flopped" face first into the water, reinjuring his eye. He was told by his ophthalmologic surgeon that he could never dive again. For this young man, who had devoted countless hours to training, travel, and competition, what was left of his self-definition required therapy to rebuild. Techniques such as reframing do not work effectively in this type of situation and only undermine the enormous efforts, mental and physical dedication, and mind-set of the athlete. In order for recovery to be complete, therapy must focus on using the drive, determination, and athlete's mind-set to create new goals and new horizons. Often we are called upon to remind the athlete to find the courage to face the adversity in spite of the potential outcome.

Neuro-feedback (EEG and EMG), thermal biofeedback, and hypnotherapy are powerful tools, which can promote healing and mediate pain, as well as improve rehabilitation rates, outcomes, and attitudes (Burte, 2002a, 2002b, 2004). Through visualization, those athletes who will eventually return to sports can mentally train and continue to develop muscle memory even while unable to perform their physical sport.

EFFECTIVE THERAPEUTIC CHANGE

Champions aren't made in gyms. Champions are made from something
they have deep inside them—a desire, a dream, a vision.

—Muhammad Ali

I have found that athletes respond especially well to interventions
such as imagery and hypnosis. This may be the result of internalized
innate abilities or because of skills they may have developed in their
training process. The T.E.A.M. concept (acronym for trust, expectations,
attitude, and motivation) that I have applied to working with athletes
was first presented by Daniel Araoz (1985) in explaining the elements
necessary for achieving a successful hypnotic experience. I have observed
that both professional and amateur athletes spend much of their time
in an alternate state. Young athletes as they step into competitive settings imagine that they are the next Alex Rodriguez, Sarah Hughes, or
Payton Manning. Older players set aside the daily stressors of life when
they step onto a court, course, field, or rink. From recreational to elite
athletes, these players share with the hypnotic subject experiences such
as time distortion, altered sense of self, the ability to disregard distraction and focus on relevant details, unconscious actions (muscle memory),
pain control, and a host of other sensations. When treating the individual
within the sports culture, the T.E.A.M. concept is always present.

Trust

The patient must be able to *trust* his therapist, coach, trainer, or parents
to provide guidance and structure. The patient must trust in the skills and
strategies employed to help obtain success, and must also trust in his or
her own prior training and preparation. For the therapist, this means that
therapeutic and clinical sport psychology skills should be employed to enhance performance. For athletes and nonathletes, focused effort and successful repetition of tasks often results in self-confidence and self-esteem.
Conversely, poor performance can represent a significant disruption in
their self-images. Therapy often focuses on helping these athletes trust in
the positive imagery associated with their typical best performances and
finding the self-confidence to dismiss negative thoughts or negative images that can lead to undesired muscle memory, while increasing positive
self-talk.

Expectations

The *expectation*s of the athletes should be realistic, attainable, and sustainable by reasonable means and interventions. For the therapist, this

means helping coaches, parents, and players set realistic goals, avoid overtraining and burnout, and allow proper recovery time and a balance of athletics and other activity. Family therapy often is a significant component in establishing appropriate expectations. Parents may set unrealistic goals, typically identified by statements expressed by the young athlete such as, "But Dad, I just want to be a kid."

Attitude

The athlete's *attitude* is critical to success, inclusive of understanding that failure, errors, and such are part of what makes the sport interesting. If she cannot fail, it is not a challenge. Embracing a range of performance as a part of playing is no less important then embracing a drive to win. For the therapist, techniques to help athletes and families include exercises that ensure failure, shame attacks, and teach learning to laugh at themselves, reframing, and reviewing the enjoyment of the competition. If an athlete cannot accept losing then he or she cannot remain competitive. The therapist must explore the issues associated with perfectionistic thinking, rumination, and a self-imposed stress response. Often problems such as the "yips" in which muscle tremors, tensing, or cognitive distraction interfere with performance are reflected by the attitude the athletes brings to competition.

Motivation

More has been written on motivation than any other topic. Maintaining motivation is critical to success. As pointed out earlier in this chapter, athletes must be willing to accept hardship (giving up going out weekend nights for practice, training, or rest) in order to remain at the top of their game. Once motivation is lost, performance often tumbles like a house of cards. For the therapist, reviewing with the client successes, goals, values, and self-established expectations, and also listening for negativistic speech, are means of monitoring if the client may be approaching burnout. Therapy should break down the areas that are demotivating and create small steps for success, help rebalance goals, and increase awareness of whether success is the parent's dream or the athlete's dream. Burnout is frequently preceded by statements such as "I forgot to do my drills," "Do we have to go to practice tonight?" or "I just want to be a kid, Dad." At these times it is critical to hear what the young athlete is asking for and recognize the need to back off the practice schedule. Family therapy is not uncommonly a part of understanding changes in levels of motivation. Therapy needs to focus on the athlete's internal locus of control. Is the athlete driven by extrinsic rewards or internal passion? For the former a cost/benefit analysis often dictates their commitment and they are less likely to succeed, where in the later case, greater stability and consistency are likely. At times significantly self-destructive behaviors may arise as a way of being heard.

However, above all else the dream and vision to be a champion drives the athlete.

It is an incredible source of energy and force of will that therapists need to utilize to overcome the unique hurdles athletes face. Murphy (2005) suggests that focusing on the value system of the athlete may be more effective in treating negative behaviors such as drug and alcohol consumption than focusing on the actual negative behaviors.

How then do we as therapists conceptualize and utilize our therapeutic skills when treating individuals who identify themselves within the athletic culture? In order to accomplish this, we as therapists need to learn the lingo, understand the demands of high-level performance, and realize that non-elite athletes may still regard themselves as legends in their own minds. It is also crucial for us to incorporate family therapy in order to better understand the pressures that young athletes may experience both outside and inside of their families and to appreciate the mindset that they exist within a culture different from those of a nonathlete.

COMMUNICATING IN THE SPORTS CULTURE

When speaking with individuals who identify with the sports culture, idioms can level the playing field, so to speak. As in social situations, knowledge of some of these may prove useful in therapy.

Tom:	Hey, what about those Yankees, they're really kicking.
Dick:	Yeah, but they're not gonna catch Boston.
Harry:	I don't know, with Jeter and Ramirez both hitting, it's gonna be close. (This goes on for 15 minutes. Then:)
Tom:	Oh, by the way, my name's Tom.
Dick:	Dick, how ya doin'?
Harry:	Harry, I'm good. Nice to meet you.

Instant Rapport

Within the domain of multicultural counseling, it is understood that knowledge of the customs for greeting, cultural idioms, and cultural styles of communication are essential to good therapeutic work (Sue &

Sue, 2008). In fact, without knowledge of the unique cultural differences between therapist and patient, one is left with a universalist mind-set that would suggest that these differences are not important and that "good therapy is good therapy."

Once we adopt such a mind-set, then we cut off multiple levels of communication critical to achieving maximal benefit in therapy. Not all individuals inculcated in the sports subculture are athletes. Indeed, I would venture to say that the majority of individuals who subscribe to the precepts of a sports culture are either former athletes or individuals who may have marginally or only recreationally participated in sports.

I have found that these individuals are gratified when they can express their identification and interest in sports either by directly discussing or by communicating in idioms and lingo. Many recognize themselves as members of the club by verbal knowledge only and are eager to initiate rapport by those means. Whereas the athlete invested in the culture is focused on her/his athleticism and issues around it, often the nonathlete enjoys flexing cerebral knowledge of stats, opinions, standing, expectations, and hopes.

> Sports are the reason I am out of shape. I watch them all on TV.
> (Thomas Sowell)

If we are to work with athletes and nonathletes enmeshed within the sports culture we should be able to recognize their shrines. Television, radio, and print such as primetime sports channels, ESPN, ESPN II, Sports Center, the sports pages, and *Sports Illustrated* are the Cable News Network, *New York Times,* religious, and entertainment sources for these individuals. Though we need not adopt their degree of devotion, as true multicultural counselors we need to be familiar with the language, rituals, and customs of that culture.

A patient came to my office and after noting my sports paraphernalia (consisting of multiple teams from multiple sports) he began to talk about his own sports interests and athletic history. Rapport was quickly established and therapy was initiated. About three sessions into treatment he started the session by saying, "You know, I wasn't sure if we could relate when I saw that signed baseball and photos of you." He then proceeded to remove his "B" cap (Boston Red Sox). For the most part individuals interested in sports welcome the rivalry, but others are invested in their culture and defend their sects (respective teams) with as much fervor as any zealot.

The athletic culture resembles the ancient religions, as opposed to the more contemporary monotheistic religions. Players are often held up as demigods. When I do therapy within this context, that perception allows me (especially with children and teens) to utilize player's lives and behaviors as ways to help my patients select values and beliefs that can create lasting constructive conduct patterns.

Comparing how athletes deal with issues, conduct themselves, or have directed themselves to achieving goals can provide a substantial set of role models, both good and bad, for many youths. Issues common to nonathletes who identify themselves within the sports culture can be easily related to those of athletes.

I believe that by accepting that the sports culture represents a clearly delineated group of individuals, and by respecting it as such, and by learning the language, terminology, and rules of the culture, one can effectively utilize the heroes and villains, and apply the values inherent in sports to everyday life. Literally, hundreds of idioms are derived from the sports culture. A brief review of sports idioms Web sites on the Internet revealed the extensive application of sports-derived terminology expressed in every facet of daily functioning.

CASE STUDY 4

Sam, a 12-year-old boy, was brought to therapy by his mother. He was sullen, withdrawn, angry, and doing poorly at school both socially and academically. Prior to the session with Sam, his mother informed me that he had seen two other therapists in the past and that he had made little or no progress with them. He was resistant to going to therapy and was giving her a hard time.

Sam came in wearing a Steelers football jersey, and a Phillies baseball cap. After a minute or two of conversation, his mother left us alone. We sat a few minutes and typical rapport building commenced.

> DR. B: You a Phillies fan or just like the hat? (Note the clipped sports speech)
>
> SAM: I'm a fan.
>
> DR. B: How do they look for next year?
>
> SAM: Good.
>
> DR. B: Did you get to watch many games last year?
>
> SAM: No.
>
> DR. B: Do you get "Extra Innings" on cable?
>
> SAM: What's that?

We talk baseball for 40 minutes. We talk baseball and football for four sessions. We agree and we disagree, but we share a culture. We talk about being a Philly and Steelers fan while living in south Florida. We talk about how he became a fan and a little about his family and his relocation.

Session 5:

DR. B: What's up?

SAM: I think my dad hates me. He doesn't talk to me unless I call him first.

This, according to Sam's mother, was the first time Sam had discussed or even mentioned his father in therapy. She also reported that he looked forward to coming during the week and would only put out the mandatory resistance because she wanted him to go and his 12-year-old hormones told him he had to rebel. He always demanded that he wear a sports jersey and cap. Sam ultimately completed therapy, worked through his anger issues, improved his grades, and joined a recreational baseball team. He came to understand his feelings about his father and how to deal more effectively with those feelings.

Okay, sports fans! Your game plan has been laid out and with no time left on the clock, the ball is now in your court.

It ain't over till it's over. (Yogi Berra)

REFERENCES

Abrams, M., & Hale, B. (Eds.). (2004). Anger: How to moderate hot buttons. In S. Murphy (Ed.), *The sport psychology handbook: A complete guide to today's best mental training techniques* (pp. 93–112). Champaign, IL: Human Kinetics Publishers.

Araoz, D. L. (1985). *The new hypnosis.* New York: Brunner/Mazel.

Burte, J. M. (2002a). Psychoneuroimmunology. In R. Weiner (Ed.), *Pain management: A practical guide for clinicians* (pp. 807–816). Boca Raton, FL: CRC Press.

Burte, J. M. (2002b). Hypnotherapeutic advances in pain management. In R. Weiner (Ed.), *Pain management: A practical guide for clinicians* (pp. 851–860). Boca Raton, FL: CRC Press.

Burte, J. M. (2004). Hypnotherapeutic advances in pain management. In R. Weiner, M. V. Boswell, and B. E. Cole (Eds.), *Pain management: A practical guide for clinicians* (pp. 741–756). Boca Raton, FL: CRC Press.

Eliot, J. (2004). Motivation: The need to achieve. In S. Murphy (Ed.), *The sport psychology handbook: A complete guide to today's best mental training techniques* (pp. 3–18). Champaign, IL: Human Kinetics Publishers.

Enns, M. W., Cox, B. J., Sareen, F., & Freeman, P. (2001). Adaptive and maladaptive perfectionism in medical students: A longitudinal investigation. *Medical Education, 35,* 1034–1042.

Guest, A. M. (2007). Cultural meaning and motivation for sport: A comparative case study of soccer teams in the United States and Malawi. *Athletic Insight,* 9(1). Retrieved September 21, 2007, from http://www.athleticinsight.com/Vol9Iss1/CulturalMeaningandMotivation.htm

Kimball, A., & Freysinger, V. J. (2003). Leisure, stress and coping: The sport participation of collegiate student-athletes. *Leisure Sciences, 25,* 115–141.

Kolt, G. S., Kirkby, R. J., Bar-Eli, M., Blumenstein, B., Chada, N. K., Liu, J., & Ken, G. (1994). A cross cultural investigation of reasons for participation in gymnastics. *International Journal of Sport Psychology, 30,* 381–398.

Koss, M. P., & Gaines, J. A. (1993). The prediction of sexual violence patterns among college populations. *Journal of College Student Personnel, 8,* 94–108.

Landin, D. K., & Hebert, P. E. (1999). The influence of self talk on the performance of skilled female tennis players. *Journal of Applied Sport Psychology, 11,* 263–282.

Murphy, S. (2005). Imagery: Inner theater becomes reality. In S. Murphy (Ed.), *The sport psychology handbook* (pp. 127–152). Champaign, IL: Human Kinetics.

Overman, S. J. (1997). *The influence of the Protestant ethic on sport and recreation.* Aldershot, UK: Avebury Publishing:

Pritchard, M. E., Milligan, B., Elgin, J., Rush, P., & Shea, M. (2007). Comparison of risky health behaviors between male and female college athletes and non-athletes. *Athletic Insight,* 9(1). Retrieved September 21, 2007, from http://www.athleticinsight.com/Vol9Iss1/HealthBehaviors.htm

Rees, C. R., Brettshneider, W. D., & Brandle-Bredenbeck, H. (1998). Globalization of sport activities and sport perceptions among adolescents from Berlin and suburban NY. *Sociology of Sport Journal, 15,* 216–230.

Reinking, M. F., & Alexander, L. E. (2005). Prevalence of disordered eating behaviors in undergraduate female collegiate athletes and non-athletes. *Journal of Athletic Training 40,* 47–51.

Rigotti, N. A., Regan, S., Majchrzak, N. E., Knight, J. R., & Wechsler, H. (2002). Tobacco use by Massachusetts public college students: Long term effect of the Massachusetts Tobacco Control Program. *Tobacco Control, 11*(Supp. 2), 20–24.

Stirling, A. E., & Kerr, G. A. (2007). Future perfectionism and mood states among recreational and elite athletes. *Athletic Insight,* 8(4). Retrieved September 21, 2007, from http://www.athleticinsight.com/Vol8Iss4/Perfectionism.htm

Sue, D. W., & Sue, D. (2008). *Counseling the culturally diverse: Theory and practice.* Hoboken, NJ: Wiley.

Wechsler, H., & Davenport, A. E. (1997). Binge drinking, tobacco and illicit drug use and involvement in college athletics. *Journal of American College Health, 45,* 195–200.

Weinberg, R., Tenenbaum, G., McKenzie, A., Jackson, S, Ansel, M., Grove, R., & Fogerty, G. (2000). Motivation for youth participation in sport and physical activity: Relationship to culture, self reported activity levels and gender. *International Journal of Sport Psychology 31,* 321–346.

Zinsser, N., Bunker, L.K., & Williams, J.M. (2001). Cognitive techniques for improving performance and building confidence. In J.M. Williams (Ed.), *Applied sport psychology: Personal growth to peak performance* (pp. 284–311). Mountain View, CA: Mayfield.

CHAPTER 16

Sports Metaphors and Stories in Counseling With Children

David A. Crenshaw and Gregory B. Barker

In the United States, parents frequently encourage their children to participate in sports. Research studies indicate that participation in athletics results in reduced delinquent behavior, improved academic performance, and better social adjustment (Kremer-Sadlik & Kim, 2007). Parents often view extracurricular sports as ways to teach social skills and to impart a sense of community to their children. By involving children in athletic activities, whether by playing in Little League baseball, joining in neighborhood pick-up games, or just by watching televised sports together, parents can promote important values. Because athletics are central to the families of many children, stories and metaphors drawn from popular sports have potential therapeutic value. This chapter does not focus on enhancing athletic performance. Instead, we hope to elucidate how the use of sports stories and metaphors in counseling promotes engagement, builds therapeutic alliances, overcomes resistance, highlights strengths, clarifies conflict and struggles, facilitates hope, and assists in the termination process.

USE OF METAPHOR AND STORIES IN COUNSELING AND THERAPY

Joyce Mills and Richard Crowley (1986) applied Milton Erickson's pioneering work to therapy with children and described the creative use of metaphor and stories with children. The first author expanded Mills' and Crowley's work to include a combination of evocative strategies, such as metaphors, stories, drawings, ancient parables, and narrative stems in child and adolescent psychotherapy (Crenshaw, 2006). Applebaum's (2000) description of evocativeness in adult psychotherapy influenced us to apply a similar framework in counseling children and adolescents.

Therapists know well the challenge of engaging children and teens to keep them interested during treatment. Bringing forth strong images, memories, and their attendant emotions can be a therapeutic ace in the hole. Evocative strategies are designed to elicit greater emotional responsiveness and meaningful involvement in the therapy process when the child is resistant or reluctant or perhaps does not know how to engage in a meaningful way. The word *evocative* means to summon forth from the depths. Evocative techniques reach a more in-depth, heart-centered place in the child and thus make therapy more meaningful and productive. Stories and metaphors evoke powerful emotions that counselors may direct toward the therapeutic goals stated in the following sections. (The word *children* in this chapter refers to both school-age children and adolescents, unless specified otherwise.)

This chapter is organized according to the use of sports metaphors and stories to pursue specific goals in counseling that roughly parallel the unfolding therapeutic process, from engagement through termination. The goals are represented in the separate main headings to follow. This chapter is organized somewhat differently from the others in this book because the authors have integrated the case studies of Josh and Gina into the goal-directed sections they best fit. This was done to make the flow of the chapter more seamless and integrated. Other goals in counseling are illustrated by the use of metaphors without detailed case material.

SPORTS METAPHORS TO FACILITATE THERAPEUTIC ENGAGEMENT AND ALLIANCE BUILDING

For a variety of reasons, children may be reluctant participants in counseling and therapy, but one key to engagement is to emphasize the collaborative process by working out a therapy contract with them. A counselor might ask, "What is it you wish to gain from counseling?" or "How can we work together to achieve these aims?"

Teamwork is essential in all but the individual sports, and even then close collaboration with a coach is vital to improving one's game. Children who show up for counseling under protest often have experienced the value of teamwork for winning in sports and probably have faced defeat as well. Using metaphors as conceptual and clinical tools enhances the counselor-client alliance and strengthens the effectiveness of therapeutic communication (Stine, 2005). Just as a poetic metaphor can convey complex emotions in remarkably few words, Stine explains that a carefully selected metaphor can be a powerful therapeutic tool, especially when it is a symbol that synthesizes multiple impulses, conflicts, fantasies, and affects.

Perhaps no coach emphasizes more the value of teamwork than Bill Belichick, coach of the New England Patriots. The Patriots are known for their exceptional success in winning three Super Bowls in recent years. Belichick does not focus on individual stars and his teams do not tolerate athletes who are not team players, no matter how much talent they possess. Tom Brady, the Patriots' outstanding quarterback in recent years, is extremely modest, always crediting his success to the outstanding teamwork of the Patriots. After their Super Bowl victories, the Patriots refused in the subsequent celebrations to be introduced as individual players, but rather as a team.

In counseling, that same teamwork can be emphasized to engage reluctant youth. The therapist can make clear that any gains will be the result of teamwork and that without teamwork, nothing substantive will occur.

Mountain Climbing

The sport of mountain climbing is useful in illustrating the collaborative process of therapy. Karen Horney (1942), one of the early psychoanalysts who immigrated to this country from Europe, used mountain climbing as a way of explaining analysis to new patients. She told her patients they could think of her as an expert mountain guide because she had climbed many metaphorical mountains, but she quickly explained that she had never climbed their particular mountain. She did not know the steep crevices, the sharp drop-offs, or the scenic views of the new mountain. She would further make clear to her patients that in order to successfully climb their mountain, she would need their help and they would need to do it together.

Shots on Goal

The following story about Josh not only engaged him in therapy, but the metaphor of *shots on goal* became meaningful in other aspects of his life.

Josh slumped in the chair as his mother began to recount the multitudinous reasons why she had called to make an appointment. As his mother described his situations at school and home, Josh slid down further, trying to lose himself in the bottom of his seat. If only Josh could have slithered through a knothole in the floor, he would have done it. Josh was a handsome and somewhat shy 17-year-old boy who was reluctant to talk as his mother dominated the initial session. She broke into tears as she described how Josh had been abandoned by his father at the age of three and how he'd never had a paternal figure in his life until she remarried when Josh was 13. Clearly, in her mind, Josh's emotional growth and confidence had been stunted by the absence of his father at so early an age. During the past year, as Josh concluded the 10th grade, his family had moved to another school district to accommodate his stepfather's new job. His mother voiced concerns about Josh's general lack of confidence and his inability to complete his school assignments.

At midterm, Josh was receiving B's and C's, and a D in history. Of more serious concern, his mother expressed fears that Josh might be following in his biological father's footsteps. At times, his mother described Josh as sullen and listless. His father had a history of depression and could never maintain a job for a sustained period of time. Further, although Josh's mother had never seen any evidence to believe her son was using alcohol or drugs, she feared he might follow in his father's self-destructive path. Josh's father, she explained, had received psychiatric treatment and was hospitalized for a dual diagnosis disorder (bipolar disorder and chemical dependency) when he was in his early 30s.

The therapist suggested to Josh's mother that he meet with her son alone at the next session and that they meet together as a family within the next month. As is often the case with adolescents, Josh was far more animated at the second session without the presence of a parent in the office. The therapist asked Josh to clarify or modify any of the issues his mother discussed at the first session. Josh could barely remember his biological father and they rarely communicated, though his father lived less than an hour's drive from him. Josh said he respected his stepfather and liked his two new stepbrothers, ages 11 and 13. For the most part, Josh did not feel there was emotional turmoil in his home.

When asked to talk about the things he enjoyed doing the most, Josh came to life. Even though he had just moved to a new school, Josh revealed that he had already made several good friends while playing soccer and lacrosse. Without a bit of conceit, Josh described his lacrosse team's current season. Apparently, Josh was the best player on the team and already had been voted to several regional all-star teams. Josh's team, however, was faltering, as it didn't have a strong enough offense to challenge some of the more skilled teams in the league. Josh said he felt pressured to take more shots on goal from his midfielder's position, but thought he would be disrespectful of his teammates if he "hogged" all of the shots. Conversely, his lacrosse coach frequently urged him to be more assertive and to take more shots. The therapist asked if there was another player with comparable skills who could carry some of the scoring load. Josh explained that lacrosse was a new sport to his school and there were simply not that many skilled offensive players on the team. The therapist then posed this simple question: if Josh's teammates realized he was their best player and if they wanted a winning record, what was keeping him from shooting more and scoring more goals for the team? Every team has its star player. Taking on that role wouldn't mean Josh was leaving his teammates behind. Rather, he'd be elevating the team to a higher level with a better record and a more competitive approach to the game.

In keeping with his coach's request, Josh and his team devised a plan for him to take 4 more shots on goal beyond his average of 10 shots in the next game. Nothing could be lost at this point and the team might just be more competitive. Not surprisingly, Josh's team won the next game as he scored 5 goals and had 3 assists in a 9-to-8 victory. Without the extra output on Josh's part, his team would likely have suffered another loss.

Soon the term *shots on goal* began to take on a whole new meaning and served as a metaphor for other aspects of Josh's life. Josh came from a working-class family and no one in his family had ever attended college. Josh thought he might like to go to college, but he had never been encouraged by teachers or family members to consider the possibility of a college education. Josh admitted he had never really put much effort into his schoolwork, as he probably wouldn't go to college anyway. There was always an opportunity to work in the family construction business after he graduated from high school.

During the next session, Josh considered his self-image and compared himself to his college-bound classmates. Josh had daydreamed about moving away from home and going off to school with kids his own age, but as no one in his family had ever gone to college, Josh felt uncomfortable entertaining any fantasies of college life. With further discussion, Josh realized he had created a scenario for himself analogous to his dilemma on the lacrosse field. Once again, Josh was reluctant to be the star in his family and to be the first one to take a shot at college. Together with his therapist, Josh decided that while his instincts to be a team player were admirable, his teammates/family would prefer him to assert his talents and to attend college. Josh clearly wanted to make a break from the family tradition and to secure a higher education. His therapist encouraged Josh to formulate a plan to get in shape to try out for college. Afterward, Josh went online and scheduled an SAT study course. He began staying after school and sought extra tutoring to raise his final grade in history from a D to a B. He spoke with teachers about writing letters of recommendation and asked his coach to contact some

Division III schools about his lacrosse potential. Josh even used the shots on goal metaphor to spur himself on to ask out a girl he had wanted to date since he had entered his new school.

Josh received several letters of interest from college athletic programs encouraging his application to their admissions departments. He became excited about the possibility of applying to several colleges on the Eastern Seaboard. Further, at the last session, Josh confided that he had worked out all summer so he could be stronger and more confident in his lacrosse skills. He hoped to lead his team to a winning record during his senior year. And, maybe, just maybe, he will lead the division in scoring the most goals.

SPORTS METAPHORS TO DEAL WITH RESISTANCE

Children are usually not thrilled with the idea of seeing a therapist, and typically it is not their idea, but that of their parents, their teachers, or a judge who decided they should seek treatment. Often what looks like "resistance" or lack of cooperation with therapy is instead a reflection of their crushed spirits. They see therapy as another sign of failure. They are reluctant to take the risk of opening up to a counselor because they fear they'll be judged. The willingness to take chances and to risk disappointment is important if one is to face life's adversities. Perhaps the story below about Babe Ruth best illustrates the maxim that you can't succeed unless you're willing to risk failure and to accept defeats along the way.

When he retired in 1935, Babe Ruth owned many of baseball's greatest records and some of its worst. The Great Bambino hit 714 home runs, easily more than any other player before him. He also had struck out 1,330 times. At the time, no one ever thought either record would ever be bested. One player finally toppled his home run mark after 65 seasons, and over 60 players have since broken his strikeout record. Babe Ruth's name has been synonymous with baseball and major accomplishments. The term "Ruthian" has come to mean a momentous feat.

At times, our clients have to make "Ruthian" efforts to overcome the psychological obstacles that might stand in their way. Perfectionistic, obsessive, and anxious children are particularly reluctant to take risks or to face the sting of possible disappointment. Children in counseling are often surprised when they learn the story of Babe Ruth because they'd never considered that so iconic a player as Ruth might have experienced his commensurate share of failures on his way to breaking many time-honored records.

We use not only legendary figures to make our point but contemporary sports heroes, particularly the child's favorite sports hero or heroine, and observe that even the most high-performing athletes have their sub-par days. How often have the kids known when Michael Jordan scored 'way below his average in a game, or periods when Alex Rodriguez went through a prolonged slump, or when Tiger Woods played poorly in major tournaments? By observing the inevitable ups and downs in performance of even the most gifted athletes, children can more easily appreciate the impossible expectations they (and sometimes their families) place on themselves. This assists them in regulating their self-esteem in a more flexible, realistic, and compassionate manner, which is an important therapeutic task. It can also improve their relationships with others because high expectations of oneself are frequently projected on others, who can never subsequently live up to those demands.

SPORTS METAPHORS TO HONOR AND HIGHLIGHT STRENGTHS

The strengths/competency-based approach has received increased emphasis in family therapy and the mental health field in general over the last decade (Allison et al., 2003). Not only has the method garnered interest in the juvenile justice system in treating both male and female adolescent offenders (Clark, 1998; Corcoran, 2005; Johnson, 2003; Pepi, 1997; Querimit & Connor, 2003), it has proven its efficacy in the residential treatment and inpatient treatment of children and adolescents (LeBel et al., 2004; Lietz, 2004; Nickerson, Salamone, Brooks, & Colbet, 2004) and in the treatment of children and youth in general (Corcoran, 2005; Helton & Smith, 2004).

The story of the "Ballistic Stallion" (Crenshaw, 2004) focuses children on times in their lives when they did something to overcome the odds, something that took courage and determination, perhaps something no one thought they could do. "The Everyday Heroes and Heroines" (Crenshaw, 2007) described in detail in Exercise 16.1 is a therapy activity to help children to identify heroes and heroines in their everyday life, including themselves. Another strategy we find useful in achieving this goal is the metaphor of "The Home Run Tape." We explain to children that when a baseball player blasts a home run, the television broadcast will replay the hit on videotape at least once. Then we engage children in a discussion of achievements they've accomplished outside of sports that could be compiled on their personal "home run tape." Of course, if they've hit their own home runs, they grasp this metaphor more vividly. Examples of home run tapes for children are "standing up to a bully," "not losing my temper when I struck out for the third time in a game," "I passed my math final after doing poorly all year," or "I told the guidance counselor that my friend was talking about suicide so she could get help."

In the early part of therapy, children may have difficulty identifying these home run tapes, but the counselor should be alert to point these out. Later in therapy, a clear sign of progress occurs when children take note on their own of their home run tapes. This metaphor observes the important principle in therapy of locating strengths in the children rather than in providing reassurance, which requires reliance on the therapist.

SPORTS METAPHORS TO ILLUMINATE CONFLICT AND STRUGGLE: THE BULL AND THE BUTTERFLY

One of the greatest boxing rivalries of all time existed between Muhammad Ali and Joe Frazier during their classic confrontations in the 1970s. In the ring, Joe Frazier was a bull who needed no red cape to be provoked. He'd charge after his opponents, head down and throwing fierce blows, in order to secure a first-round knockout.

His relentlessness made Frazier the perfect foil for his nemesis, Muhammad Ali. In their three classic bouts, the contrasting styles of the two fighters were highlighted. Ali was considered the more scientific fighter who could "float like a butterfly and sting like a bee." Unlike Frazier, Ali did not seek to knock out his opponents immediately, but rather to use his prodigious speed and boxing skills to wear down his opponent. When the time was right, Ali would inflict the coup de grace.

Every family member has a signature style when communicating and interacting with one another. Often there is a misunderstanding as to why people assume contrasting styles.

Gina was a 15-year-old ninth-grade girl who came to a first counseling session with her mother and stepfather. Gina's mother, Kay, also had a 12-year-old daughter from a previous marriage. The two girls' father had moved to another state, but maintained regular contact with them by phone and they visited him during holidays from school.

In the preceding month, Gina had broken the family curfew on three occasions. Much to her parents' dismay, she'd begun dating an 18-year-old boy who was about to graduate from high school. During this time, Gina's mother and her stepfather, Brett, began to suspect that Gina was engaging in sexual relations with her new boyfriend. Further, they had noticed alcohol on her breath when she returned from parties on the weekends. Every time they confronted Gina about any of these issues, she erupted in anger and retreated to her bedroom. Gina's mother would try to reason with her daughter about their differences, but Gina would refuse to entertain any discourse whatsoever.

The interactions between mother and daughter only served to incense Gina's stepfather. Although he had no children of his own, he was sure that Gina should not be running roughshod over everyone else in the household. When Brett felt his wife was failing to make any progress in discussing issues with Gina, he would step in and lay down the law. The subsequent groundings and punishments only led Gina to further withdraw from both her mother and stepfather. Gina likened her home to Nazi Germany and compared Brett to Adolf Hitler.

During the third session, the therapist mentioned how he used to watch the fighting styles of Ali and Frazier while he was in college. Naturally, Gina knew very little about the history of these boxing greats, but the counselor persisted in describing the fierce competition that existed between the two legends and some of the reasons why the rivalry caught the world's attention at the time. The therapist explained that each fighter used a style that best suited his physical abilities and personality.

The story continued about how Frazier was always the aggressor in the bouts, constantly forcing the action. Boxing commentators commonly assumed that if the fight should last into the later rounds, Ali would have the advantage due to his superior boxing skills. Frazier was a puncher who wanted to inflict damage upon Ali in the first few rounds and hoped to knock him out early in the fight. Frazier intimidated most of his opponents with his aggressive style. Boxing pundits assumed Frazier realized his skills were inferior to Ali's, so Frazier compensated for his weaknesses with a ferocious punching onslaught.

Gina's therapist observed there are people whom we meet in life who appear to be secure in their assertive and aggressive nature, but, in actuality, these "bulls" disguise deep primal fears about their ability to answer the boxing-round bell. Sometimes people who are seemingly assured and confident in nature move forward assertively because they fear losing and revealing their inadequate skills. "Bulls" must intimidate others to reach their goal. It may seem improbable, but the "bulls" in life are actually scared and afraid to alter their style. They are uncertain and struggle to get up on their toes to bob and weave.

Gina immediately grasped the significance of this metaphor, seeing herself as Ali and her stepfather as Frazier. However, she could not play the role of Ali just yet. In the therapist's opinion, Ali went through rigorous hours of arduous training before he could assume the title of The Greatest. Before Gina should begin to dodge her stepfather's onslaught and aggressive discussions, she needed to go to her "gym" and start training to hone her skills.

During the subsequent sessions, Gina and her therapist began to role-play different approaches she might take when her stepfather and mother infuriated her with their punishments and seemingly unreasonable restrictions. Gradually, Gina gained confidence in the more sophisticated and mature approaches she could assume with her parents. In fact, she no longer ran to her room to seek refuge from the oncoming "bull." Gina realized her stepfather was not really a dictator, but rather a figure that lacked some of the skills to negotiate and reason. She understood her stepfather's approach, as he had never known any other style. How could he take on another role? Gina's stepfather never had children of his own and therefore he had no previous training in the child-rearing "gym" in his life.

As Gina became more skillful at dodging her parents' arguments, the divisiveness in their home diminished gradually. She ceased retreating to her room during times of tension. Discussion replaced confrontation. Gina's parents felt much less desperate in their attempts to convey their concerns and to control her social life. A new arrangement developed between the parents and their child, with each feeling more respected and validated. As Gina developed better communication skills and gained more control over her behavior, she ceased making unsophisticated stinging assaults on her parents and began to "float like a butterfly."

SPORTS METAPHORS TO FACILITATE HOPE

Floyd Patterson, the late former heavyweight boxing champion, told the story of a teacher who went out of her way to recognize his intelligence, and he credited that brief interaction as a turning point in his life. Patterson was in a school for troubled boys at the time. One day his teacher announced she would ask a question and the boy who gave the right answer would get a prize. When she asked her question, Floyd's hand went up, but another boy raised his hand at the same time. The teacher called on the second boy, who gave the correct answer. In a rage, Patterson stormed out of the room. When his teacher followed him out into the hallway, she found Patterson crouched on the floor with a tear rolling down his face. She knelt down, put her arm on his shoulder, and said, "Floyd, I knew you had the correct answer, so I have a prize for you also."

Probably the teacher never gave this exchange another thought, but Patterson credits her willingness to go out of her way to help him and validate him (she knew he had the correct answer) as a pivotal moment in his life. Patterson explained that his teacher had faith in him, believed in him, and made him want to try harder, and so he did. He became the heavyweight boxing champion of the world.

The first author of this chapter met Floyd Patterson in 1975 when Patterson came to a residential treatment center for troubled children after a fire destroyed the boys' dormitory and school building. Patterson offered to speak to the children after hearing that the boys had lost their possessions in the fire and were being housed in temporary quarters, sleeping on cots in a gym at another facility. Patterson gave them encouragement and hope that difficult times in life can be survived and can make the survivor stronger.

Not only did Patterson distinguish himself on a world stage as a boxer, but he displayed the kind of compassion his teacher showed to him in the school hallway, the moment that changed his life. Patterson fought to regain his heavyweight crown after losing it in the first of three matches with Ingemar Johannson of Sweden on June 20, 1960. Patterson was well prepared for the challenge, fought fiercely, and by the fifth round, Johansson lay unconscious on the canvas. Patterson, however, rather than be jubilant, was appalled at the damage he had done and "knelt on the canvas cradling Johansson's head in the crook of his arm and promised his still unconscious opponent a third rematch" (Garner & Costas, 1999, p. 20). Patterson also won the third fight by a knockout, but it was a fierce battle, with Patterson being knocked down twice in the first round. Later on, in 1982, Patterson and Johannson both ran in the New York City Marathon.

In the ring, there was no competitor fiercer than Floyd Patterson. The surprising expression of his gentler inner self makes us wonder if after the second fight, when in compassion he knelt down and cradled his opponent's head in his arms, and later when he came to a residential center after a devastating fire to offer hope and encouragement to a group of troubled boys, he was passing on the compassion shown by his teacher in that brief exchange that turned his life around. The teacher will probably never know, but Floyd Patterson's story is an object lesson on how a small act of kindness or compassion can make a huge difference in the life of another human being.

In addition to the message of hope that this story imparts, it also beautifully illustrates how giving to others elevates the spirit. Too often children feel they have nothing to offer, to give, or to contribute. Our sense of belonging is reinforced by contributing, whether to a team, to a friend, to a classmate, or someone who really needs a friend.

SPORTS METAPHORS TO FACILITATE
TERMINATION IN COUNSELING

One of the most poignant moments in sports history was Lou Gehrig's farewell speech at Yankee Stadium on July 4, 1939. After being diagnosed with the incurable disease that has since become known as Lou Gehrig's disease, he stepped to the microphone and told the overflowing crowd that he was "the luckiest man on the face of the earth." Manager Joe

McCarthy called Gehrig, known as the "Iron Horse" because he played in 2,130 consecutive games (a record that stood for over 50 years), "the finest example of a ballplayer, sportsman, and citizen that baseball has ever known" (Garner & Costas, 1999, p. 17). Babe Ruth was one of many former teammates on hand to give the courageous Gehrig a big hug. There probably were very few men or women in the crowd who were not tearful on that emotional, unforgettable day.

Parting is hard, particularly for those who have suffered more than their share of losses. The end of counseling may be another loss for some children, depending on the length of the therapeutic relationship and the meaning that the connection has for the child. Some children may be more than ready to end the counseling process and need little or no preparation, while others may need to be sensitively prepared for the termination. Lou Gehrig, over his 15-plus seasons with the Yankees, shared many positive and heartbreaking moments with his teammates. Since most counseling is brief and problem-focused, the degree of attachment will not usually rival the bonding or shared history that Lou Gehrig experienced with his teammates. We should not, however, trivialize the ending for children for whom the attachment has been significant and meaningful.

One of the important goals of therapeutic termination is to help children take ownership of the gains they have made in counseling. It would be a good time to review the child's home run tapes during the course of counseling. If children are unable to remember or identify any home run tapes, the counselor can remind them of their successes. The therapist can also write a letter to the child and give it to him at the last session, describing these home run tapes and other things the therapist regards as special about working with that child. This may help to further reinforce these gains.

Michael Jordan, in a TV interview before his final retirement from basketball, discussed how he had learned something different and valuable from each of the coaches he had during his career. He explained that he took a piece of what each had given him and made it his own, but each coach, in his own way, had contributed to Jordan's success. This brief lead-in can be a springboard for children to discuss what they have gained from counseling that they now own and can take with them as they move on with their lives.

Another way to accentuate and consolidate the gains the child has made is to talk about courageous comebacks. Many children will be surprised to learn that Michael Jordan was cut from his high school basketball team in Wilmington, North Carolina as a sophomore (Garner & Costas, 1999). In his junior year, however, Jordan made the team and began a career that arguably made him the most famous basketball player ever. There have been dramatic and amazing comebacks in sports history that can serve as a springboard to discuss the courageous comebacks the child has made during the course of the counseling process.

We want the child to leave counseling confident that their changes are credited to them and are not dependent on the continuing presence of the therapist. Sports metaphors provide a source of clarification for the child transitioning out of the counseling process.

SUMMARY

Because athletics play such a huge role in our culture and in the recreational life of children, sports metaphors tend to strike a responsive chord in youngsters receiving counseling. The goal of the sports metaphors illustrated in this chapter is not to optimize athletic performance (which is covered in the chapter by Jan Burte), but to create a bridge of communication that can penetrate to the heart of a child's emotional dilemma and possibly provide solutions to the child's struggles.

Metaphors may facilitate therapeutic engagement, form alliances, break down resistance, honor and highlight strengths, illuminate conflict and struggle, foster hope, and prepare the child for counseling termination. The use of sports metaphors or stories will not appeal to every child or teen in therapy or counseling, nor will they appeal to every therapist or counselor. However, the authors find that many younger clients resonate with the language of sports metaphors and stories. With guidance, many children can be helped to understand how the principles of sports can be effectively applied to resolving their own therapeutic issues. When the timing is right for therapists to take their shots on goal, the tools in this chapter may assist in reaching the net, often a well-defended net—the heart of a child or teen.

Exercise 16.1: Structured Therapeutic Activity: Everyday Heroes and Heroines

Purpose: The goal of "The Everyday Heroes and Heroines" is to honor courage and determination in the circle of people that make up the child's day-to-day life. This activity is one of the therapeutic techniques in the Heartfelt Feelings Coloring Card Strategies (HFCCS), which is designed to structure the therapeutic communication so that children can more easily communicate heartfelt feelings and address emotionally significant matters (Crenshaw, 2007). The HFCCS consists of 20 Expressive Cards and 20 Relational Cards and specific directives contained in the HFCCS Clinical Manual that are intended to explore deeply held feelings and the child's important relationships.

The cards are designed like greeting cards with the heart shape on the front of the card, and the inside panels of the cards contain directives that explore specific emotions and the relational world of the child. This activity, which uses the metaphor of sports heroes as a lead-in, reinforces the relational resources available to the child and celebrates the strengths within self as well.

BACKGROUND

An "Everyday Hero" was introduced as an evocative projective drawing and storytelling strategy in *Evocative Strategies in Child and Adolescent Psychotherapy* (Crenshaw, 2006). The following lead-in is offered to the child: "It would be nice if we all could play in the NFL and make the game-winning touchdown, or play in the NBA and hit the game-winning jump shot just at the buzzer, or play baseball in the major leagues and hit the walk-off home run in the bottom of the ninth inning" (2006, 181–182). "While we may never have the opportunity to be a sports hero or a brave firefighter or policeman who rescues a person or saves a life, we still may be heroes or heroines as a result of everyday acts of courage. Do you remember the first time you jumped off the high diving board? Do you remember when you were learning to ride a bike and you told your dad to let go and you were on your own? Do you remember standing up to a bully? These are everyday acts of courage and heroism.

"Now, please think about the people in your everyday life, including your parents, your family, including grandparents, aunts and uncles, cousins, your friends, your teachers, your coaches, and others in the community, and identify as many as you can who have been heroes or heroines for you. You can also include yourself because it is important to recognize your own heroic courage and determination. Think about something you've done that perhaps others didn't think you would be able to do, but you did—a time when you were heroic.

"Draw each of the people you can identify who in some way has shown courage and determination and is a hero or heroine in the heart on the front of the cards and then write on the inside of the card a note to each one or tell the story of why you picked each of these persons."

SYMBOL WORK WITH "EVERYDAY HEROES OR HEROINES"

The therapist can build on the HFCCS in honoring the courage and determination of the everyday heroes or heroines by asking the child to pick a symbol from an assortment of miniatures to represent each of the heroes and heroines (including the self) and place the symbols on top of the corresponding cards. Then the child can be asked to arrange the cards with the symbols on top in any configuration he or she chooses. The child can be asked about the chosen alignment or configuration of the cards/symbols as a way of expanding the therapeutic conversation.

The child can also be asked to make up a story about the group of heroes and heroines now represented not only by the cards but by symbols picked for each one by the child. Finally, the therapeutic dialogue can be extended by asking the child why he or she chose the particular symbol for each of the selected everyday heroes or heroines.

RESOURCES FOR THE CLINICIAN FOR THIS THERAPEUTIC ACTIVITY

Crenshaw, D. A. (2006). *Evocative strategies in child and adolescent psychotherapy.* Lanham, MD: Jason Aronson/Rowman & Littlefield Publishing.

Crenshaw, D. A. (2007). *The Heartfelt Feelings Coloring Card Strategies (HFCCS) Kit* can be obtained from the Coloring Card Company, LLC, 120 Main St., Flemington, NJ 08822. Tel. #: 908–237–2500; Fax #: 908–284–0405; e-mail@coloringcardcompany.com; Web site address: www.coloringcard company.com. The kit contains a Clinical Manual, 20 Expressive Cards, and 20 Relational Cards. Additional sets of the cards can be ordered from the Coloring Card Company.

REFERENCES

Allison, S., Stacey, K., Dadds, V., Roeger, L., Wood, A., & Martin, G. (2003). What the family brings: Gathering evidence for strengths-based work. *Journal of Family Therapy, 25,* 263–284.

Applelbaum, S. A. (2000). *Evocativeness: Moving and persuasive interventions in psychotherapy.* Northvale, NJ: Jason Aronson.

Clark, M. D. (1998) Strengths-based practice: The ABC's of working with adolescents who don't want to work with you. *Federal Probation, 62,* 46–53.

Corcoran, J. (2005). *Building strengths and skills: A collaborative approach to working with clients.* New York: Oxford University Press.

Crenshaw, D. A. (2004). *Engaging resistant children in therapy: Projective drawing and storytelling strategies.* Rhinebeck, NY: Rhinebeck Child and Family Center Publications.

Crenshaw, D. A. (2006). *Evocative strategies in child and adolescent psychotherapy.* Lanham, MD: Jason Aronson/Rowman & Littlefield Publishing.

Crenshaw, D. A. (2007). *The heartfelt coloring card therapy strategies.* Rhinebeck, NY: Rhinebeck Child and Family Center Publications.

Garner, J., & Costas, B. (1999). *And the crowd goes wild*. Naperville, IL: Sourcebooks, Inc.

Helton, L. R., & Smith, M. K. (2004). *Mental health practice with children and youth: A strengths and well-being model*. New York: The Haworth Press.

Horney, K. (1942). *Self-analysis*. New York: Norton.

Johnson, N. G. (2003). On treating adolescent girls: Focus on strengths and resiliency in psychotherapy. *Journal of Clinical Psychology, 59*, 1193–1203.

Kremer-Sadlik, T., & Kim, J. L. (2007). Lessons from sports: Children's socialization to values through family interaction during sports activities. *Discourse & Society, 18*(1), 35–52.

LeBel, J., Stromberg, N., Duckworth, K., Kerzner, J., Goldstein, R., Weeks, M., et al. (2004). Child and adolescent inpatient restraint reduction: A state initiative to promote strength-based care. *Journal of the American Academy of Child & Adolescent Psychiatry, 43*, 37–45.

Lietz, C. A. (2004). Resiliency based social learning: A strengths-based approach to residential treatment. *Residential Treatment for Children & Youth, 22*, 21–36.

Mills, J. C., & Crowley, R. J. (1986). *Therapeutic metaphors for children and the child within*. New York: Brunner/Mazel.

Nickerson, A. B., Salamone, F. J., Brooks, J. L., & Colby, S. A. (2004). Promising approaches to engaging families and building strengths in residential treatment. *Residential Treatment for Children & Youth, 22*, 1–18.

Pepi, C. L. (1997). Children without childhoods: A feminist intervention strategy utilizing systems theory and restorative justice in treating female adolescent offenders. *Women & Therapy, 20*, 85–101.

Querimit, D. S., & Conner, L. C. (2003). Empowerment psychotherapy with adolescent females of color. *Journal of Clinical Psychology, 59*, 1215–224.

Stine, J. J. (2005). The use of metaphors in the service of the therapeutic alliance and therapeutic communication. *Journal of the American Academy of Psychoanalysis and Dynamic Psychiatry, 33*, 531–545.

PART VII

Innovations in the Use of Popular Culture

CHAPTER 17

Using Pop Culture Characters in Clinical Training and Supervision

Alan M. Schwitzer, Kelly E. MacDonald,
and Pamela Dickinson

Effective treatment in today's mental health world depends on using a valid framework to assess and make sense of client needs (Hinkle, 1994; Seligman, 2004). Conceptual skills provide the clinician with a rationale for his or her work with clients. Further, with today's emphasis on brief counseling methods and eclectic psychotherapy models, efficient client evaluation, diagnosis, conceptualization, and treatment planning have become essential (Budman & Gurman, 1983; Mahalick, 1990; Neukrug, 2001). This chapter explains how to use "practice clients" drawn from pop culture—literature, popular fiction, television, movies, and virtual media—as a tool for professional training and clinical supervision to reduce practitioner discomfort, increase familiarity and comprehension, provide intermediate experiences for skill development, enhance confidence, avoid ethical problems of working within one's competencies, and cast a wide net for a diverse and challenging "caseload."

The chapter first reviews the importance of developing sound clinical thinking skills in order to function successfully in today's professional mental health world, and defines the role of clinical training and supervision in skill development. Next, the use of pop culture clients to assist trainees and supervisees to develop case conceptualization, diagnosis, and treatment planning skills is explained. Then, two case illustrations drawn from pop culture are provided. And finally, specific supervision and training strategies, clinical and ethical considerations, and methods for bringing pop culture clients alive, are discussed.

CLINICAL THINKING SKILLS: NATURAL HELPING VERSUS PROFESSIONAL COUNSELING AND PSYCHOTHERAPY

Individuals who choose a career as a mental health professional—including counselors, social workers, psychologists, and psychotherapists—very often describe themselves as "natural helpers" (Neukrug & Schwitzer, 2006, p. 5). They might enter the mental health field because earlier in life, in their families of origin, in their neighborhoods, and among their friends and peers, they commonly found themselves in the role of the good listener, intelligent analyzer, and effective problem solver when those around them encountered life's difficulties. However, the demands of professional mental health work and professional skills required that they go beyond the qualities needed by natural helpers. Natural helpers such as friends and relatives rely on intuition, familiarity, personal opinions, and natural inclinations as they spontaneously listen, support, analyze, encourage, push, and make hopeful suggestions. By comparison, professionals rely on purposeful skills and systematically attempt to guide the counseling relationship through a sequence of organized stages, intentionally aiming to achieve specific client outcome goals (Neukrug & Schwitzer, 2006).

To accomplish this shift from natural helper to counseling professional, a set of tools is needed with which to gain an understanding of the client's situation and needs, describe the person's functioning, identify goals for change, and determine the most effective interventions for achieving these goals. These clinical thinking skills are required competencies for today's mental health professionals (Seligman, 1996). Included are case conceptualization, diagnosis, and treatment planning.

Case conceptualization refers to the ability to observe and make sense of client behaviors, thoughts, feelings, and physiology (Neukrug & Schwitzer, 2006). Diagnosis refers to use of the *DSM-IV-TR* system to identify and describe the clinically significant patterns associated with clients' distress, impairment in functioning, or significantly increased risk of distress or impairment (American Psychiatric Association [APA], 2000). In turn, treatment planning refers to plotting out the counseling process to form a road map that can be followed to help achieve goals for change (Seligman, 1993, p. 288, 1996, p. 157). When employed by trained professionals, the treatment plan follows directly from the diagnosis and case conceptualization.

Feeling Overwhelmed

Learning to use these important clinical thinking skills can be overwhelming for beginning counselors and trainees (Neukrug & Schwitzer, 2006). The current *DSM-IV-TR* edition alone contains about 300 separate diagnoses, is nearly 900 pages, and weighs more than 4 pounds! Beginning clinicians often experience ambiguity and feel confused when they start the process of forming a reliable framework for conceptualizing, diagnosing, and treatment planning in response to each new client situation they encounter (Loganbill, Hardy, & Delworth, 1982; Martin, Slemon, Hiebert, Halberg, & Cummings, 1989). Over the years, students in training sites (Robbins & Zinni, 1988) as well as newly employed therapists (Glidewell & Livert, 1992) consistently have reported lacking confidence in their clinical thinking skills and abilities. In fact, Hays, McLeod, and Prosek (2007) recently found that even many experienced practitioners lacked sufficient diagnostic abilities. Further, professional debate about the dilemma of clinical assessment and treatment formulation still continues (Lopez et al., 2006).

Clinical Training and Supervision

To assist with the progression from natural helper to mental health professional, the use of clinical supervision is vital to counseling and psychotherapy practice. Supervision is an intensive, interpersonal relationship in which a more experienced, more advanced professional facilitates the development of therapeutic competence in another professional or developing professional (Loganbill et al., 1982). Furthermore, supervision is important across the professional life span. Students tend to rely on supervisors for intensive support and challenge, as well as extensive expert advice, as they begin the process of learning to be a practitioner. For students, supervisors often take the lead (and the liability) for assessment, case conceptualization, and treatment planning, and for implementation of the intervention process. Interns, residents for licensure, and others who are new to the field tend to rely on supervisors for moderate support, intensive challenge, and solid expert advice as they build on the foundations of their early training and clinical experiences. Likewise, even licensed and other experienced clinicians continue to rely on supervision for expert consultation, to add new approaches to their repertoire, for guidance with specialized populations, and to deal with personal dynamics when they interfere with one's professional work. Generally speaking, earlier in one's training, supervision focuses on basic skills and case content, while later in one's development, it focuses more on personal functioning in the professional role. Over the course of one's professional development, the responsibility for assessment, case conceptualization, and treatment planning gradually shifts from supervisor to supervisee (Loganbill et al., 1982; Neukrug & Schwitzer, 2006).

For the most part, experienced competent clinicians have learned to systematically apply abstract, general frameworks to the task of conceptualizing various client concerns, whereas novice and less well trained professionals tend to engage more extensively in repetitive, case-specific conceptual work for each new client situation; however, gaining more experience gradually equips emerging professionals with the cognitive skills needed for efficient, accurate clinical assessment and treatment planning (Martin et al., 1989; Schwitzer, 1996). Therefore, counseling and psychotherapy educators and clinical supervisors can benefit from teaching and training methods to enhance learning and professional development in this skill area. That's where pop culture "clients" come in.

USING POP CULTURE CLIENTS TO BUILD CLINICAL THINKING SKILLS

Clinical thinking is complex and can seem daunting. As with the proverbial route to Carnegie Hall, becoming equipped with good case conceptualization, diagnosis, and treatment planning skills requires "practice, practice, practice." The use of practice cases drawn from pop culture can assist novice clinicians and their supervisors. In fact, training programs such as those for psychiatric residencies and psychoanalysts traditionally have relied on "clients" drawn from popular cinema and other pop culture sources to illustrate case conceptualization (Greenberg, 1993). Using "cases" drawn from historical figures, literature and fiction, movies and television, fairy tales and cartoons, or Web-based and virtual sources has several specific training benefits (Neukrug & Schwitzer, 2006; Schwitzer, Boyce, Cody, Holman, & Stein, 2006).

First, popular characters provide an expanded, and a more diverse, caseload than typically might be available in real-life training sites and mental health workplaces. Pop characters provide an ample, easily accessible supply of clinical cases with which to practice conceptualizing client dynamics and needs, diagnosing apparent symptoms, and planning hypothetical treatment. Furthermore, even in settings with extensive real-life caseloads, pop clients can supplement everyday clinical practice with characters who are more diverse according to ethnicity, culture, geography, religious identity, sexual orientation, age, or developmental life phase—and who present a much wider range of presenting concerns and etiologies—than might be experienced otherwise.

Second, unlike real-life client cases, advanced skill at conducting intakes and facilitating clinical interviews is not required to obtain the information needed to begin case conceptualization. When working with real clients, the chance to work on case formulation skills is dependent on the clinician's existing skills at data collection (APA, 2000; Loganbill et al., 1982; Martin et al., 1989). Further, with real clientele, client information may become available only over the long haul of the counseling relationship; clients vary in their ability and willingness to share all of the information that might inform case formulation; and an agency's intake and recording procedures sometimes are added constraints. By comparison, when a practice client comes from a media source, all of the available information appears right away for immediate use.

Third, some ethical problems are avoided with pop clients. Most importantly, the ethical problem of working within the limits of one's existing competencies (American Counseling Association, 1995; American Psychological Association, 2003; National Association of Social Workers, 1999) is mitigated. With real clients, the main obligation is concern about the effects of one's clinical thinking products on the client's welfare. Supervisors often must closely monitor trainees' work and its application. With popular characters, the clinician has the room and flexibility to practice and strengthen these skills without concern about an actual impact on a client's actual well-being. In addition, the ethical problem of confidentiality is circumvented. Whereas ethical guidelines limit the extent and nature of client information that can be shared outside of the clinical and supervision relationships for training purposes, the "clinical data" pertaining to pop culture clientele can be openly and freely discussed or debated in case staffings, group supervision, classrooms, professional development workshops, and elsewhere.

All in all, popular culture clients offer an extensive, potentially diverse caseload, with all available data immediately presented, for whom ethical constraints are circumvented.

POP CULTURE CLIENT PRACTICE CASE METHOD

Schwitzer and colleagues (Neukrug & Schwitzer, 2006; Schwitzer et al., 2006) outlined the details of the pop-culture-client practice-case method. The method has been used in classroom teaching, supervision, and professional development workshops. When practicing with pop clients, a full practice case exercise can be completed, or a partial exercise (for example, trying out just a diagnosis or just a solution-focused treatment plan) can be used. As it has been previously described (Schwitzer et al., 2006), the full case method exercise requires developing all of the following elements for the character—that is, client-selected.

Introducing the Popular Character

The character selected as client is briefly introduced and described in everyday language, as compared with the clinical language and professional vocabulary to be used in all of the subsequent sections. The character is described as he or she fits in his or her media context, important pieces of the story line are given, and the stage is set for the clinical thinking to follow.

Basic Case Summary

The case summary comprises 5 short sections: (a) identifying information, (b) presenting concerns, (c) background, family information, and relevant history, (d) previous problem and counseling history, and (e) goal for counseling and course of therapy to date (LaBruzza & Mendenz-Villarrubia, 1994; Seligman, 1996). Because specific mental health settings vary so widely in their records, a generic basic case summary approach is used.

Case Conceptualization: Applying Theory to Practice

Case conceptualization is seen as a clinical thought process that is a bridge between theory and practice. Four steps are employed (Schwitzer, 1996; 1997). These steps are:

1. casting a wide net to identify client concerns
2. organizing concerns into logically or intuitively meaningful themes and groupings
3. making theoretical inferences about client concerns and client symptom themes
4. making narrowed theoretical inferences about deeper client difficulties

Multiaxial *DSM-IV-TR* Diagnosis

Tentative diagnostic impressions of client symptoms are provided.

Treatment Plan

A treatment plan is built based on the case summary, diagnostic impressions, and conceptualization. Either a solution-focused or a theory-driven treatment plan (or both) is developed. To gain experience employing one of the commonly available professional treatment planning reference books (Jongsma & Peterson, 2003), a solution-focused treatment can be formulated to address immediate presenting concerns. A solution-focused treatment plan directly addresses the symptoms recorded in Step 1, and/or the constellations of symptoms organized in Step 2, of the Case Conceptualization. To gain experience applying one or more theories of counseling and psychotherapy to a specific client situation, a theory-driven treatment plan can be designed. A theory-driven treatment plan addresses presenting concerns, etiological factors, and sustaining factors according to the assumptions of the clinical orientation that is applied. It targets the theoretical inferences shown in Step 3, and narrowed theoretical inferences shown in Step 4, of the Case Conceptualization. Both types of plans comprise goals for treatment, interventions to be employed, and outcomes (including measures of change).

TWO CASE ILLUSTRATIONS

Two case illustrations follow: Gollum of *The Lord of the Rings* (Jackson, et al., 2001; Tolkien, 1991) and E. Lynn Harris's John Basil Henderson (1998, 1999, 2001, 2003).

Case 1: Gollum

Introducing the Character

The central figures of *The Lord of the Rings* (Jackson, et al., 2001; Tolkien, 1991) fantasy story, hobbits, live in The Shire, a rural, preindustrial community in Middle Earth, where life revolves around planting and harvesting, weddings, children, parties, and good food and companionship. In this rather utopian society, few hobbits ever ventured far from home. Bilbo Baggins was the notable exception. Seventy-five years before the opening of *The Lord of the Rings*, Bilbo had a great adventure involving long-distance travel, great peril, and dragons. In his travels, Bilbo was nearly eaten by a loathsome creature named Gollum but won his freedom in a riddle contest, secretly taking a golden ring found in Gollum's lair as his prize. Many years later, Bilbo's nephew, Frodo, is summoned to a secret meeting where he learns that Bilbo's souvenir actually is a powerful talisman, thousands of years old, which grants its bearer power over all creatures. The ring's creator, Sauron, has finally located the Ring and intends to destroy all the inhabitants and places of Middle Earth to retrieve his lost weapon—unless Frodo can keep the Ring out of the enemy's control by throwing it into a far-away volcanic pit.

However, the Ring is tainted by an evil magic and therefore has an intoxicating effect that is irresistible to all creatures (although hobbits less than most), and anyone who sees, touches, or wears the Ring falls captive to its power. During the ensuing quest by Frodo and his allies to destroy the ring in the volcano, they encounter a malevolent presence stalking their footsteps: the creature, Gollum. Gollum has endured tortuous difficulties and now is pursuing his treasured Ring. In fact, Gollum once had been a pleasant creature much like a hobbit, named Sméagol; however, he had been compelled to murder to obtain the Ring, then had possessed it for 500 years, and had grown enslaved to its intoxicating power before finally losing it to Bilbo. Although elements of Sméagol begin to emerge within the being of Gollum as he assists Frodo's quest, it is unclear whether the power of the Ring has created a yearning in Gollum so deep that it will permanently consume him.

Gollum has been involuntarily admitted for a psychological evaluation after being detained for swimming in a forbidden pool, and on suspicion of spying, during the quest.

Basic Case Summary

Identifying Information. Sméagol is the given name of a male, hobbit-like client captured trespassing at a secure location. He also responds to the name "Gollum," an onomatopoetic reference to an unexplained choking or coughing sound he makes repeatedly when under stress. Historical records indicate the client is between 500 and 600 years of age. At the time of detainment, the client was working as a private travel guide for two hobbits.

Presenting Concern. Gollum has been involuntarily admitted for a psychological evaluation while awaiting questioning on charges of spying. The arresting Captain noted in his report that he was "alarmed by the creature's suspicious, skulking demeanor and an ill-favored look." The same notes describe Gollum's exaggerated and immature emotional display, anguishing shrieking, keening, and sobbing, upon being lightly restrained. Once the restraints were removed, the client curled into a fetal position, rocked, clutched his arms in a self-soothing manner, and began responding to condemnatory auditory hallucinations with alternating cries of self-criticism and self-defense.

Background, Family Information, and Relevant History. The client responded to questions about his background in a distant, hesitating manner, claiming he has neither family nor home. Additional information was obtained through interviews with Gollum's hobbit traveling associates. They reported that Gollum once was called Sméagol and was a member of a community of Stoors, one of three races of hobbits. It is reported that at some time in the distant past Gollum returned home bearing a magic Ring and wounds suggesting recent involvement in an altercation, just before his best friend was found murdered. The hobbits who were interviewed reported that Sméagol's fascination with the Ring increased until he began "acting strangely," shunning contact with his neighbors and acting increasingly suspicious, angry, and secretive, eventually resulting in his being ostracized from his community. Alone, he appears to have withdrawn into a private world where little but the Ring mattered. Over the past 500 years, the evil power of the Ring has led Sméagol to transform into the untrustworthy and dangerous creature called Gollum.

Problem and Counseling History. The client, Gollum, reports no previous counseling experience. The relative unavailability of mental health resources in Middle Earth also makes it unlikely the client has received any previous mental health treatment despite numerous indications of probable psychopathology.

Goals for Counseling and Course of Therapy to Date. Two information gathering sessions have been conducted with the client. At intake the client was uncomfortable with all social interaction, remaining agitated, fearful, and reluctantly communicative. Currently, Gollum remains unable to devote sustained attention to any topic other than the impending destruction of the Ring. He does not recognize the physical and psychological dependence he has developed for the power exerted by this object. Goals for treatment include: (a) establishment of a therapeutic relationship; (b) client acknowledgment of the dysfunctional nature of his behavior; (c) acceptance of his dependence on the Ring; (d) client agreement to enter a supervised treatment facility; (e) elimination of hallucinations and other psychotic features; (f) reduction of antisocial behaviors; and (g) establishment of a functional level of social interaction.

Case Conceptualization: Applying Theory to Practice

Step 1: Casting a Wide Net to Identify Client Concerns. Cognitive, affective, behavioral, and physiological symptoms and concerns include: lying, stealing, murderous behavior, obsession with obtaining and retaining the Ring, periods of rage, violent outbursts, paranoid beliefs, agitation, plural references to self ("we" instead of "I"), manipulation, verbal tics ("gollum" sound), social avoidance, auditory hallucinations, physical and psychological "craving" for Ring, gives up activities to use/ protect access to intoxicating effects of the Ring, malnutrition, physical deterioration, torture survivor, erratic sleep patterns, extreme distrust, flashbacks, extreme self-sufficiency, poor personal hygiene, intolerance of bright light, absence of empathy, lack of guilt or remorse.

Step 2: Organizing Concerns Into Logically or Intuitively Meaningful Themes and Groupings. The thoughts, affect, behaviors, and physiological symptoms observed were logically organized into four groups on the basis of shared phenomenology, that is, according to areas of dysfunction: *substance dependence* (drawn from obsession with substance acquisition, living in isolation to facilitate use, continued use despite physical deterioration, malnutrition, physical effects of unnatural lifespan, alteration of physical structure, continued Ring-seeking behavior despite known danger, agitation, sleep difficulties, and withdrawal symptoms), *antisocial behaviors* (drawn from violence, lying, stealing, rage, manipulation, lack of empathy, and feeling little shame or guilt), *thought disturbances* (drawn from auditory hallucinations and plural self-references), and *posttraumatic stress* (drawn from being a torture survivor, flashbacks, paranoid ideation, extreme fear, rage, violence, and vigilance).

Step 3. Making Theoretical Inferences About Client Concerns and Client Symptom Themes. The clinical orientation applied by the clinician to the client themes developed in Step 2 was addiction theory. It was determined that enthrallment with the Ring had an effect similar to intoxication. At first glimpse of the Ring, Gollum was compelled to possess it. Intoxication facilitated neglect of others, and resulted in the client's own suffering, yet he continued to wear the Ring. The client preferred to live in isolation and protect access to the Ring rather than relinquish it and pursue a normal life. Regarding his antisocial behaviors, he resorted to theft, violence, and murder to acquire the Ring for his own; lying began with a need to hide the methods used to acquire the Ring; and lack of empathy, guilt, or remorse reflect his powerlessness in the need to possess the Ring and are necessary conditions to maintain access to the Ring at all costs. The pursuit, capture, and torture he endured—which led to posttraumatic stress symptoms—were inflicted by enemies to whom he would not disclose the Ring's location, despite the obvious dangers to self. Rage, agitation, sleep difficulties, and violent outbursts may reflect withdrawal from the effects of the Ring. Hallucinations of a condemnatory "self" are echoed by Gollum's use of the plural self-reference and—according to addiction theory—may be explained by one or more of the following: substance intoxication; substance withdrawal; the strain of living in total isolation to enjoy the addictive pleasure of the object; the physical, emotional, and cognitive stress resulting from prolonged exposure to the Ring; or guilt and shame resulting from the murder of his friend.

Step 4: Making Narrowed Theoretical Inferences About Deeper Client Difficulties. Beginning with widely identifying client symptoms in Step 1, then organizing these symptoms into themes according to shared phenomenological areas of dysfunction in Step 2, and in Step 3, applying conceptual inferences drawn from addiction theory to these themes, the clinician inferred that: the Ring magically exerts a potentially addictive influence and explicitly induces dependence in its wearer; long-term contact with the Ring and the need to maintain access to the object of dependence produces antisocial and psychotic behaviors enhanced by dependence-related issues of guilt and shame; and the client's posttraumatic stress features could be attributed to previous torture and efforts to protect access to the substance. At Step 4, deeper or narrowed inferences were drawn, on which addiction theory-driven treatment might be planned: intoxication has subdued almost all other physical, emotional, and social needs; substance-seeking behaviors have taken precedence over almost all other activities; and consequences have offered little deterrence.

Tentative Diagnostic Impressions

Axis I.	304.90 Ring (other substance) dependence, with physiological dependence
	292.12 Ring (other substance) withdrawal, with hallucinations
	309.81 Rule out posttraumatic stress disorder
Axis II.	301.70 Antisocial personality disorder
Axis III.	Malnutrition, advanced age
Axis IV.	Extended social isolation, repeated incarcerations, fugitive lifestyle, torture
Axis V.	GAF = 25 (at intake)

Treatment Plan: Addiction Theory Treatment Plan

The clinician used addiction theory as a basis for building a theory-driven treatment plan. An addiction theory-based treatment plan was expected to address Gollum's concerns by targeting the theoretical inferences shown in Step 3, and narrowed theoretical inferences shown in Step 4, of the case conceptualization (see Table 17.1).

Case 2: John "Basil" Henderson

Introducing the Character

John "Basil" Henderson is the central character in a series of popular culture novels by author E. Lynn Harris. Included among these novels are *If This World Were Mine* (Harris, 1998), *Abide With Me* (Harris, 1999), *Any Way the Wind Blows* (Harris, 2001), and *A Love of My Own* (Harris, 2003). These daring examples of contemporary African American fiction have as their main story line the experience of male homosexuality and bisexuality—which ordinarily are taboo subjects in African American culture. In the novels, Harris's various characters pursue college experiences, engage in African American romantic relationships, and are affected by the presence of AIDS. However, one main effect of the books

Table 17.1 Gollum: Addiction Theory Treatment Plan

Goal	Objectives	Intervention	Outcome Measures (What Client Will Do)
Treat physical and psychological dependence on Ring.	Acknowledge dependence on power provided by Ring.	Have client describe life before finding the Ring.	Enumerate early pleasures of life.
		Discuss needs served by possession of the Ring.	Compare benefits to losses.
	Prepare for addictions treatment.	Discuss relationships and interests relinquished to indulge fascination with Ring.	State surrender of free will made to keep Ring.
Reduce or eliminate psychotic features.	Decrease perceived sources of threat.		Submit willingly to treatment.
Reduce antisocial behaviors.	Increase capacity for trust.	Discuss acceptance of these losses to retain possession of Ring.	Engage in fewer violent outbursts, and demonstrate reduction in hallucinations.
		Move from prison to residential treatment facility.	Reduce plural self-references by 10% per week.
		Refer for medical evaluation of psychotic and violent behavior.	Demonstrate decreased activation of flight or fight response.
		Begin speech-language therapy.	

Demonstrate readiness for reduction in level of supervision.	Accept responsibility for behavior. Increase independent functioning.	Practice evaluation skills. Strive toward acclimation to others in treatment facility. Establish Middle Earth chapter of Alcoholics Anonymous. Practice trust-related actions. Reward nonviolent interaction. Encourage group disclosure of dependence-related behaviors. Discuss sacrifices made to obtain, protect, or find Ring. Accept maintaining access to Ring as behavioral motivation. Explore history of antisocial behaviors, and identify behaviors that have endangered or ignored the rights of others.	Show less fear in small groups of residents or staff. Attend group sessions. Increased sustained eye contacts per session. Increase frequency of client-initiated social behaviors or verbalizations. Make disclosures without excessive anxiety, and increase participation within group. Discontinue previously maladaptive behaviors. Suggest life changes possible without Ring dependence. Decreased statements rejecting or diffusing responsibility for actions. List at least 3 actions that have negatively affected others.

(continued)

Table 17.1 Gollum: Addiction Theory Treatment Plan (*Continued*)

Goal	Objectives	Intervention	Outcome Measures (What Client Will Do)
		Confront client defenses such as denial, minimization, and rationalization.	Make necessary amends with offended individuals, and verbalize appropriate feelings of remorse.
		Discuss responsibility as willingness to admit wrongdoing, request forgiveness and make atonements for hurtful deeds.	Maintain perfect attendance.
		Promote increased responsibility at AA chapter.	Welcome and support newcomers.
		Describe methods of modeling positive habits.	Verbalize goals for Post-Ring Era.
		Prepare for destruction of Ring and acute withdrawal.	Pre-arrange for medical needs.
		Prepare for physical deterioration when Ring is unmade.	Appreciate benefit of new learning and social connections.
		Review and optimize support system to facilitate recovery.	

is to challenge readers to consider their own attitudes and behaviors regarding sexuality, especially homosexuality and bisexuality in the African American context.

Basil Henderson is portrayed as an intelligent, physically attractive, sophisticated, and sexually compelling young adult. Initial impressions are that Basil, who is wealthy and charming enough to successfully pursue the women of his choice, would be an ideal relationship partner—the perfect guy! However, readers soon learn that below the surface, Basil has misogynistic attitudes, has a history of sexual promiscuity with women and men, and brings with him a history of past sexual abuse. In fact, like many real-life clients, one result of Basil's past sexual abuse experiences is that today he is confused about his own sexual identity. As the story lines develop in the novels, E. Lynn Harris examines Basil's tenuous parent-child relationships, his past traumas and current confusion about these experiences, his hostile feelings toward women, his deeper sexual desires and fantasies, and defining love relationships with one important man and one important woman during his life.

Basic Case Summary

Identifying Information. John "Basil" Henderson is an African American male in his early to middle 30s. He works as a partner in a prestigious New York City sports agency, where he serves as an agent for professional athletes. He lives in an upper Manhattan penthouse, which has been described as lavish. Based on his appearance in the interview, he would be described as physically and socially attractive. He reports that his attractiveness and social skill are important aspects of his everyday life.

Presenting Concern. Basil came in for assistance following the recent ending of a romantic relationship. He reports that he unexpectedly ended his engagement to a "beautiful" theatrical actress on the morning they were to be wed. Basil reported coming to counseling to gain an understanding of his decision to end the relationship in spite of his strong love feelings for his former fiancée, and to address his significant guilt feelings.

Background, Family Information, and Relevant History. The client is a former professional football player who currently resides alone in New York City. He was raised in a single-family home by his biological father and reports he has never known his biological mother. Basil apparently grew up believing his mother to be a "terrible" person who deliberately abandoned his father and him. He has felt long-standing resentment toward his mother, and retains hostile ambivalent feelings toward women generally. Basil recently learned of a younger sister from his biological mother, and has established a relationship with his sister. Since establishing positive relationships with the sister and fiancée, he reports rethinking his negative beliefs about his mother and women generally. His mother now is deceased. A second traumatic aspect of Basil's childhood was being sexually abused in the form of penetration by his paternal uncle, who was a frequent visitor at the house. Basil reports despising his uncle and has developed anger toward his father for failing to protect him from the abusive uncle.

Basil characterizes both his mother's absence, and his childhood sexual victimization, as vividly traumatic; he attributes his current feelings of anger and confusion to these experiences. He admits a history of negative, hostile feelings toward girls and women, and reports frequently "using them for sex." He also admits a history of "despising" homosexual males; verbally abusing gay men in his environment; and feeling frustrated by his own attraction to men. He minimizes his sexual acts with men by suggesting, "It's only sex." He stated that he is not gay, and cited as evidence the attraction women commonly express for him.

The client's own thoughts and feelings about himself appear to be overridingly more important to him than the thoughts or feelings of others.

Problem and Counseling History. The client, Basil, sought professional counseling once previously, about 2 or 3 years ago, to address his traumatic childhood experiences and their impact on his adult sexuality. He ended counseling unsuccessfully.

In our initial session, Basil used vulgar language to describe his uncle as having stolen his manhood. He also described some of his thoughts and feelings about his mother and women generally. He explained that whenever his previous therapist suggested confronting his uncle or father about his abusive past (in the form of a written letter), he would become enraged. He eventually did send such a letter to his uncle; however, the uncle died prior to receiving it. Basil has not yet addressed the subject with his father.

Basil described ongoing difficulties resolving his feelings about his physical attraction to men. He reports being romantically rejected by a former male partner, which compounded his confusion and ambivalence about romantic attractions. He reported having difficulty discussing the topic, and said this, in part, led to the ending of his previous counseling relationship. He reported that his previous therapist suggested that Basil end his engagement to his fiancée until he clarified his own sexual identity, and when Basil refused, the therapist ended their counseling work.

Basil now is experiencing similar anger and confusion regarding his feelings toward men and women, and he reports that unresolved feelings regarding his childhood abuse also have resurfaced. He reported breaking off his engagement at the last moment out of fear of commitment in light of his identity confusion, and because as the wedding became closer he found his attraction to men resurfacing. He reports having not disclosed to his former fiancée either his past sexual experiences with men, or his childhood trauma. He reports currently feeling a combination of low mood, guilt, and also relief.

Goals for Counseling and Course of Therapy to Date. Basil has come in for an initial intake interview. During the session, he expressed depressed mood, anxiety, and frustration. He was open, able to verbalize his thoughts and feelings, and used profanity to underscore his points. Basil reports as his main goals the following: increase self-awareness; clarify and accept his sexual orientation; accept his past sexual abuse; and resolve feelings toward his mother. He reported wanting to make a commitment to ongoing psychotherapy to address these goals. Following the intake, Basil appeared more relaxed. At the end of the meeting he also expressed interest in writing a letter of apology and explanation to his former fiancée, and in confronting his father about the childhood abuse he experienced.

Case Conceptualization: Applying Theory to Practice

Step 1: Casting a Wide Net to Identify Client Concerns. Cognitive, affective, behavioral, and physiological symptoms were identified. Basil was experiencing problematic thoughts including: "I miss Yancy"; "My uncle took my manhood"; "I hate the way I feel about liking men"; "Something is wrong with me"; "I look too good to have to deal with this mess"; "I miss my mother; why did she leave me?"; "My Dad let my uncle hurt me"; "Why can't I be normal?"; "Most women are good only for sex"; and "Who am I?"

Problematic feelings included: anger, confusion, depressed mood, abandonment, guilt, selfishness, arrogance, loneliness, fearfulness, feelings of being abnormal, resentfulness, self-consciousness, and dissatisfaction.

Behaviors included: breaking off engagement; history of failure to make romantic commitments; sexual attraction to both men and women; avoidance of present-day interactions with biological father; inability to clarify his sexual orientation; inability to disclose with history of abuse or sexual confusion outside of the counseling relationship; verbally degrading gay men; excessive boasting and bragging (for example, about his wealth, his physical attractiveness, and his sexual prowess); history of sexual promiscuity; history of perceiving and utilizing women as objects for sex; relying on vulgar language; avoiding former lovers; and avoiding locations where he might interact with gay males.

Physiological symptoms included: increased irritability and diminished ability to concentrate.

Step 2: Organizing Concerns Into Logically or Intuitively Meaningful Themes and Groupings. The thoughts, affect, behaviors, and physiological symptoms observed were logically organized into four groups on the basis of shared phenomenology, that is, according to areas of dysfunction:

1. *Sexual abuse and identity confusion* (drawn from cognitive and affective symptoms in Step 1 pertaining to his childhood abuse history; and from his mixture of current thoughts, feelings, and sexual activities in Step 1 pertaining to his sexual identity questions)
2. *Relationship difficulties* (drawn from breaking off engagement, inability to make romantic commitments, long-standing problematic thoughts and feelings pertaining to abandonment by his mother and hostile feelings toward women generally, etc.)
3. *Deepened anger* (drawn from hostile objectification of women; dehumanizing hostility toward gay men; anger toward father, uncle, and mother; feelings of resentment and dissatisfaction; use of vulgar language, etc.)
4. *Narcissism* (drawn from excessive boasting about his positive qualities, excessive bragging about his sexual prowess, overemphasis on physical attractiveness, etc.)

Step 3. Making Theoretical Inferences About Client Concerns and Client Symptom Themes. The clinical orientation applied by the clinician to the client themes developed in Step 2 was cognitive-behavioral therapy. It was determined that his sexual abuse symptoms and identity confusion, relationships difficulties, anger, and narcissistic symptoms could be explained and, in turn, treated by identifying faulty thoughts and the problematic feelings and behaviors that resulted. For example, Basil appears to catastrophize: he perceives himself as irreparably harmed and inadequate due to his childhood trauma. Further, he maintains irrational thoughts: he blames his father for not protecting him. He believes his mother intentionally abandoned him and inflicted pain on him. He believes that had his mother been present, the abuse would not have occurred. Regarding dysfunctional behaviors, he avoids relationships and confrontations pertaining to the abuse; engages in faulty denigrating behaviors toward women and gay men; withdraws from commitment in intimate relationships; and inappropriately sexualizes relationships. Taken together, a set of faulty beliefs stemming from his earlier experiences appears to sustain his current symptom themes.

Step 4. Making Narrowed Theoretical Inferences About Deeper Client Difficulties. Beginning with widely identifying client symptoms in Step 1, then organizing these symptoms into themes according to shared phenomenological areas of dysfunction in Step 2, and in Step 3, applying constructs from cognitive-behavioral therapy, the clinician inferred that:

Basil's sexual identity concerns, sexual abuse concerns, hostile anger, and narcissism stem from catastrophizing, irrational thinking, cognitive distortions, and dysfunctional behaviors resulting from his earlier past experiences. At Step 4, a deeper inference was drawn that the client was experiencing deep, compound beliefs that were faulty. These faulty foundational beliefs were: something must be terribly wrong with him, his sexual desires and behaviors are unacceptable to him because society and his culture denigrate them, and there is a grave conflict between his external perfection and the dark secrets he holds and must not share. Starting with exhaustively listing symptoms, then forming themes, and next applying cognitive behavioral theoretical constructs to infer etiology and sustaining factors, a case conceptualization is formed on which cognitive behavioral treatment might be planned.

Tentative Diagnostic Impressions

Axis I.	309.81 Rule out posttraumatic stress disorder, chronic
	995.53 Sexual abuse of a child (focus of clinical attention is on the victim)
	302.90 Sexual disorder not otherwise specified
	V61.20 Parent-child relational problem
Axis II.	V.71.09 No diagnosis on Axis II
	Narcissistic personality traits
	Borderline personality traits
Axis III.	None
Axis IV.	Problems in primary support group: sexual abuse, neglect of a child, disruption of family by estrangement, death of family members
	Problems related to the social environment: loss of fiancée, loss of friends
Axis V.	GAF = 55 (at intake) GAF = 61 (highest past year)

Treatment Plan: Cognitive Behavioral Treatment Plan

The counselor used cognitive behavioral therapy as a basis for building a theory-driven treatment plan. A cognitive behavioral treatment plan was expected to address Basil's concerns by targeting the theoretical inferences shown in Step 3, and narrowed theoretical inferences shown in Step 4, of the case conceptualization (see Table 17.2).

APPLICATIONS AND LIMITATIONS

The cases of Gollum and Basil Henderson illustrate the use of pop culture characters as theoretical practice clients. Both showed the

Table 17.2 John Basil Henderson Cognitive Behavioral Treatment Plan

Problem Area	Long-Term Goals	Short-Term Outcomes (What Client Will Do)	Interventions
Sexual abuse: self-report of being sexually abused with clear, detailed memories; pervasive pattern of promiscuity and sexualization of relationships.	Work through issues related to being sexually abused with consequent understanding and control of feelings.	Tell the entire story of the abuse encountered. Demonstrate increased ability to talk openly about the abuse, reflecting increased acceptance.	Actively build level of trust in individual sessions with Basil necessary to help him increase his ability to identify and express his thoughts and feelings.
	Recognize and accept the sexual abuse history without sexualizing current relationships.	Decrease secrecy in his family by informing key nonabusive family members regarding abuse (e.g., father, fiancée, sister).	Encourage Basil to verbally express and clarify feeling associated with the abuse experienced.
	Begin process of moving from perception of self as victim of sexual abuse and toward perception of self as survivor of sexual abuse.	Verbalize the ways the sexual abuse has impacted his life.	Guide Basil in role-play in which he practices disclosing to key nonabusive family member about the abuse and its effects.
		Read assigned books to assist him in overcoming irrational shame caused by abuse.	Have Basil create a list of the ways the sexual abuse has impacted his life and process this with him in sessions.

Sexual identity: remains conflicted regarding sexual preference.	Identify and accept sexual orientation.	Assign sections of *Healing the Shame that Binds You* (Bradshaw), *Shame* (Kaufman), *Facing Shame* (Possum & Mason) and process key concepts in sessions.
Romantic relationship conflicts: broken off engagement; lack of communication and trust in romantic relationships; pattern of repeated conflictual and broken relationships due to faulty beliefs, avoidance, and sexualizing behaviors.	Develop new behaviors needed for effective, open communication in relationships. Increase accurate self-perceptions regarding own role in relationship conflicts.	Complete cognitive behavioral forgiveness exercises and process in sessions.
	Increase feelings of forgiveness for self, perpetrator (uncle), and other connected to abuse (father). Discuss all past sexual encounters, thoughts and feelings about sex, etc., to help make rational decision regarding his sexual orientation.	Help process these thoughts, feelings, and past sexual behaviors to increase self-awareness.
	Identify his sexual orientation in therapy. Prepare to identify his sexual orientation to someone close to him.	Encourage Basil to be open and honest regarding sexual orientation, confront irrational beliefs, offer support and positive reinforcement.
	Accurately identify causes for past and present conflicts in relationships. Identify a pattern of repeatedly forming destructive intimate relationships.	Offer suggestions for approaching the disclosure, address rational and irrational fears, offer support.

(*continued*)

335

Table 17.2 John Basil Henderson Cognitive Behavioral Treatment Plan (*Continued*)

Problem Area	Long-Term Goals	Short-Term Outcomes (What Client Will Do)	Interventions
Problematic affect: mild depression; deepened anger; abandonment feelings.	Develop healthy cognitive patterns and beliefs about himself and the world that lead to alleviation of mild depression symptoms.	Discuss level of closeness or distance desired in relationships and how this is related to irrational intimacy fears.	Assist Basil by having him keep journal of conflicts and process in sessions.
		Identify patterns of sexual behaviors, attitudes, and beliefs learned in family or origin.	Assist Basil in identifying his family of origin history to determine faulty assumptions and destructive behavioral patterns being adopted in current relationships.
		Verbally express an understanding of relationship between his depressed mood and his irrational beliefs, and repression of feelings such as hurt.	Assist Basil to explore fears and thoughts associated with becoming too close or feeling too vulnerable to hurt, rejection, or abandonment.
		Keep a daily record of all dysfunctional thinking, situations in which this occurs, behavioral and mood outcomes.	Assist Basil by completing genogram that identifies patterns of sexual behaviors, activities, beliefs among family members.
			Encourage Basil to share feelings of hurt, etc., regarding pain inflicted in childhood, and resulting in current thoughts and depressed mood.

Problem	Goals	Objectives	Interventions
Narcissism: arrogance and preoccupation with self when interacting with others; degradation of others while promoting self.	Decrease overall intensity and frequency of angry feelings and increase ability to recognize and appropriately express angry feelings when they occur.	Replace negative and self-defeating self-talk with verbalizations of realistic and positive self-cognitive messages.	Review and process record of dysfunctional thought in session, and confront irrational beliefs with rational alternative thoughts.
			Positively reinforce Basil when he uses positive self-talk.
	Alleviate control of abandonment feelings on present-day behaviors.	Identify targets and causes of anger.	Assign Basil to keep daily record of persons, situations, etc., that cause him anger, irritation, or disappointment.
	Develop ability to view self and others as being equally worthy of respect, care, or love; and engage in respectful, caring, or loving behaviors when interacting with others.	Identify pain and hurt from his past, and resulting thoughts and expectations that fuel current angry reactions.	Assist Basil to clarify his feelings and thoughts of hurt and anger that are tied to past traumas.
		Verbalize feelings of anger in a controlled, assertive way.	Process Basil's recent angry feelings and demonstrate more rational alternative behaviors.
		Identify thoughts, feelings, and beliefs regarding his mother leaving the home and how her absence has affected him.	Process these thoughts, feelings, and beliefs; offer validation and support; and confront Basil to move forward with present life.
		Recognize that his mother's absence was not his fault.	

(continued)

Table 17.2 John Basil Henderson Cognitive Behavioral Treatment Plan (*Continued*)

Problem Area	Long-Term Goals	Short-Term Outcomes (What Client Will Do)	Interventions
		Identify his negative beliefs and behaviors and their effects on others, while keeping all negative or degrading comments about others unspoken. Demonstrate increased empathy and increased use of respectful behaviors when interacting with others.	Help Basil to identify more rational alternative thoughts for the causes of his mother's leaving the family. Assist Basil in identifying and processing these beliefs and behaviors and their effects on others; confront beliefs and behaviors in sessions. Engage in role-plays that allow Basil to practice appropriate and caring interactions with others.

progression from introducing the clients using everyday descriptions of their story line and context, to clinical description in the form of a basic case write-up, and then on to formal clinical thinking in the form of diagnostic impressions, case conceptualization, and treatment planning. With just two such cases, issues of addiction, confinement against one's will, multicultural considerations, influences of family experiences including parental abandonment and childhood sexual abuse, sexual identity confusion, applications of addictions theory and cognitive behavioral treatment, and the specific question of gay and bisexual behavior in the African American community—"living on the down low"—all emerged. All of the information needed to assess these clients was immediately available in the books and movies from which they were taken. Ethical responsibilities were mitigated. For some clinicians, these clientele probably offered a broader, more diverse caseload than found in daily practice. Taken together, these two illustrations show the benefits of using pop culture clients in training, supervision, and professional development. (See Exercise 17.1 for a therapeutic exercise.)

There are several uses for the pop culture client training experience. First, it is an effective method for use in clinical supervision, case staffing exercises, workshops, and similar professional development formats. An individual student or clinician can prepare and present a case for consideration and feedback from peers and colleagues. Or, several individuals can prepare the same case for presentation—allowing greater opportunity to "expose differences in professional viewpoints and to uncover differences in . . . assumptions about the characters" (Schwitzer et al., 2006, p. 75). Differences in professional judgments about primary concerns, etiology and sustaining factors, diagnoses, treatment options, individual factors, and sociocultural influences might be processed. This can be especially useful in multidisciplinary professional settings. As a nuts-and-bolts exercise, students and beginning clinicians can use the exercise for the straightforward purpose of practicing the various clinical thinking skills—such as writing a treatment plan or deciding on a diagnosis. In addition to individual supervision and case staffings, the method works well in formal classrooms, too (Neukrug & Schwitzer, 2006; Toman & Rak, 2000).

The approach also has limits. The method is useful in supervision pairings and group settings when all the participants are equally familiar with the pop characters being used. However, differences in background, culture, or interests can sometimes limit the pop culture common ground shared by participants. For example, Schwitzer et al. (2006) described discovering belatedly that international students participating in practice sessions were unfamiliar with the American Disney cartoon characters being highlighted as clients. Similarly, not every supervisor and supervisee will be equally familiar with *The Lord of the Rings* and Gollum, or will have read the pulpy fiction where Basil Henderson resides. The method allows consideration of gender, ethnicity, socioeconomic status, sexual orientation, and other diverse characteristics experienced by clients. However, it must be noticed when pop culture illustrations reinforce, rather than illuminate, inappropriate characterizations or stereotypes. The movies, fiction and literature, television shows, cartoons, games, and other sources of pop clients must be carefully examined for the pitfalls in how they portray characters as well as for their strengths. For example, two topics for discussion might be the portrayal of Basil's histrionic-narcissism in the context of gay male stereotypes, and the portrayal of Gollum, who is dealing with a substance dependence disorder, as a shady person of suspect character. In another often-seen example, the common characterization of fairy-tale stepmothers as evil must be confronted when these popular culture media are used, especially given today's prevalence of blended families. Finally, although the interesting variety of pop characters inhabiting the pop cultural world make great practice clients, they are not a substitute for real-life supervised experiences with actual clients and their sometimes all-too-real concerns and dynamics.

Exercise 17.1: Exercise: Using Popular Culture In Clinical Supervision

First, select a character that interests you and might make a compelling client. The character might be drawn from a favorite current or old television show, a movie or art film, pulpy fiction or high-brow literature, drama, mainstream cartoons or anime, games, or elsewhere. The character might even be other than human!

Second, write a brief description of the character in everyday language. Include information about the character, his or her media context, the main story line, and anything needed to understand him or her.

Third, prepare a Basic Case Report. Include the following sections: (a) identifying information, (b) presenting concerns, (c) background, family information, and relevant history, (d) previous problem and counseling history, and (e) goal for counseling and course of therapy to date. This should be a chance to apply clinical language and professional vocabulary, in contrast to the everyday language employed in the brief character description.

Fourth, formulate a case conceptualization. Include the following steps: (a) casting a wide net to identify client concerns, (b) organizing concerns into logically or intuitively meaningful themes and groupings, (c) making theoretical inferences about client concerns and client symptom themes, and (d) making narrowed theoretical inferences about deeper client difficulties. The case conceptualization is a bridge between theory and practice. It provides the road map from clinical orientation to a plan of action.

Fifth, prepare a multiaxial *DSM-IV-TR* diagnosis to describe the client's symptoms.

Sixth, build a solution-focused treatment plan, and theory-driven treatment, or one of each. For each plan designed, include the following: goals for treatment; interventions to be employed; and measurable outcomes.

Finally, share your client formulation with colleagues, discuss with a supervisor, and continue to "Practice! Practice! Practice!"

REFERENCES

American Counseling Association. (1995). *Code of ethics and standards of practice for counselors.* Alexandria, VA: Author.

American Psychiatric Association. (2000). *Diagnostic and statistical manual of mental disorders* (4th ed., text rev.). Washington, DC: Author.

American Psychological Association. (2003). *Ethical principles of psychologists and code of conduct.* Washington, DC: Author.

Budman, S., & Gurman, A. (1983). *Theory and practice of brief therapy.* NY: Guilford Press.

Glidewell, J. C., & Livert, D. E. (1992). Confidence in the practice of clinical psychology. *Professional Psychology: Research and Practice, 23,* 362–368.

Greenberg, H. R. (1993). *Screen memories: Hollywood cinema on the psychoanalytic couch.* NY: Columbia University Press.

Harris, E. L. (1998). *If this world were mine: A novel.* New York: Random House.

Harris, E. L. (1999). *Abide by me.* New York: Random House.

Harris, E. L. (2001). *Any way the wind blows.* New York: Random House.

Harris, E. L. (2003). *A love of my own.* New York: Random House.

Hays, D. G., McLeod, A. L., & Prosek, E. A. (2007). *Diagnostic variance among counselors and counselor trainees.* Manuscript submitted for review for publication.

Hinkle, J. S. (1994). The *DSM-IV:* Prognosis and implications for mental health counselors. *Journal of Mental Health Counseling, 16,* 33–36.

Jackson, P. (Director), & Walsh, F., Boyens, P., Sinclair, S., & Jackson, P. (Screenplay). (2001). *The lord of the rings: The two towers* [Motion picture]. United States: New Line Productions.

Jongsma, A. E., Jr., & Peterson, L. M. (2003). *The complete adult psychotherapy treatment planner* (3rd ed.). New York: Wiley.

LaBruzza, A. L., & Mendez-Villarrubia, J. M. (1994). *Using DSM-IV: A clinician's guide to psychiatric diagnosis.* Northvale, NJ: Jason Aronson.

Loganbill, C., Hardy, E., & Delworth, U. (1982). Supervision: A conceptual model. *The Counseling Psychologist, 10,* 3–42.

Lopez, S. J., Edwards, L. M., Teramoto Pedrotti, J., Prosser, E. C., LaRue, S., Vehige Spalitto, S., & Ulven, J. C. (2006). Beyond the *DSM-IV:* Assumptions, alternatives, & alterations. *Journal of Counseling & Development, 84,* 259–268.

Mahalick, J. R. (1990). Systematic eclectic models. *The Counseling Psychologist, 18,* 655–679.

Martin, J., Slemon, A., Hiebert, B., Halberg, E., & Cummings, A. (1989). Conceptualizations of novice and experienced counselors. *Journal of Counseling Psychology, 36,* 395–400.

National Association of Social Workers. (1999). *Code of ethics of the National Association of Social Workers.* Washington, DC: Author.

Neukrug, E. S. (2001). *Skills and techniques for human service professionals: Counseling environment, helping skills, treatment issues.* Pacific Grove, CA: Brooks/Cole.

Neukrug, E. S., & Schwitzer, A. M. (2006). *Skills and tools for today's counselors and psychotherapists: From natural helping to professional counseling.* Belmont, CA: Thompson Brooks/Cole.

Robbins, S. B., & Zinni, V. R. (1988). Implementing a time-limited treatment model: Issues and solutions. *Professional Psychology: Research and Practice, 19,* 53–57.

Schwitzer, A. M. (1996). Using the inverted pyramid heuristic in counselor education and supervision. *Counselor Education and Supervision, 35,* 258–267.

Schwitzer, A. M. (1997). The inverted pyramid framework applying self-psychology constructs to conceptualizing college student psychotherapy. *Journal of College Student Psychotherapy, 11,* 29–48.

Schwitzer, A. M., Boyce, D., Cody, P., Holman, A., & Stein, J. (2006). Clinical supervision and professional development using clients from literature, popular fiction, and entertainment media. *Journal of Creativity in Mental Health, 1,* 57–80.

Seligman, L. (1993). Teaching treatment planning. *Counselor Education and Supervision, 33,* 287–297.

Seligman, L. (1996). *Diagnosis and treatment planning in counseling* (2nd ed.). NY: Plenum Press.

Seligman, L. (2004). *Diagnosis and treatment planning in counseling* (3rd ed.). New York: Plenum Press.

Tolkien, J. R. R. (1991). *The lord of the rings* (1-volume ed.). New York: Houghton Mifflin. (Original works published 1954–1955)

Toman, S. M., & Rak, C. F. (2000). The use of cinema in the counselor education curriculum: Strategies and outcomes. *Counselor Education and Supervision, 40,* 104–114.

CHAPTER 18

The Therapeutic Use of Popular Electronic Media With Today's Teenagers

Scott Riviere

Today's teenagers are more tech-savvy than ever before and life without technology and the new media is quickly becoming a fading memory. It is rare to walk through a shopping mall, coffee shop, or high school campus without seeing teenagers carrying some type of electronic device to help them stay connected to their world and each other. Whether it is with a cell phone, text messaging, instant messaging, or e-mail, today's teenagers are more electronically connected to their counterparts than ever before.

In this chapter, I am going to explore how teenagers use the various electronic media in both their everyday lives and in psychotherapy. I will discuss the advantages and disadvantages of communicating with e-mail, instant messaging, text messaging, software programs such as Microsoft PowerPoint™, as well as explore the use of photo editing and the Internet.

It is important to acknowledge that while much has been written about the dangers of the Internet and the disconnect that technology can create (Appleman, 2004; Criddle, 2006; Jantz & McMurray, 2000; Johnson, 2004; Willard, 2007), this chapter will focus on the constructive use of some of these technologies in helping teenagers overcome obstacles in their life and reconnect with each other in a powerful and positive way.

A TECHNOLOGICALLY LITERATE POPULATION

Look around at where adolescents hang out and what they do. They go to school, congregate at malls, coffee shops, and smoothie bars, visit friends' houses, and may even spend time at home. All the while, technology is impacting their lives. Computers, cell phones, text messages, MP3 players, digital cameras, and Internet access are all parts of this generation's norm. Computer applications and keyboarding are all part of most school curricula beginning as early as elementary school. Adolescents are familiar with most software programs including word processing and presentation programs. While Microsoft Word™ and Power Point™ might be the most well-known software programs, there are several others on the market that are familiar to many teens such as RoughDraft™, EasyOffice™, Astound™, Keynote™, and Writer™. It is not uncommon to walk into a shopping mall and find teenagers walking side by side, both of them talking on their cell phones—to other people. With the advent of MP3 players, teenagers download music from the Internet and are frequently seen exercising, walking from class to class, or even talking to others with earbud headsets dangling out of their ears. It is also common to see adolescents using their digital cameras or camera function on their cell phones and then immediately posting those images and videos to You Tube™ or on their MySpace™ account, so that others can see what's going on in their life. The proliferation of media and technology in the lives of adolescents can be traced to a number of influential factors.

Affordability

Technology seems to become less and less expensive as time goes on. Prepaid cell phones, free shareware programs, affordable digital cameras, free wireless access points, and inexpensive MP3 players are common in the marketplace. When cellular phones were initially marketed, they were housed in a 5-pound bag, had limited battery life, and offered prohibitively expensive limited-minutes plans. Internet plans started at $30 a month with limited usage, and wireless Internet technology was not yet invented. Two megapixel cameras cost hundreds of dollars, compared to current models that are five times as powerful and a fraction of the cost. Now, older teenagers can usually afford their own cell phones even if parents do not provide one, and it is easy to find free Internet access points at the local library. Free "shareware" software that mimics the functions of almost every major software brand on the market is available online, and the price of a one-gigabyte MP3 player is now under $30. With all of these options readily available, it is no wonder that technology is making its way into everyday life.

Easy Access

In most major American cities, free Internet access is available at fast food restaurants, public libraries, and sports arenas, to name a few. Most public and private schools have access to computers as well as online capabilities. If the teenager does not have access to his own cell phone, a willing peer is readily available to share. New vehicles are factory-equipped with MP3 players and external ports to plug in favorite tunes from one's iPod. Everywhere you go, access to these technological advances is becoming easier and easier.

Quick and Efficient Communication and Anonymity

America's fast pace naturally lends itself to technology. Text messages are quick and efficient kernels of information that can be quickly passed from one person to another. Cell phones with multiple-recipient speed dialing virtually guarantee that someone somewhere will be available when we need to talk. Additionally, and thanks to specialized calling and receiving options, excuses abound for screening and ending calls—for the conflict avoidant. With the advent of Caller ID, Caller Block, and Private Numbers, technology allows the individual to take a literal and psychological step back from face-to-face conversation and deal with others from an emotionally safer place, or one of complete anonymity. Clever, technologically sophisticated teens can and often do forge entirely new identities online and may completely misrepresent themselves to others.

Autonomy

Independent. Individual. iPod™, iPhone™. All of these resoundingly resonate with the letter "I." All shout autonomy (or perhaps narcissism) to the world. Today's generation of youth is frequently referred to as "Generation Me" due to its self-centered attitude. Adolescents have always searched for individuation and separation from parents and others, and technology plays a big part in the process. Anyone can have his own screen name, e-mail account, social network profile, and Web site without anyone else's permission! How is that for independence?

THE MORE THINGS CHANGE, THE MORE THEY REMAIN THE SAME

Despite the popularity, ubiquity, and availability of technology, the issues that challenge today's teenagers, and those that they confront, are in many ways similar to those faced by previous generations of teens. They still grapple with responsibility, connection, emotional regulation, identity formation, and autonomy. However, today's teenagers also face new and unforeseen developmental obstacles.

WHAT HAS NOT CHANGED

Above all else, teenagers are humans, and as such, invariably struggle. Today's teenagers still struggle in their quest to remain connected while moving toward independence. They seem surprisingly capable of bridging emotional and social divides with the assistance of their electronics. Today's teenagers still have to make decisions regarding sexuality, morals, values, responsible decision making, peer pressure, choices in their relationships, performance at school, and about the place in their lives for drugs and alcohol. Peer pressure is ever present and impacts on all of these important decisions. Apart from the inclusion of technology, today's teenagers still have to make these decisions on their own with the input of those around them. The following are aspects of the developmental processes of adolescence, and how teenagers have grappled with the changes that occur during this stage of life.

Cognitive Growth

Piaget (1952, 1954) theorized that the primary adolescent cognitive change was in their ability to think on a more abstract level. The formal operations stage of cognitive development enables most teenagers to engage in logical reasoning and abstract thinking. Countless teenagers ponder the meaning of life and anxiously await the sharing of what they perceive as deep insights with friends and family. This cognitive shift allows teenagers to develop insight into themselves and the world around, and leads to many exciting and sometimes painful discoveries. This is also an area that can lead to confusion. Teenagers struggle to reconcile black and white lessons of parents and teachers with the grays of reality, as they also attempt to consider multiple solutions to their problems.

Connection With Others

Another primary need in this stage of life is to have a relationship (Riviere, 2005). Regardless of whether this relationship is in the form of a friendship or an intimate connection, it still has the primary importance in an adolescent's life. It is easy to remember the joy that came from having a close network of friends and the pain that arose from rejection, isolation, and loneliness. Teenagers are perhaps the most vivid examples of this. How many people were you willing to cram in your parents' van to attend prom? The more, the merrier! Or the manic joy that came from a girlfriend who said yes to the question of "going with" you, only to be outdone by the deep depression that resulted when you broke up and vowed, "I will never go out with anyone else!"

Regulation of Emotions

Another characteristic of this stage is that an adolescent's emotional maturity tends to lag behind physical, sexual, and intellectual development. How many parent/teen arguments start with the parent saying "Stop yelling at me," only to hear the teenager scream back, "I'm not yelling!" Because this process takes several years to master, helping parents to be patient with the process can help alleviate many escalations. Riviere (2005) indicates that the evolution of communication in adolescence is enmeshed with intensity of emotion. Parents often complain that the roller coaster of emotions that is so typical of this developmental stage is one of their biggest struggles.

Creating a Meaningful Existence

Psychosocial development theory identified the key adolescent conflict as one between forming a cohesive identity and avoiding role confusion (Erikson, 1950). A successful resolution of this stage incorporates the acceptance of self, a positive attachment in relationships, and the belief that one has the ability to provide, give back to the world, and discover one's vocation in life. During this stage, emotional approval shifts toward peers. Parents frequently request counseling during this time because they feel as if their children are pulling away from them. Helping the adolescent maintain his or her identity within the context of the family is often a request of parents. Mental health professionals can frequently help families navigate through this transitional period so that the teenager can develop a sense of self and maintain his or her attachment to family.

WHAT HAS CHANGED

Adolescents still ponder the meaning of life, connect with others, strive to master their emotions, and seek to create a meaningful existence. The impact of technology on these processes is evident in virtually every setting. Technology is being used in the classroom, at home, in relationships, and on the go. Two technologies that have a major impact on the daily life of adolescents are the multifunction cell phone and the widespread access to the Internet (Goodstein, 2007). These advances play such a big role in everyday life for today's teenager, that to take away their cell phone or Internet access for 24 hours is likely to feel to them as if they have been placed in solitary confinement. Cell phones have proven to be a reliable, cost-efficient, and common way for humans to communicate with one another. Long gone are the days of having to wait until someone returned home to talk. Answering machines and pagers have been replaced by modern cell phones that are equipped with cameras, text messaging, voicemail, and Bluetooth™ technology for a truly hands-free experience. Adolescents often use the rationale that parents can get in touch with them "whenever you want" to justify mom and dad purchasing a cell phone. Regardless of the reason, cell phones and adolescents are becoming as synonymous as teenagers and risk taking. Adolescents have always enjoyed talking on the phone for hours. Thanks to unlimited-minutes pricing plans from most cellular providers, parents can rest easy as well. Text messaging and social networking sites are quickly becoming the preferred method of communication between adolescents. Texting is quick, easy, and efficient and comes in handy when talking on the phone may not be appropriate or feasible. Social networking sites typically include blogs and comment sections to communicate with multiple people at once. The downside of all of this is the increasing impatience if someone is not available when we want to talk!

The widespread access to the Internet also has a profound impact on this generation. For teenagers, the Internet is also a place where practical needs are met with increasing frequency (Kelsey, 2007). They connect with each other and learn more about each other via the use of surveys and questionnaires (see Exercise 18.5). Surveys and questionnaires can be found all over the Internet just by doing a simple search. These allow teenagers an opportunity to be asked questions that they may have never thought of asking themselves before. Often, these questions require adolescents to reflect insightfully, and also open their minds to possibilities that they may have never thought of before. Teenagers frequently search the Internet for sites of various personal interests. It is not uncommon for parents to complain how often their children stay on the computer just simply surfing (randomly exploring Web sites).

Today's teenagers also use the Internet to search for information regarding topics that they may not be comfortable discussing with anyone else. Many teens do not have people they feel comfortable confiding in regarding issues such as sexuality, drug use, abuse, neglect, and various other issues that they as teenagers face. The Internet can provide them an opportunity to access information where they can begin to explore options to overcome these obstacles.

Instant messaging and e-mail are today's equivalent to the handwritten note or letter that used to have to be delivered by mail. Free online access and wireless Internet connections are becoming more common at places where people hang out, especially teenagers. There are several methods for adolescents to communicate/connect with each other via the Internet. E-mail and instant messaging remain the most common, but message boards, open and private chat rooms, and blogs are becoming more popular (Richardson, 2006). These "virtual rooms" are online forums where they can talk with select groups of individuals with similar interests.

Another aspect of the Internet is the ability to join social networking sites such as MySpace™ and FaceBook™. These sites are quick and easy to set up and are free for anyone wanting to join. Most teenagers access these sites as a way of making new friends, as well as posting information on their daily life. Some adolescents are even tech savvy enough to create their own personal Web site, which they can design and use to express various ideas about their personality, their family, or any other things that are going on.

Blogs are another common technology to today's teenagers. A blog is an electronic journal through which an individual can chronicle the events of the day or give an opinion about any particular subject. Blogs can be charged with a high degree of emotional energy, and it is not uncommon to hear an adolescent rant and rave about the various injustices that have happened over the course of their day.

Adolescents are so familiar with technology that it's hard to imagine, from their point of view, a world that does not include Web sites, e-mails, instant messaging, chat rooms, log discussions, message boards, text messaging, and the up-and-coming video era of the Internet. These advances in technology require a new layer of *tools* and *information* for the modern therapist to utilize in assisting this population. These tools are designed to assist adolescents to work through the various obstacles and struggles that they may be experiencing in life, reconnect with family and friends, find their confidence in themselves, and move forward to a more productive and fulfilling life. As we proceed through the remainder of this chapter, we will reexamine the important adolescent developmental issues noted above, but focus on how modern teenagers use technology to navigate these challenges.

Self-Discovery

Today's teenagers use several electronic mediums to discover and explore the age-old question of "Who am I?" Most teenagers today own some type of Internet-based Web profile, whether that is a social networking site such as MySpace™, FaceBook™ or others, or their own personal Web page (Collier & Magid, 2006). Their sites or Web pages can be customized to their own personalities, as well as interests. Whether it be through customized music, graphics, and various other add-ons (frequently called "pimping"), or through posting photographs that have been edited by various software editing programs, or even answering surveys that they find online, today's teenagers are continuing to connect and explore the formation of their identity.

Cognitive Growth

The primary cognitive change that develops during adolescence is the ability to engage in logical reasoning and abstract thinking (Piaget, 1952, 1954). This can be seen very clearly in an adolescent's ability to answer the various surveys that they receive online. By answering open-ended questions, the teenager begins to leave the concrete thinking of the latency age years and begins to form values and beliefs that have been independent of things they may have been taught. All of these things are fascinating to teenagers and they frequently write of their experiences online through their Web blogs or online journals. In this context, there are several online survey sites that encourage adolescents to answer questionnaires or surveys that are designed to help them think on an abstract level, as well as aid in their own self-discovery and in self-exploration of their own values and beliefs. Xanga.com™ is a popular Web site frequented by teenagers that offers free personal blogs and questionnaires to users with a valid e-mail account (see Exercise 18.1).

Connection With Others

Adolescents yearn to belong to something and be somebody, and today's technology allows them to connect with teenagers literally from around the world who have similar interests, values, and ideas. Nowhere else do we see this more than in the increased popularity of social networking sites, where teenagers frequently communicate with each other in an attempt to connect and form friendships and relationships. Most social networking sites now incorporate a comment or blog section in which members of the community can write messages to each other. It is in this way that teenagers can stay connected with each other without having to engage in an immediate two-way conversation.

Another aspect of this stage is that teenagers seek fulfillment in a love relationship. Teenagers today use technology to connect socially and develop intimate relationships. Text messaging, e-mail, and instant messaging are all ways that teenagers open up lines of communication between them and people they are interested in going out with. Most social networking sites allow members to approve or deny another member's profile so that you can learn more about an individual without that individual having full access to your profile.

Regulation of Emotions

Although most communication between teens and their peers is known to be emotionally charged, it is also common for teens to vent their frustrations in cyberspace. Daily online journals are common tools where adolescents process their emotions and give and receive feedback from others. This cathartic process of venting and receiving consolation and/or challenges from others can help an adolescent learn to better manage and express emotions.

Creating a Meaningful Existence

Along with all of the positive feedback that one can receive from a supportive network of family and friends, technology can assist teenagers in learning more about their talents and gifts. It is easy to explore intellectual abilities via online intelligence tests, and online sites are available that can give the teenager some insight into possible personality traits that can be helpful or damaging in their relationships. Vocational and aptitude questionnaires are also available for the adolescent to explore. A simple Google™ search provides the needed access.

POTENTIAL EFFECTS OF TECHNOLOGY

Technology's greatest impact seems to be in the availability to teenagers of tools and resources for self-expression, connection, and self-understanding. However, the effect of these advances is becoming clearer as some of the dust settles. Suler (2004) identified one of these effects and coined the term *online disinhibition effect*. He reports that the use of online and electronic media has allowed today's teenagers to disconnect from each other in a real way in order to experiment with identity formation, explore various roles in life, and engage in relationship enhancement on a psychologically safe level. He identifies several elements that are a part of this disinhibition effect. These include *dissociative anonymity*, or in other words, "You don't know me." Adolescents can easily change their identity on the Internet, or claim a different age or a different city or state where they live, and they have the ability to work anonymously. The second element he coins is the *dissociative imagination*. This phenomenon occurs when an adolescent looks at his or her behavior as just a game or "playing" on the Internet. People can create an online persona that can be very different than their real-life personality. In this way, the teenager can explore with different ways of relating to other people. Another component of this online disinhibition effect is invisibility. Prior to video conferencing on the Internet, most communication between teenagers occurred through text. This allowed the teenager to be invisible to the other person regarding their physical appearance, tone of voice, facial expressions, and various other aspects that are so beneficial to communication. Asynchronicity, another component of the disinhibition effect, occurs when a teenager's communication with others is not in real time, as it is with a telephone call or face-to-face conversation. There are several times in which a message may be sent and not responded to for minutes, hours, or even days. Minimizing authority is the final component of this effect. Teenagers may lose the inhibition they have when talking with older people or authority figures. They may say things or act in a way that is much different than they would if they were in a face-to-face interaction. In any event, teenagers will test out various behaviors online that they may not otherwise feel comfortable expressing.

Taken in whole, this disinhibition effect can have both a positive and negative impact. On the positive side, teenagers frequently reach out to others, affirm people they barely know, and practice random acts of kindness and generosity. Adolescents will frequently communicate thoughts and feelings in an online forum that they might be too anxious or uncomfortable expressing in a face-to-face conversation—whether it be in their blogs, message board, or even through e-mail. They can also explore possible personality characteristics online that they don't feel comfortable expressing in a social setting. On the negative side, teenagers can verbally abuse and threaten others, access inappropriate content, and engage in illegal activity.

TEEN TECHNOLOGY TOOLS FOR THERAPISTS

How can today's mental health professional use technology in the counseling process? Start by not being afraid of or intimidated by technology. Several big cities and small towns offer free classes for learning the basics of today's technology. College campuses, professional workshops, and online learning are all available to anyone interested in learning more. This is truly an investment in the future, so begin by learning now. Fortunately, most of your teenage clients are more than ready and willing to help answer any particular questions you may have. A therapist can also develop his or her own site on the Internet. Web sites require an annual maintenance fee and registration of your Web site name. Register.com™ and GoDaddy.com™ are two of the sites that can be visited to find out if the name you select is available. MySpace™ and FaceBook™ are both free sites that can be joined in a matter of minutes simply by following the instructions on the screen.

E-mail is a faster convenient way of communicating with today's teenagers. It is recommended that mental health professionals develop a confidentiality clause to be included in every e-mail (Exercise 18.2). It is always a good idea to get parental consent for your clients to communicate via e-mail, Web site comments, and text messaging (Exercise 18.3). Most of the parents I have worked with are comfortable with this situation, as they realize today's teenagers are becoming more and more technologically savvy. Therapists can develop and even send their own electronic questionnaires to teenagers. Sometimes, teenagers are more comfortable opening up over the Internet than they may be in your standard office setting. Therapists frequently are able to use technology to help parents and teenagers communicate. Using music, lyrics. and songs that accurately communicate their feelings can be a powerful tool in helping adolescents to express themselves. Encouraging parents to communicate with their teens through e-mails or even text messages can also be beneficial. You may consider adding wireless Internet access in your lobby or incorporating a computer software program in your sessions. Purchasing a stereo that plays MP3 or WMA formatted music and includes an external jack for the personal MP3 players can also be beneficial. Teenagers frequently bring in a song that describes them best and music can easily be incorporated into the therapy process.

The bottom line is that technology is already incorporated into the life of today's teenager, and along with all the bad that we hear about on a frequent basis, technology can also have a positive impact in the therapeutic relationship. Technology is not meant to take the place of the emotional connection that exists between two individuals, yet it can supplement the many ways in which we communicate and reach out to one another. The following case studies are examples of technology and the positive impact it has on the therapeutic process with three different clients.

CASE STUDIES

Jenny

Thirteen-year-old Jenny was referred for individual counseling due to panic attacks and recent discharge from a residential treatment center. During the initial assessment period, she was disengaged and would answer questions with the customary shoulder shrug or one-word answer.

She had seen several other therapists in the past and had a high level of distrust in the counseling process. She was a child of a divorce who was being raised by a single mother who had limited time due to employment obligations. She was frequently left to tend to herself and was quite independent and cautious of developing an attachment to others. She indicated a history of sexual experimentation, drug and alcohol use, overtly defiant behavior, and poor social skills. Jenny was very knowledgeable about technology and arrived to sessions frequently listening to her MP3 player or talking on her cell phone. She was also quite talented with digital photography and photo editing software.

Several sessions went by before she began to open up. On one occasion, I had my laptop computer under my chair and she asked if she could check her MySpace™ account for messages. I gave consent and she quickly booted up the computer and went online to check her account. At one point, she inquired, "Don't you have your own MySpace™ page?", to which I quickly replied, "No." She then proceeded to set up an account for me in less than a few minutes. She set herself up as one of my first MySpace™ "friends" and would frequently send e-mails and comments regarding how her day was going or simply to complain about punishments she had been given. This was a tremendous help to the counseling process because it enabled me to be aware of the day-to-day struggles that Jenny was having. She would also use her digital camera and photo editing software to enhance and post pictures onto her site that would help her to explore her identity and influence others' perceptions. We would frequently look at the pictures that she had posted on her site and process her thoughts and emotions regarding her self-image. Jenny was able to acknowledge parts of her physical appearance that she found unattractive by examining the angle of the camera as she took self-portraits. We would also process what possible perceptions or assumptions others would make when looking on her site. Over the course of our work, Jenny developed several insights regarding her life and role within the family. Technology continued to be an ongoing part of our sessions together, and in looking back, it has been gratifying to see the many changes that have occurred since our first meeting.

Emily

Fifteen-year-old Emily was referred to counseling for oppositional behavior at school and home. Her family history was positive for addictions, bipolar disorder, and anxiety disorders. Emily was a willing participant in treatment and had actually asked her parents for counseling in order to help with her mood swings and to more effectively cope with problems at home and at school. She was an honor roll student and was involved in school activities and community organizations. The family had previously received drug and alcohol treatment for an older sibling who had relapsed several times and the parents were somewhat resistant to the counseling process based on previous experiences.

Technology was incorporated into our first session when Emily asked if she could answer a cell phone call! She was quick to engage, but the conversations were superficial and avoidant. She would frequently indicate, "It's hard for me to talk about personal stuff." When asked if she talked to anyone about her problems, she indicated that she often wrote in her Xanga™ account and got feedback and support from her network of online friends. She allowed me access to her sites and indicated that it was the best way to keep in touch with how she was doing on a daily basis. She would frequently send questionnaires that she had answered about herself. These questionnaires offered me invaluable insights into how she perceived her life and also opened up doors to topics that I would have never been aware of. During the course of treatment, a friend of Emily's died in a tragic car accident. She was able to write several comments to her deceased friend's MySpace™ account in order to help her gain closure on this event. It was at this time that I realized how beneficial these sites could also become for a family that is suffering from grief. I have included a copy of the comments that were posted in just one day. (See Exercise 18.4.)

It was comforting to know that teenagers from around the world empathized with Emily's loss and were able to offer support and love to her family. Unfortunately, shortly after this experience, the family discontinued counseling and I was disappointed that neither I nor she had the opportunity to gain closure on the therapeutic process at the time. However, approximately 2 months later, I received an e-mail comment from her Xanga™ account and we both had the opportunity to process what she had gained from the counseling process as well as what she would have wanted to be different. It also gave me the opportunity to say good-bye and honor all of the progress that she had made. This particular teenager still sends an occasional update when we are both online!

John

Fifteen-year-old John was referred for counseling due to poor performance in school and oppositional behavior at home. This teenager indicated that he had been depressed for the last few years of his life and thought that the root of his depression stemmed from the abandonment by his father. His parents had never been married; his father traveled frequently and was currently living in another country. John had very little contact with his biological father over the course of his life and had never confronted the situation. His mother married his father when he was 5 years old and no major behavioral or academic problems were reported during his latency years.

After approximately 2 months of individual counseling, John decided to confront his father about being abandoned. We spent two sessions exploring options for confronting his father, which included inviting him to a counseling session, contacting him over the telephone, creating a video, or writing him a letter. He came up with the idea of creating a Power Point™ presentation that he could e-mail to his father. He had been learning about the program at his high school and felt capable of creating a presentation that could accurately communicate the multiple effects of his father's choices on his life. We spent approximately two sessions deciding what he wanted to communicate to his father. He used his knowledge of the software program to develop a slide show that included text, music, and pictures.

Upon completion of this project, we developed a list of desirable outcomes that could result from sending the file to his father. John decided that he would not expect a return e-mail from his father and would send the file on two separate sessions to ensure that it was received. At our next session, we e-mailed the file and spent the remainder of the session processing his emotions around the experience. He reported feeling proud of confronting this issue in his life and remarked, "It was a lot easier than I expected. I still can't believe I sent him a PowerPoint™!" We sent the e-mail attachment again on the next session because he had not yet had a response from his father. I made the request that he send his father a short e-mail along with the file outlining what he wanted and what decisions he would make if his message was not responded to. Here is the text portion from John's e-mail:

Dad,
    I am not surprised that you have not written me back. As I stated in the PowerPoint™, you have let me down more times that I can count. I have blamed myself for you not being a part of my life but that will stop today. A simple "I'm sorry" would have been good enough but I don't think I really need that anymore. I am not sure what the future holds but I am letting go of stressing out about you being a part of my life. I will appreciate my step dad more and be glad that he is willing to raise me as his own. I will not be contacting you after this email and will leave the ball in your court to make the effort. After I turn 18, I will make an attempt again but if you do not make an effort to be part of my life I cannot say that I will be willing to let you back in. I wished things would have been different but we don't always get what we want, right? Anyway, hope to hear from you.
                                                                    Your son.

We spent the remainder of the session exploring the content of his e-mail and John indicated that it felt like he was saying good-bye at a funeral. We met only a few more times after this session and both client and family saw a tremendous change in his attitude, emotions, and behavior. We were fortunate enough to complete a closing celebration with John and his family to acknowledge all of the hard work that he had completed and to affirm what a great person he truly was becoming. I can't say how much technology impacted the outcome of the case, but John found the confidence to confront his father in his ability to create an accurate and meaningful message through computer software. Since this session, I now include it as a standard option for confronting people or issues in an adolescent's life.

Postscript to John

Another option that I have recently discovered is the Web site www.post secret.com. Every Sunday, this site displays selected postcards that have been received on the Web site. Others are compiled and used to create books that can be purchased at most major bookstore chains. The postcards tend to be very raw, creative, provocative, genuine, and even sometimes humorous. Although some of the cards may contain content that some may find objectionable, I have found it to be a very healing experience for clients to discover that they are not the only person struggling with a particular issue. The therapist can also help the client create a postcard detailing the effects of an event on his life and mail it to Post Secret.com. This Web site was created to assist individuals in self-disclosure of secrets that have been either destructive to or productive in their life. The act of confronting a past memory can be a very healing experience for some teenagers, as is seeing that others share similar struggles.

CONCLUSION

All things considered, it is difficult to argue that technology is not impacting the way in which humans relate to each other. Because mental health professions tend to deal directly with people on a daily basis, we are in a prime position to gauge the changes that are happening in the everyday lives of the people we help. There may be times where we are challenged by our adolescent clients to expand our definitions of *relationship* and *communication* and to go beyond traditional weekly verbal interchanges that are the hallmark of face-to-face counseling and psychotherapy. Whether good or bad, technology is a part of the contemporary adolescent experience, and while intimidating for some of us not-so-tech-savvy clinicians, it can also be quite exciting. In spite of the many wonderful uses to which I have put technology in my clinical work, I am still a bit of a traditionalist in believing that face-to-face contact will always be the core of the human (and clinical) experience. There is a basic truth in the following sentiment recently shared by a teen: "I don't care about all of this technology crap. When you're hurting, nothing can replace a good face-to-face talk with a friend."

Exercise 18.1: Questionnaire From www.xanga.com

What would you do if . . .

I smelt like raw fish?
Everyday I took a walk to the moon?
I had AIDS?
I never told any of you guys what I was feeling?
I never spoke?
I didn't have a little brother to obsess over and I found something else but really weird to obsess about?
Everyday I took horsepills to hopefully someday maybe transform into a hedgehog?
I wasn't wasting my time online making this questionnaire?
I wasn't a liberal?
I didn't like donuts?
I obsessed over creepers while the whole time I didn't even know what a creeper was?
I had an incurable disease?
I had a curable disease?
I called you a slob?
I smoked cigarettes?
I told you I abused animals and killed babies in my spare time?
I finally had the courage and soulless heart to tell a dead baby joke?
I didn't make this damn questionnaire so long?

Exercise 18.2: Sample E-mail Confidentiality Clause

Confidentiality Notice: This message, including any attachments, is for the sole use of the intended recipient(s) and may contain confidential and privileged information. Any unauthorized review, use, disclosure, or distribution is strictly prohibited. If you are not the intended recipient, please contact the sender by reply e-mail and destroy all copies of the original message.

Exercise 18.3: Sample Parental Electronic Communication Confidentiality Release

Therapist Name
Electronic Consent Form
Address
City, State, Zip
Phone

RELEASE OF INFORMATION

RE:_____

I hereby authorize *Therapist Name* to communicate via electronic methods (cell phone, text messages, e-mail, Web-based comments, blogs, and attachments, etc.).

TO _____

For the specific purpose listed: Continuity of care
This consent shall be valid for 1 year.

I understand the legal issue of informed consent. I understand the nature of the contents to be released, the need for the information, and that there are statutes and regulations protecting the confidentiality of authorized information. I hereby acknowledge that this consent is truly voluntary and is valid until such request is fulfilled. I further acknowledge that I may revoke this consent in writing at any time except to the extent that action based on this consent has been taken.

_____   _____
Patient Signature   Signature of Witness

_____   _____
Date   Date

_____
Legal Guardian in case of Minor

Exercise 18.4: Sample Comments From www.myspace.com. All Identifying Data Removed

May XX, 200X 11:43P

I'm just so tired
Won't you sing me to sleep

And fly through my dreams
So I can hitch a ride with you tonight
And get away from this place
Have a new name and face
I just ain't the same without you in my life
Late night drives, all alone in my car
I can't help but start
Singing lines from all our favorite songs
And melodies in the air
Singin' life just ain't fair
Sometimes I still just can't believe you're gone
And I'm sure the view from heaven
Beats the hell out of mine here
And if we all believe in heaven,
Maybe we'll make it through one more year
Down here
Feel your fire,
When it's cold in my heart
And things sorta start
Remindin' me of my last night with you
I only need one more day
Just one more chance to say
I wish that I had gone up with you too
And I'm sure the view from heaven
Beats the hell out of mine here
And if we all believe in heaven
Maybe we'll make it through one more year
Down here
You won't be comin' back
And I didn't get to say goodbye
I really wish I got to say goodbye

xxxx

May XX, 200X 11:07P

hey baby girl.
i know i know i left you a comment already.
but hunni i miss you.
it still hasn't really hit me.
but we will meet again sweetheart.
and look how much you are going to be missed. i am praying for your
   family.

i know you are in a better place now, so watch over your friends and
family baby girl.

i miss our crazii lil times when i first startes going to la. lol=)

you came out in the bug with us.

and when i went pick you, xxxxxx and xxxx up it was 8 of us in my
lil car.

i miss you girl.

but i'm sure you will meet my cousin kevin and if you do please tell
him i love him and i miss him.

we will meet again someday sweetheart.

i love you!

love alwayss,

XXXXXX

May XX, 200X 10:25P

—hey ariel.

—how are you?

—when i saw you in that casket today, it was so unreal.

—like it wasn't suppose to happen this way.

—it was un-exspected.

—& so hard to live with and accept.

—but i should be happy for you.

—your in a wonderful place now.

—your watching over me.

—i know it.

—i'll see you some day again.

—by the way, i have your boots.

—lol.

—ily.

May XX, 200X 8:41P

hey ariel me and you never really talked alot but ima still miss
you. . . . . at least ur in a better place now. . . .ily. . . . . .

May XX, 200X 7:13P

Ariel,

I love you so much, and I am gonna miss you alot. It seems so hard to
believe that you're gone. I remember when you came to my birthday
party in sixth grade, and gave me that gag gift. I still have them. I love
and miss you, and I always will.

Love you,

XXXXXX

May XX, 200X 5:38P

ARiiEL,
gosh girl . . . it seems just the other day you came to my house for
the first time to swim with xxxx && them. i had soo much fun that
day. your a great girl && its not fair you didnt get the chance to
show the world that. at least your in a btter place right now. i know
your watching over all of us right now. i love you && i will miss you
greatly. you will always be in my thoughts . . . ill never forget you
PiP
XXXXXX

May XX, 200X 2:21P

Just a few weeks ago we were haggin out and chillin, its very hard for
me to belive you are gone . . . rest in peace ariel, watch over us
XXXX

May XX, 200X 10:32A

hey my little angel,
i know i done left you a comment,
but you know me.. :)
today will probably be the hardest
day on me & all of us.. its so hard
to see you gone. it still doesnt seem
realistic. i think when it starts to
hit me, it'll hit me hard.. i can't
wait to see you again one day.
i just CAN'T! i miss you so much
already. i wish i could've at least
said 'i love you' before the wreck
but God has his reasons for why this
happened.. your family will always be
in my prayers.. in fact, i went to
maw's yesterday, and practically
almost bawled in tears to see everyone
& all i can think about was how me and
you always went there to eat, and when
we ate, WE ATE! and how that one time
me, you, silver, & a few others stayed
up the whole night and when the sun
came out, we hurried and ran our white
butts down the road to see the sun.

but now you have a better view than
any of us! brat! :P i love you!
love always + forever,
XXXX

Exercise 18.5: Developing a Questionnaire

Most adolescents are familiar with online questionnaires and are read-ily available to respond with insightful answers. Questionnaires are easy to design and often consist of open-ended questions on a variety of topics. Start by typing up to 20 questions that you would be interested in knowing the answers to. Questions could be concerning family, perceptions of self, friendships, dating, drug/alcohol use, future plans or dreams, or opinions on current events. Questions can be phrased in order to elicit a "yes" or "no" answer, then followed up with a "why?" Once the questionnaire is developed, copy and paste the questionnaire into an e-mail and send it to the adolescent. If you know their social networking site screen name and have access to their account, you can also paste the questionnaire to their site either as an e-mail or comment. It is common for the adolescent to an-swer the questionnaire and then send it back with the expectation that you will answer the questions and forward the responses back to him or her.

The following are questions that I frequently use in questionnaires.

1. How honest of a person are you? Rate 1 to 10 (10 being most honest)
2. What do you do for fun?
3. What event of your childhood had the most positive impact on your life?
4. What event of your childhood had the most negative impact on your life?
5. How attractive do you think you are? Rate 1 to 10 (10 being most attractive)
6. If you had one hour to live, what would you do?
7. If you had a magic wand what would you change?
8. Have you ever broken any laws?
9. Which member of your family is the most caring?
10. Which member of your family is the most selfish?
11. How have you changed in the past year?
12. How have you remained the same?
13. When do you pretend to be someone you are not?
14. How would your friends describe you?
15. How would your family describe you?
16. If you could do something over, what would you choose?

17. Have you ever been drunk or high?
18. Where do you want to be in 5 years?
19. Complete the sentence. Something I really need is.
20. If you won a million dollars, what would you do with it?

REFERENCES

Appleman, D. (2004). *Always use protection: A teen's guide to safe computing.* Berkeley, CA: Apress.

Collier, A., & Magid, L. (2006). *MySpace unraveled: A parent's guide to teen social networking.* Berkeley, CA: Peachpit Press.

Criddle, L. (2006). *Look both ways: Help protect your family on the Internet.* Washington: Microsoft Press.

Erikson, E. H. (1950). *Childhood and society.* New York: Norton.

Goodstein, A. (2007). *Totally wired: What teens and tweens are really doing online.* New York: St. Martin's Griffin.

Jantz, G., & McMurray, A. (2000). *Hidden dangers of the Internet: Using it without abusing it.* Colorado Springs, CO: Harold Shaw.

Johnson, S. (2004). *Keep your kids safe on the Internet.* New York: McGraw-Hill.

Kelsey, C. (2007). *Generation MySpace: Helping your teen survive online adolescence.* New York: Marlowe & Company.

Piaget, J. (1952). *The origins of intelligence in children.* New York: Norton.

Piaget, J. (1954). *The construction of reality in the child.* New York: Basic Books.

Richardson, W. (2006). *Blogs, wikis, podcasts, and other powerful web tools for classrooms.* Thousand Oaks, CA: Corwin Press.

Riviere, S. (2005). Play therapy techniques to engage adolescents. In L. Gallo-Lopez & C. E. Schaefer (Eds.), *Play therapy with adolescents* (pp. 121–158). Lanham, MD: Jason Aronson.

Suler, J. (2004). The online disinhibition effect. *CyberPsychology and Behavior, 7,* 321–326.

Willard, N. (2007). *Cyber-Safe kids, cyber-savvy teens: Helping young people learn to use the Internet safely and responsibly.* San Francisco: Jossey-Bass.

Index

SPRINGER PUBLISHING COMPANY

Using Superheroes in Counseling and Play Therapy

Lawrence C. Rubin, PhD, LMHC, RPT-S, Editor

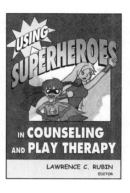

"There is something democratic about a therapy that can respond empathically to the experiences that patients enjoy and feel that they understand emotionally."
—From the Foreword by **John Shelton Lawrence,** PhD
Morningside College, Emeritus

With an incisive historical foreword by John Shelton Lawrence and insight from contributors such as Michael Brody, Patty Scanlon, and Roger Kaufman, Lawrence Rubin takes us on a dynamic tour of the benefits of using these icons of popular culture and fantasy in counseling and play therapy. Not only can superheroes assist in clinical work with children, but Rubin demonstrates how they can facilitate growth and change with teens and adults. Early childhood memories of how we felt pretending to have the power to save the world or our families in the face of impending danger still resonate in our adult lives, making the use of superheroes attractive as well to the creative counselor.

In presenting case studies and wisdom gleaned from practicing therapists' experience, the book shows how it is possible to uncover children's secret identities, assist treatment of adolescents with sexual behavior problems, and inspire the journey of individuation for gay and lesbian clients, all by paying attention to our intrinsic social need for superhero fantasy and play.

List of Contributors:

Leya Barrett	Harry Livesay	Karen Robertie
Michael Brody	William McNulty	Lawrence C. Rubin
Jan Burte	Cory A. Nelson	Jennifer Mendoza Sayers
George Enfield	Jeff Pickens	Patty Scanlon
Roger Kaufman	Robert Poole	Ryan Weidenbenner
John Shelton Lawrence	Robert J. Porter	Carmela Wenger

2007 · 368 pp · Hardcover · 978-0-8261-0269-0

11 West 42nd Street, New York, NY 10036-8002 • Fax: 212-941-7842
Order Toll-Free: 877-687-7476 • Order Online: www.springerpub.com

SPRINGER PUBLISHING COMPANY

Psychological Masquerade

Distinguishing Psychological From Organic Disorders, Third Edition

Robert L. Taylor, MD

When faced with a patient whose psychological symptoms may stem from an organic, or medical, condition rather than from a psychological condition, how does the practitioner determine exactly which is the true case? To facilitate this process and give psychologists, social workers, and nurses a useable guide to assessment, Robert Taylor created *Psychological Masquerade* and has updated it to be the most complete handbook you will ever need in the field.

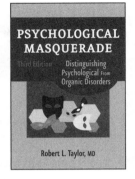

New chapters on violent behavior, amnesia and dementia, sex obsession, and Munchausen-by-Proxy fill out the guide and numerous case studies help clarify diagnostic criteria and provide a welcome hands-on approach to caring for clients in this delicate balance. As a further enhancement of the text as assessment tool, self-tests for hypothetical cases are included as are specific clinical tests that aid in clue gathering.

This is the perfect clinical guide for any practitioner who is likely to come into contact with psychological masquerade among clients and will be a welcome addition to the practitioner's toolbox.

Table of Contents:

2007 · 304 pp · Softcover · 978-0-8261-0247-8

11 West 42nd Street, New York, NY 10036-8002 • Fax: 212-941-7842
Order Toll-Free: 877-687-7476 • Order Online: www.springerpub.com